Teaching STEM with Confidence:
Practical Tips and Strategies for New and Experienced Teachers

by Beverly Simmons

Edited by Alex Wayne Stripling, Jr.
Published by Printing Futures, Vancouver WA

ISBN 978-1-942357- 58-2
Hardcover Version

Photo permissions and authors, illustrators, designers, photographers available for download at the URL. http://www.PrintingFutures.com

Printing Futures
Publishing in Oregon

Teaching STEM with Confidence:
Practical Tips and Strategies for New and Experienced Teachers

Dedicated to Jeannie and Wayne who share my passions, pleasures, and problems with unconditional love and resilience, and to Hannah, who inspires me to share my stories!

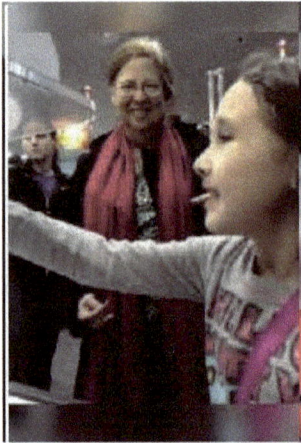

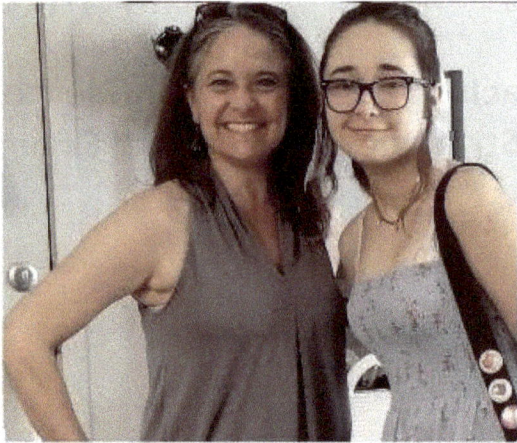

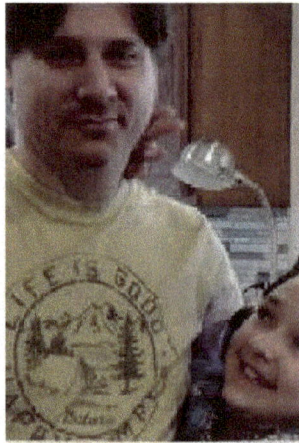

Table of Contents

Forward: Meet a Passionate STEM Educator

This forward is written by Jeannie Ruiz, Executive Director, iNSL.

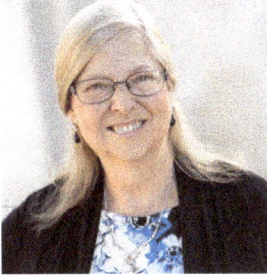

Beverly Simmons, a dedicated mother of three from a small town in southern GA, embarked on an inspiring journey to forge a fulfilling career in education and beyond. As a visionary and award-winning classroom teacher, she defied norms by creating an acclaimed program that integrated subjects in a multi-aged setting using data and analysis of project-based learning to teach a common core education, usually defined by non-integrated, stand-alone subjects. Beverly and her ground-breaking team employed innovative ideas such as using racing and remote-control cars to teach core subjects, while also innovating using computer-based mathematics to teach algebra years before they were common place in schools.

Development

Development: Early in her career, Beverly's innovative ideas were recognized by the Georgia Institute of Technology School of Computing and she was entrusted with leading the first year of the NSF funded Learning by Design curriculum project. Her success in this program led to her recruitment by Ford Motor Company, where she and her new company of engineers and educators established a Ford Technology Showcase Center next to the renowned Henry Ford Museum. Following this accomplishment, she and her engineering partner were selected by the Detroit Science Center Board to spearhead the design, build-out, and opening of the NEW Detroit Science Center Building, Exhibits, IMAX

Theater and Planetarium. It is on time and under budget opening captivated 32,000 visitors within its first 48-hour grand- opening. Beverly accepted the position of Vice President for the first year, staffed and managed sixty-five persons, and initiated the long-term program strategy for the venue.

Beverly's company of educators and engineers achieved significant milestones and awards. The team worked with owner, Gary Eaker, to design and build the AeroDYN Wind Tunnel in NC as they pioneered NASCAR's groundbreaking STEM Initiative, Ten80 Student Racing Challenge. The US Army shifted its sponsorship focus to scaling Ten80 Racing Challenges after recognizing their impact from working with Beverly's team as Ryan Newman's NASCAR sponsor.

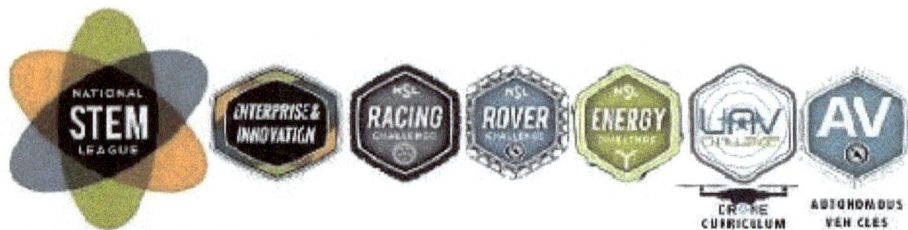

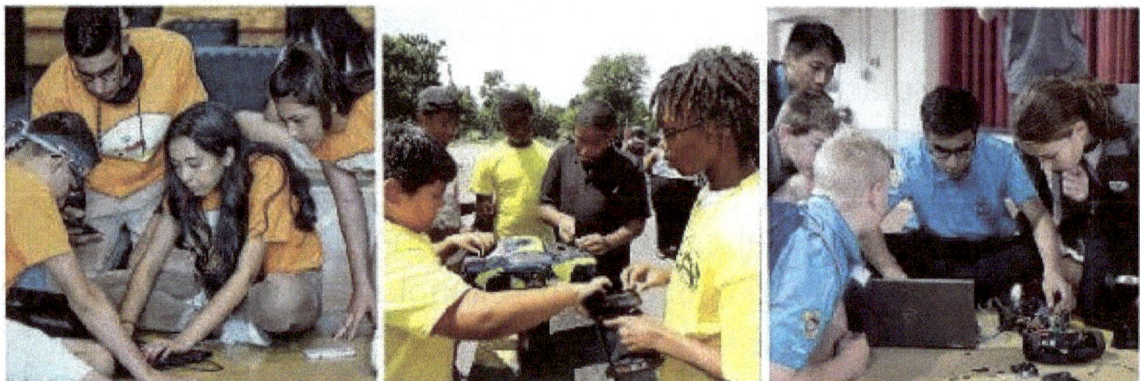

Over seven years, from 2012-2019, the US Army/Ten80 Innovators in Training STEM Tour hosted over 60,000 students for one day STEM events held in 10-12 cities annually, scaling the Ten80 National STEM League.

Recognized by President Obama's 'Change the Equation' initiative as Exemplary STEM initiatives ready for broad implementation, the Ten80 Student Racing Challenges and three other programs garnered national acclaim within the business and education fields.

The Racing Challenge National STEM League is in its 17th year as a classroom, camp and competition for middle and high school students. There is an elementary version called Driving STEM that has improved the math scores of students in grades 3-6 for over twenty years using small radio-controlled cars and technology made for classrooms. During Covid, as students were forced to work from home and outside activities were limited with respect to using radio-controlled cars, autonomous vehicles, or drones, Ten80 Foundation renamed itself as The International STEM League (iNSL) to reflect its flagship program. Working with Beverly to lead the organization through this difficult time, Executive Director, Jeannie Ruiz, helped iNSL harness the power of Esports and Sim Racing in collaboration with iRacing.com, Eisengard.AI, and Rx5 CyberUnity, to keep students "on track" racing, collecting data and maximizing performance.

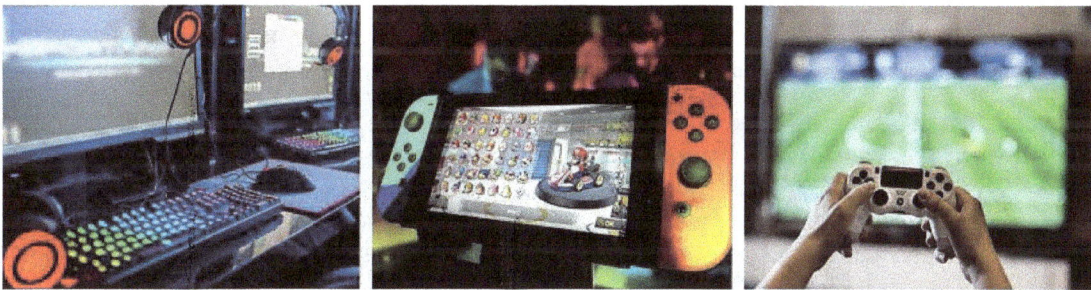

PreK - Pro Programs Engaging 1000s of Students

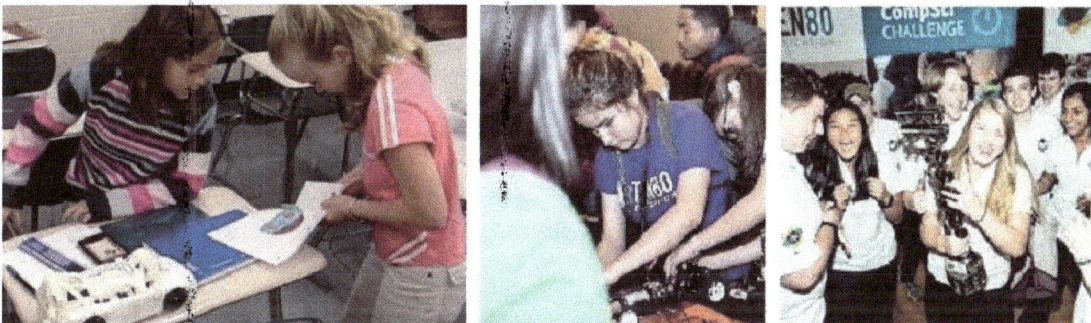

Beverly's accomplishments earned her a place among STEMconnector's prestigious inaugural 100 Women Leaders in STEM. Beverly also became a US State Department STEM speaker where she has provided keynotes and professional development across the US and in 8 countries.

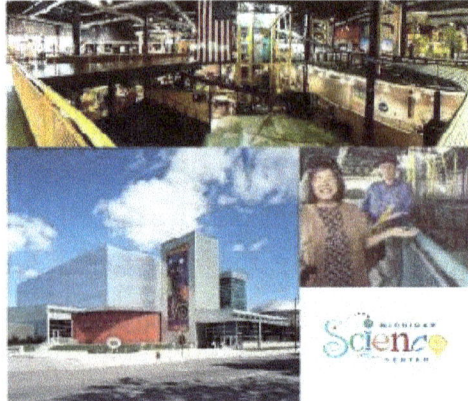

Training teachers to embrace a STEM mindset and teach it with confidence is how we can bring sySTEMic change that lasts! Beverly enjoyed raising her children and teaching other children. Now, she dedicates her time to passing on what she has learned to other teachers

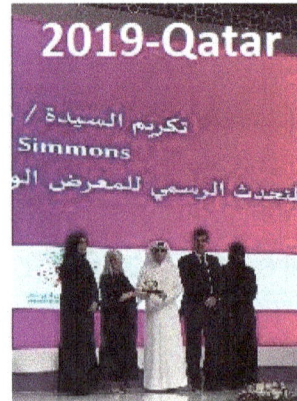

Beverly Simmons

FOUNDER AND CO-CHAIR OF BOARD OF DIRECTORS TEN80 FOUNDATION

Beverly Simmons has been recognized as Teacher of the Year, GA Middle Grades Team of the Year and as a GA finalist for Presidential Awardee for Excellence in Science and Mathematics Teaching. Her informal science experience includes Spirit of Ford Conference Center, and the NEW Detroit Science Center. Simmons is Co-founder of Ten80 Education and currently serves as Founder and Co-Chair of Ten80 Foundation Board of Directors. Programs developed through her work with Ten80 include the Ten80 Student Racing Challenge: NASCAR STEM Initiative, a version of which has recently partnered with the US Army.

I. Igniting the Spark
Empower Educators to Unleash the Power of STEM

As we step into a future propelled by technology and innovation, the significance of STEM education grows ever more profound. STEM, an acronym for science, technology, engineering, and mathematics, forms the bedrock for equipping students with the necessary skills to thrive in today's workforce and the ability to thrive in the unpredictable workforce of the future.

Jobs in STEM fields are in high demand, and they offer some of the highest-paying and most exciting career opportunities available. However, many jobs will be created in the next decade that do not even exist today; Therefore, STEM skills must be presented to students in ways that teach them more than a list of algorithms in math or facts in science. While these core skills are necessary, their true value lies in the fact that they are the starting grid for creativity and innovation. Encourage students to cultivate a STEM mindset, fostering curiosity, questioning, and creative thinking, instead of solely seeking the "correct answer." Teachers should embrace lessons and activities that may not always have a definitive "key" to solutions, promoting a comfortable learning environment.

STEM skills are essential for success in all areas of modern life, and they are particularly important for students who are interested in pursuing careers in science, technology, engineering, or mathematics.
As we move into a world that is increasingly driven by fast-paced innovations in technology, it is becoming more important than ever before for students to have a strong foundation in STEM subjects. The emergence of Artificial Intelligence is not a surprise. However, few people not in the IT field expected it to make such an accessible and dramatic entry into daily life as it has in recent months. This should serve as a wake-up call to educators that we must start infusing the STEM

mindset into all classrooms to better serve the students in our care. Too many students find that they are ill-equipped to choose a career when they enter college. Their pathway is often blocked by their level of comfort and expertise in mathematics. By providing students with a strong foundation in science, technology, engineering, and mathematics, teachers can help to build the skills and mindset that students need to be in a position to have more options and opportunities with respect to their careers.

What Does it Mean to Teach STEM with Confidence?

This series of articles is based on the author's recently published book, Teaching STEM with Confidence: Practical Tips and Strategies for New and Experienced Teachers, a guide that provides practical advice and strategies for teachers to confidently integrate STEM into any subject classroom. The book is designed for both new and experienced teachers who are looking for effective and practical ways to feel confident teaching STEM.

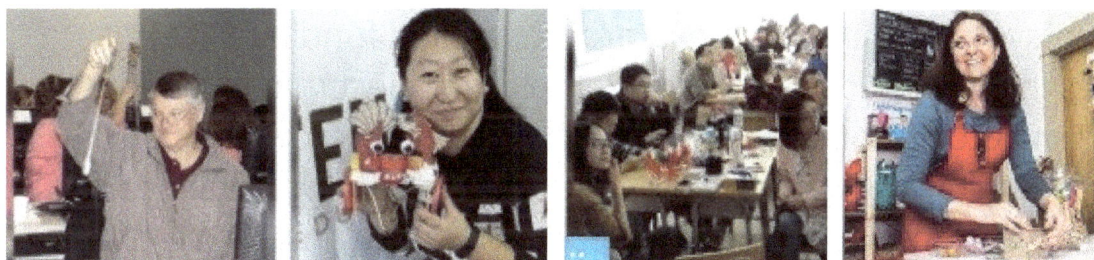

II. What is STEM?

STEM education refers to an interdisciplinary approach to teaching science, technology, engineering, and mathematics in an integrated and cohesive manner. It aims to develop critical thinking, problem-solving, and collaboration skills while encouraging creativity, innovation, and curiosity among students. STEM education is essential in today's world as it prepares students for the challenges of the 21st century and provides them with the necessary skills to succeed in the workforce. STEM education is not only about teaching these four subjects individually. It is about integrating them into a single learning experience.

The National Science Foundation (NSF) began using the term "STEM" to refer to science, technology, engineering, and mathematics in its reports and publications in the early 2000s. The exact date of its initial usage by the NSF may vary, but it was during this time that the term gained traction and recognition within the educational and research community. The NSF has been a strong advocate for STEM education and has played a significant role in promoting and funding STEM initiatives in the United States. For example, a project that involves building an autonomous vehicle or a robot requires knowledge of various STEM concepts such as programming, mechanical engineering, and electronics. By integrating these concepts, students can see the connections between them and how they work together to achieve a common goal.

In STEM education, teachers encourage students to explore and experiment with new ideas and concepts. They also help students develop a growth mindset, which is essential in STEM fields. A growth mindset means that students believe that their intelligence and abilities can be developed through hard work, dedication, and perseverance. This mindset is critical in STEM fields as it encourages students to take risks, learn from their mistakes, and persist in the face of challenges. STEM education is not only beneficial for students but also for teachers. It provides teachers with an opportunity to collaborate and learn from each other. STEM education is a relatively new field, and there is always something new to learn.

As recently as 2012, only a decade ago, teachers attending the National Science Teachers Convention were learning about STEM. At this convention, groups of teachers came by booths with the word STEM in their company or program titles because their administrators had told them to bring back something "STEM" related. The questions they asked ranged from, "What does that even mean?" to "Do you have any STEM furniture?" and "I was told to bring something STEM back. Help?"

What, then, is the first step in this journey? Educators, many never having been exposed to the inner workings of careers outside of academia, can start by becoming comfortable with an idea that drives innovation in industry: "Fail fast, fail often." The underlying idea behind "fail fast, fail often" is that failure is not something to be feared or avoided but rather embraced and used as a stepping stone towards improvement and innovation. It encourages a mindset of resilience, adaptability, and continuous learning, fostering an environment where experimentation and creativity can thrive.

While a "STEM" class is often an exceptionally good class for students taught by an imaginative STEM literate person, it is not the embodiment of what STEM should be in our schools.

Reflections: Across the Curriculum

Some of you may remember a movement known as "Reading Across the Curriculum" that acknowledged the importance of reading as a fundamental skill that is applicable and beneficial across different disciplines. It facilitated the integration of reading skills and literacy development across various academic subjects beyond just English/language arts classes. English/language arts classes. Integrating a STEM mindset across the curriculum can help students develop critical thinking, problem-solving, and collaboration skills, which are essential for success in any field.

When I taught middle school, I always reminded myself how surprised I was on the day that I realized my students could not set up a simple graph. I walked immediately to our math teacher's room to say we had to do something differently. Jackie was also astonished because her walls were covered in graphs like the ones our students could not create in my science classroom. We will revisit this because it was my first real lesson on what it means to generalize learning.

Embrace the Role of STEM in a Country of Innovators!

America's ability to innovate is what other countries are trying to emulate. STEM skills and mindset are at the heart of innovation. Our team uses an image we created and named the STEM Innovation Arrow to drive curriculum toward STEM pathways. We will revisit it later in the book but the first thing to notice is that content and skills are at the core of innovation.

America's ability to innovate is what other countries are trying to emulate. STEM skills and mindset are at the heart of innovation. Our team uses an image we created and named the STEM Innovation Arrow to drive curriculum toward STEM pathways. We will revisit it later in the book but the first thing to notice is that content and skills are at the core of innovation.

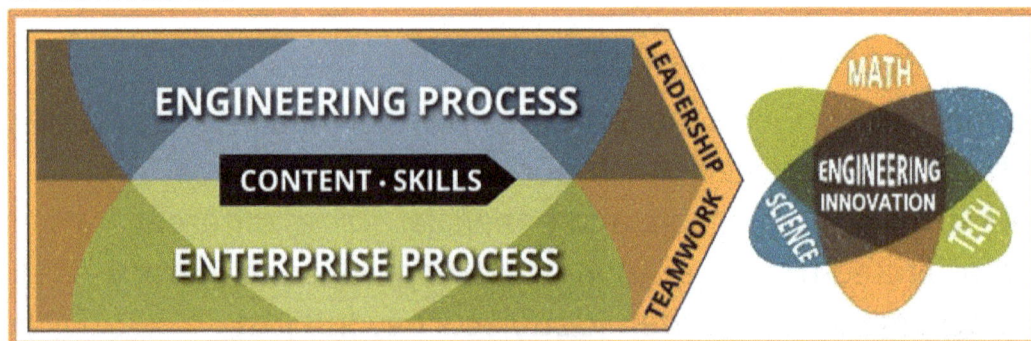

Innovation thrives when a critical mass of individuals come together in close proximity, whether physically or through virtual collaboration, to tackle shared or similar challenges. Singular contributions do not singularly birth innovations into the world. Sustaining a nation's innovative prowess in the contemporary landscape necessitates a consistent influx of individuals equipped with a foundational educational toolkit rooted in science, technology, engineering, and math (STEM) skills. This collective cohort should mirror the cultural and ideational diversity inherent within their society. Notably, a key factor in America's role as an innovation vanguard stems from the rich diversity permeating our populace.

Women and minorities are traditionally underrepresented in STEM. STEM Education plays a pivotal role in bridging the gender and underrepresented minority gaps in K-12 achievement.
Despite accounting for around half of the employed US workforce, in 2023, the gender gap in STEM remains significant, with women making up only 28% of the STEM workforce. Only 24% of the STEM workforce are members of underrepresented minority groups. By encouraging students from diverse backgrounds to pursue STEM careers, we can create a more inclusive workforce, which will benefit society.

Too often, career-focused studies are relegated to Career Technology Education (CTE) classrooms which use a set of career pathways to prepare students for further education or post-secondary jobs. While CTE plays an important role in overall STEM education, it falls in the category of "necessary, but not sufficient".

Anyone listening to the news or social media has heard the term "labor shortage." More accurately, America is experiencing a "skills mismatch" where there is a discrepancy between the skills and qualifications possessed by job seekers and the skills demanded by employers in an ever-changing and technology-driven labor market.

Addressing this skills mismatch which can have negative consequences for both job seekers and employers requires a combination of efforts from educational institutions, employers, and policymakers. This includes aligning curriculum with industry needs, offering training and apprenticeship programs, promoting lifelong learning, and fostering effective collaboration between educational institutions and businesses.

A Hechinger Report/Associated Press analysis of CTE enrollment data from forty states reveals deep racial disparities in who takes these career-oriented courses. Black and Latino students were often less likely than their white peers to enroll in science, technology, engineering, and math (STEM) and information technology classes, according to the analysis, which was based primarily on 2017-18 data.

Meanwhile, they were more likely to enroll in courses in hospitality and, in the case of Black students in particular, human services. The median annual salary for cooks is $27,500 annually, while chefs and head cooks earn $56,000, according to the Bureau of Labor Statistics. Meanwhile, the typical engineer makes $100,000. For computer programmers, annual earnings are $92,000.

From 2021 to 2031,
STEM Occupations are Projected to Grow Faster Than Others

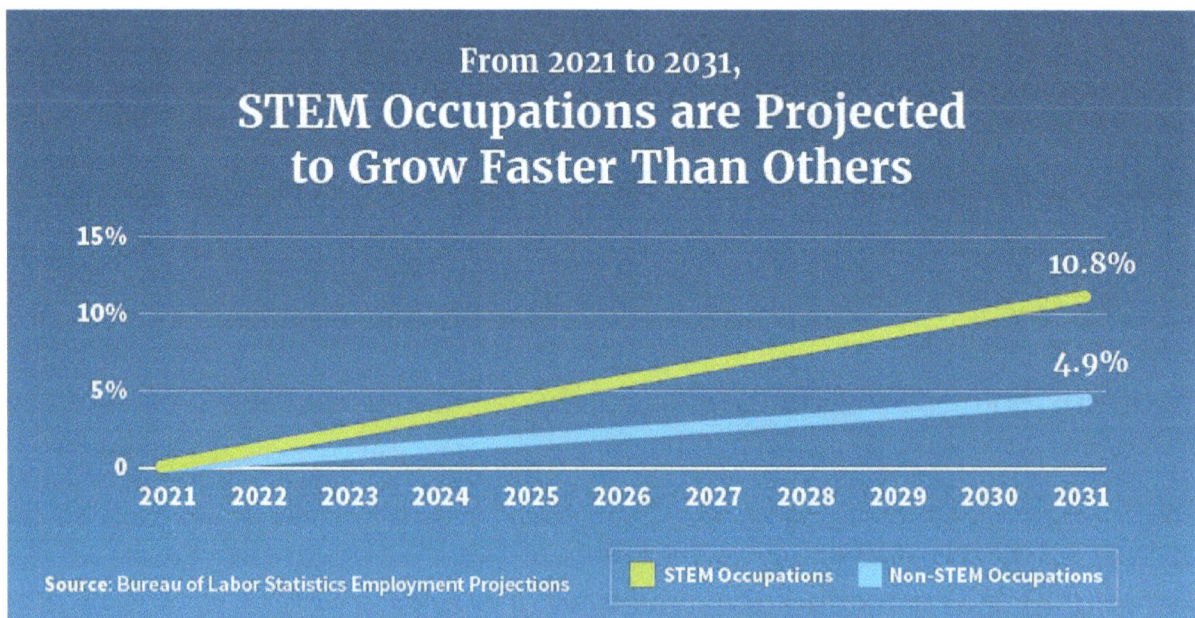

Source: Bureau of Labor Statistics Employment Projections   STEM Occupations   Non-STEM Occupations

Michael Dawson, who runs Innovators for Purpose, an after school STEM program based in Cambridge, Massachusetts, said schools do not do enough to expose students to different careers or nurture those with a passion in STEM. One of his former students, who loved math and science, was placed in carpentry classes, Dawson said. "I'm not sure if there's a lot of people that are really guiding these students into the types of classes that they really need to get to," Dawson said. "The counselors are busy."

Nationwide, counselors serve an average of 430 students each. At this moment, in my Vancouver WA home district, educators are striking and some of the major issues include the need for more planning time, emotional support staff, and counselors to manage the needs of students which have multiplied in complexity since COVID-19.

Across K-12 classrooms, it is imperative to harness every teaching environment—going beyond solely CTE or STEM classrooms—to ensure that the skills imparted hold real-life relevance for students and possess applicability for holistic problem-solving. STEM education serves as a conduit for instructing students in systematic and rational problem-solving approaches, equipping them with the ability to employ data-driven and evidence-based reasoning to surmount intricate challenges.

The acquisition of STEM skills confers an advantage adaptable to any forthcoming career trajectory. Conversely, an absence of these skills creates an insurmountable barrier, limiting numerous students from pursuing their desired professional paths.

Teach Resilience and Growth Mindset with STEM
The concept of "Growth Mindset" was introduced by psychologist, Carol S. Dweck, in her book titled "Mindset: The New Psychology of Success."

The book was first published in 2006. In it, Dweck explores the idea that individuals can have either a fixed mindset or a growth mindset when it comes to their abilities and intelligence. Mindset became widely influential and popularized the concept of growth mindset, leading to its widespread adoption in educational and organizational settings.

Cultivating a growth mindset stands as a pivotal element in approaching the instruction of STEM subjects with confidence. A growth mindset is rooted in the conviction that intelligence and capability evolve through diligent effort, unwavering commitment, and unyielding perseverance. It stands in stark contrast to a fixed mindset, which presupposes that intelligence and aptitude are inherent and immutable traits. This shift entails not only reevaluating our conventional emphasis on attaining the "correct solution" and pursuing an "A" grade, but also expanding and reshaping these notions to promote the development of a growth mindset. Instances where a project prototype falters still yield invaluable learning encounters. The assessment should encompass more than the capacity for rote memorization and retrieval. While not novel, this concept has yet to be fully embraced in manners that truly mirror the progressive trajectories of contemporary education.

What does it look like when educators begin to encourage a growth mindset within STEM? What kind of projects lead students in this direction? What role do "real world" problems play in an effective STEM classroom?

Only a small number of our students will find themselves employed to solve complex equations. There is simply an expectation that they possess the ability to tackle such problems and discern which equations are relevant for finding solutions. Their employability often hinges on their aptitude for handling practical tasks, the results of which may not be predetermined. Instances of "real-world challenges at a professional level could encompass:

- This electric car needs batteries that last longer on each charge and are light enough to make production of this car feasible.
- We have heavy trucks and light cars and bikes riding over the same road. What combination of materials should be used to maximize the life of our roadways?
- All young people care about is good music and wi-fi in their cars. Can we make a self-driving car that has great social technology in it?
- What material is best for my baby's sleepwear?
- And, my baby is always turning over his cereal bowl. Can't someone produce a solution to that?

This list does not begin to address the challenges faced in fields like Particle Physics and Astrophysics and Meteorology. These "real world" problems are messy and require multiple kinds of expertise and technology to formulate a workable and often compromise solution. However, the optimal solution is what one seeks. Successful STEM professionals can collaborate with a team to organize such problems, isolate variables, and identify which variables are on the critical path to a successful solution. As expert analytical people, STEM professionals, understand the limits placed on them by nature and physics and can work within the constraints placed on them by budget and material properties as well. They identify creative opportunities for improvements and sometimes market-disrupting innovations along the way.

The person who can function in this high-energy, high-stress, high-expectations workplace is the one we must be educating in our classrooms today. While not everyone will have these kinds of careers, no one should be excluded because they lack STEM literacy. To equip our students with the aptitude and outlook essential for a professional setting geared towards resolving genuine challenges, educators must acquire the ability to formulate classroom predicaments that are not only solvable but also applicable.

Problems can mimic the real world, but must be manageable versions of those to be of use in a classroom. Good projects are often set up to maximize some performance relevant to opposing variables. Setting up the investigation using "Good Investigation Procedures" (GIP) and learning to coax the story from data are the objective. As these skills are learned and practiced, the problems can become "messier."

Crafting a Project-Based Learning (PBL) curriculum that is both captivating and efficacious is as demanding to mastering any art form. This endeavor demands practice and must be facilitated by an educator at ease with the principles of a growth mindset. Teaching STEM with confidence does not require that every educator becomes a curriculum developer. Every educator needs to learn to identify and facilitate lessons that are appropriate for their students.

Reflections About Excellent and Scalable Stem:

Through Ten80 and the International STEM League, I have engaged with expert STEM professionals to develop award winning curriculum. There was a learning curve over many years, and it is not something every teacher should be expected to do. When I hear that teachers are "creating curriculum" I am sorry that their time is being diverted from their real goal: teaching.

I spent three years following industry analytical people to understand the way problems are really solved in the workplace. That experience led to the formation of the International STEM League which is designed to be a practice league for future STEM professionals. It is based on how much I learned from those experiences that I did not learn in school. It is based on all the times these expert problem solvers said, "I wish I had .... when I was in school."

The US STEM Team of the US Army funded our program to expand after President Obama's evaluation initiative endorsed our programs as Excellent STEM and Ready to Scale. Only four programs nationally reached that level of endorsement.

Over six years, our "Innovators in Training" Tour reached over one thousand students each month in one-day events that led to significant positive shifts in students' perceptions of STEM's importance in their lives and future careers. The impact was measured through independent evaluations. Moreover, these experiences spurred the formation of teams engaging with ourTen80 STEM programs, classes, and competitions.

Those first students are now in their mid-twenties and are making their mark on STEM fields. Recently, iNSL, our nonprofit organization, formalized an agreement with a Cloud Technology startup, founded by a former student. This Tech CEO introduced me to another alumnus from their TN team who has a BS in mechanical engineering and a Doctor of Education (Ed.D.) in Educational Leadership. He spearheads international STEM education strategies for a 22,000-member industry association. These are just two of many alumni who are changing the ecosystem in tech for traditionally underrepresented minorities.

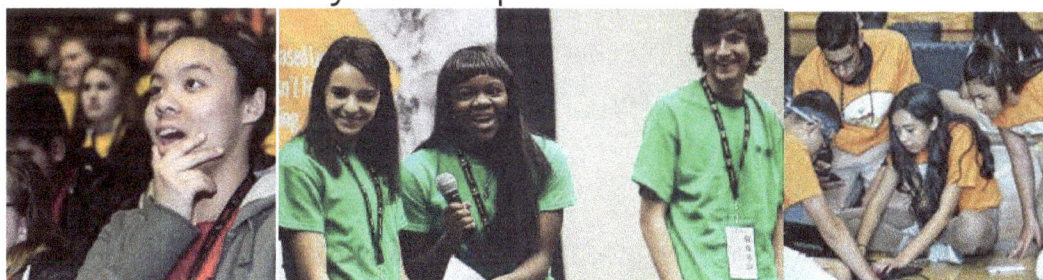

III: Innovation Matters

"If invention is a pebble tossed in the pond, innovation is the rippling effect that pebble causes. Someone has to toss the pebble. That's the inventor. Someone has to recognize the ripple will eventually become a wave. That's the entrepreneur."
— (Tom Grasty, PBS Idea Lab)

Innovation tends to happen when a critical mass of people are in close proximity - physically or virtually collaborating - working on the same or similar problems. In our educational systems, we often emphasize individual innovators and their "aha" moments or screams of "Eureka," celebrating their brilliance and achievements. In doing so, we frequently miss the crucial opportunity to place these moments in the broader context of their times.

It is essential to teach students that innovation is not solely the domain of the exceptional few. With rare exceptions, it results from a collaborative process influenced by the societal and intellectual currents of the era.

Industry 4.0, alternatively known as the Fourth Industrial Revolution or 4IR, represents the forefront of digitizing the manufacturing sector. Fueled by disruptive trends such as the exponential growth of data and connectivity, advanced analytics, human-machine interaction, and significant advancements in robotics, Industry 4.0 has ushered in a remarkable acceleration of technological innovation.

In this rapidly evolving technological landscape, the pace of innovation is unparalleled. What once took years to develop now unfolds in mere weeks, reshaping not only the digital realm but also the physical world. Yet, the journey from idea to realization within this swift current is far from simple. Contrast this with the past, where technological change advanced at a glacial pace, and the technologies our ancestors embraced in their youth remained central throughout their lifetimes.

Today, educators must equip students for success in a 21st-century workplace marked by extraordinary technological velocity. This demands a willingness from teachers and administrators to adopt fresh teaching methods and innovative curricula.

With nearly 1.35 million tech startups worldwide, a staggering global internet penetration rate of 63% as of 2022, and an anticipated 463 exabytes of data production by 2025, we witness an exponential rise in connectivity and information exchange. With approximately 5 billion internet users and their numbers continually surging, the dynamics of innovation have shifted from solitary brilliance to the collective efforts of a global community. (Amardeep Pundir, 2023)

In this era, the transformative power of technology is not limited to the few but is accessible to those willing to collaborate, adapt, and contribute to the accelerating wave of progress. We have seen the power of collaboration in driving innovation since the beginning of the Scientific Revolution.

Unfolding primarily in Europe during the late 1500s and 1600s, this was a period of profound transformation in our understanding of the natural world, and stands as an early testament to the power of collaboration. It marked a seismic shift in human understanding. Scientific inquiry challenged long-held religious beliefs, moral principles, and the traditional scheme of nature. This period of questioning and discovery was facilitated by the collaborative efforts of scientists, mathematicians, and thinkers from various disciplines.

Optics, the study of light and its properties, provides one of many compelling examples of how collaboration fueled innovation during the Scientific Revolution. The work done in optics during this period laid the foundation for our modern understanding of light, vision, and the behavior of electromagnetic waves.

Scientists like Johannes Kepler, René Descartes, and Isaac Newton made significant contributions. Kepler's work on the optics of lenses, Descartes' development of the law of reflection, and Newton's groundbreaking experiments with prisms all built upon each other's ideas. Individually, these scientists were not prone to collaborative efforts. However, their society was changing due to technologies such as the printing press.

Another key element that facilitated collaboration during the Scientific Revolution was the establishment of scientific societies. These organizations were created to discuss, validate, and disseminate new discoveries. Scientific societies brought together scholars, thinkers, and practitioners, fostering an environment of shared knowledge and collaboration.

Scientific papers emerged as vital tools for communicating complex ideas comprehensibly. They allowed scientists to share their discoveries, hypotheses, and methodologies with their peers. The newly emerging scientific method allowed scientists to test and verify the conclusions of their peers. Shared papers underwent rigorous scrutiny, which encouraged further refinement of ideas and experiments. This collaborative approach accelerated the progress of science and the development of ever improved technologies.

The influence of scientific collaborations during the Scientific Revolution extended beyond the realm of science and directly impacted all areas of society, such as art. One fascinating example is the connection between the renowned Dutch painter Johannes Vermeer and the scientific instrument known as the camera obscura. Vermeer's work serves as a striking testament to the interplay between art and science during this transformative period.

The camera obscura, which translates to "dark chamber" in Latin, is an optical device that projects an image of the external world onto a surface inside a darkened room. During the Scientific Revolution, the camera obscura was not just a scientific curiosity. It also became a tool for artists and curious minds. It allowed for the accurate depiction of perspective, proportion, and light in ways that were previously challenging to achieve. Vermeer, like many artists of his time, is believed to have used the camera obscura to aid in his artistic process.

Vermeer's paintings are renowned for their exquisite rendering of light and its interplay with objects and spaces. The camera obscura can produce a focused image with depth, similar to how Vermeer's works often have a sense of depth and focal accuracy. The camera obscura can create soft-focus areas and smooth gradations often seen in Vermeer's artworks. This mastery of light in his works aligns closely with the principles of optics and the scientific understanding of light emerging during the Scientific Revolution.

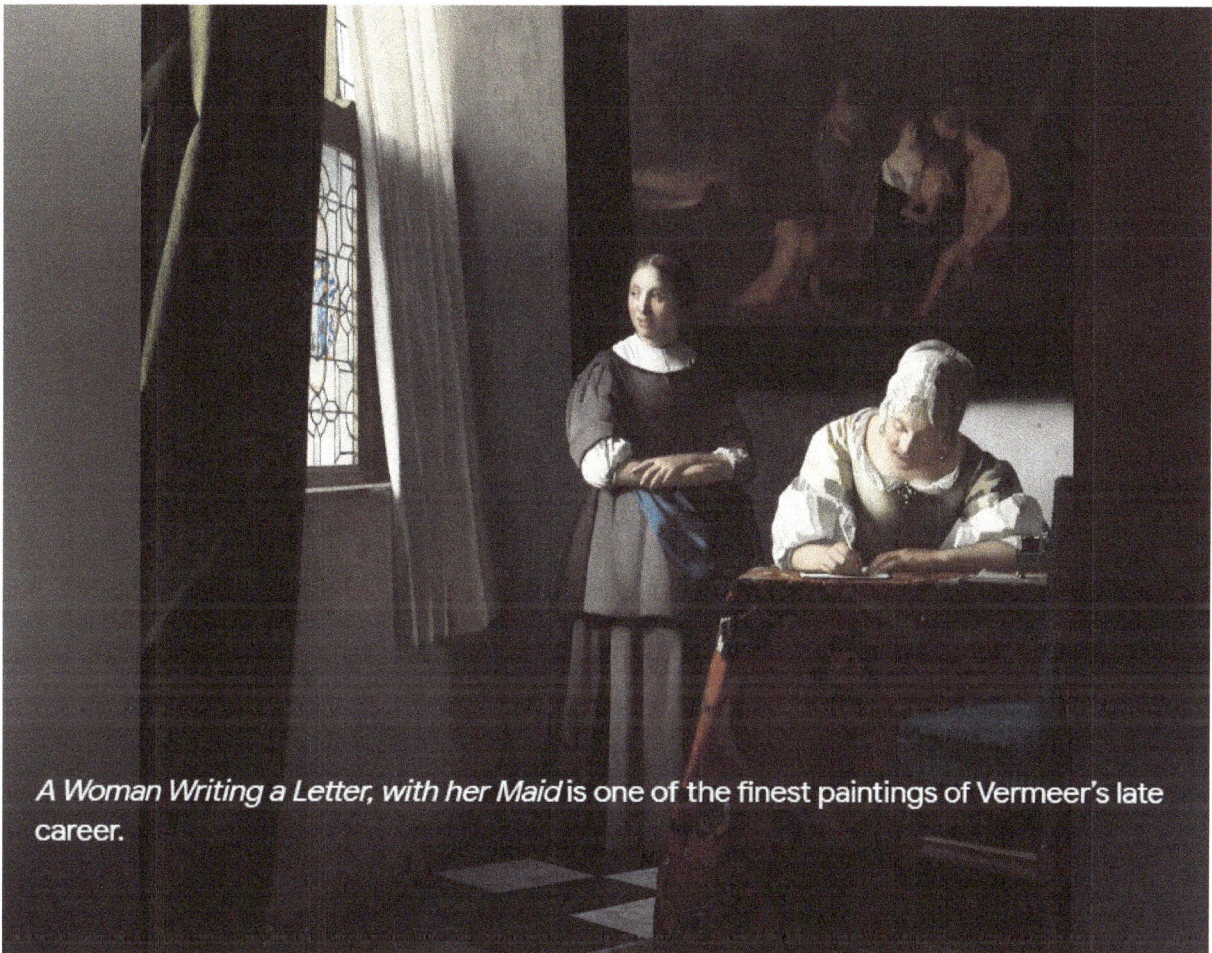

A Woman Writing a Letter, with her Maid is one of the finest paintings of Vermeer's late career.

The story of Johannes Vermeer and his use of the camera obscura serves as a compelling example of how scientific collaborations and innovations influence every facet of society. Vermeer's ability to capture light and perspective in his paintings was enhanced by his engagement with the scientific discoveries of his era.

this story underscores the idea that during times of great intellectual ferment, boundaries between disciplines blur, leading to a rich cross-pollination of ideas and creativity.

It is clear that such connections are happening in our world today. Young artists are often more adept at drawing with digital software than a pencil, marker, or charcoal. Ai is helping graphic arts take great leaps in what can be created and altered. Movies are often created by actors in front of green screens using CGI.

Innovation today is not limited to one industry or one facet of society. The connected world is one in which we are living and one in which we must, as educators, thrive if we are to confidently lead our students to succeed in this high-tech workplace.

The speed of technological innovations in the 21st century owes much to the rapid communication enabled by the worldwide internet system. Scientists and mathematicians from around the globe can now collaborate in real time, 24/7.

While concerns about secrecy within organizations persist, the benefits of having more minds working on a problem far outweigh the drawbacks. The internet has become the modern equivalent of the scientific societies of the past, connecting experts and enabling collaborative problem-solving.

STEM Ecosystems have grown across the country in the past few years as educators attempt to support one another's understanding and supplement one another's resources in much the same way as the scientific community has done since the Scientific Revolution began. As STEM teachers, we should also engage students intrigued by the intersection of art and science, sometimes called STEAM. As novel techniques, software, and technologies emerge regularly, the dynamic interplay between art and science undergoes constant and evolving transformations. We should teach about these intersections of subjects and society so that learning is less siloed. It is not enough to know the names and a few facts about early scientists. It does not help one understand how early innovations actually happened and it fosters the belief in students that scientist are all white men with wild hair. The idea that only a select few are smart enough to be innovative is an idea that is not appropriate for modern times.

Innovation is what makes America a country to be envied and emulated. All students can be part of that today if they understand the role that technology can play to even playing fields. It is imperative that we, as educators, stay informed and knowledgeable about this ever-changing landscape and work to grow our own collaborative network of like-minded STEM focused teachers.

The International STEM League (iNSL) is pioneering an award-winning approach to STEM education that views it as a "performing art" demanding practice, dedication, and enthusiasm. We believe that being innovative is not just about what you know but about forging new paths, shifting perspectives, and envisioning transformative solutions. It is a thought process cultivated from our earliest experiences, where imagination takes root. The richness of these neural pathways, fostered through interdisciplinary learning, not only reinforces concepts but also cultivates creativity, critical thinking, and problem-solving skills.

Rather than compartmentalizing knowledge and skills, an integrated approach connects STEM subjects within a relevant context, aligning with real-world applications. We understand that educators should have the flexibility to customize and adapt STEM programs to their students' unique learning styles and needs. We advocate for teachers to be equipped with the tools and insights necessary to unveil the evolution of big ideas in science and technology, reinforcing the relevance of their teachings.

By instilling STEM awareness and a project-based learning mindset, teachers can spark systemic change in education, nurturing the creative and innovative thinking essential for our students to thrive in an ever-evolving world. In the end, It is not just about imparting knowledge; It is about empowering our future "Innovators in Training" to shape a brighter tomorrow through the dynamic world of STEM.

Reflections – Camera Obscura

Lesson Overview
Materials needed per student or pair of students:

- Empty Pringles can (or similar can, like an oatmeal can)
- push pin
- 1 foot of aluminum foil
- scissors
- tape
- waxed paper or tracing paper

I recommend this as one of many great lessons on making camera obscuras.

https://annex.exploratorium.edu/science-explorer/pringles_pinhole.html

Reflections – Where's the Math?

In 1995, pre-digital cameras, a visiting engineer, helped me and my students have our first interaction with integrated STEM projects. We used a video camera to record students dropping egg carriers from an 8-foot ladder. We created a release mechanism to control the drops and placed a tape with measurements on the wall behind the drop area. The last step was to use a stop frame VCR (look it up:) to play back the videos on the classroom TV with a clear acetate sheet on the TV surface. When each video started, students used a Sharpie to mark the position of the egg carrier on the acetate.

The video played at 30 frames per second, so we stopped it every three frames and marked where the carrier was after one-tenth of a second. We could all SEE that the carrier dropped a greater distance with each tenth of a second than in the previous tenth of seconds.

For the first time, my students SAW acceleration, the speed change due to gravity's pull. Things fall farther in the same time as gravity accelerates the object. Later, we would drop things from the ladder on the local fire truck and SEE what terminal velocity meant as dropped items stopped accelerating. Because we had a tape measure in the background, we could tell how far it fell in each tenth second. We could see how the activity of the carrier's parachute reacted during the fall and map it to the speed and acceleration of the carrier.

When students graphed the data and compared carrier designs, they made their first data-driven decisions. They won the state competition for three years in a row. By the third year, they were shocked that the other schools never seemed to have any numbers to support their designs.

This lesson today can be taught using digital cameras and counting frames is much simplified. It can also be taught with online simulators from groups like Phet. However, there is a worthwhile learning experience in having students see the egg crate they built on the screen, marking its acceleration on top of it, and internalizing that experience with both their hands and their minds

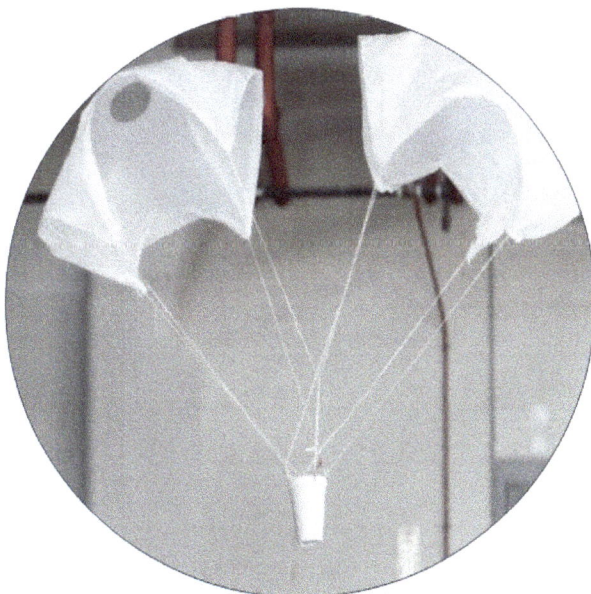

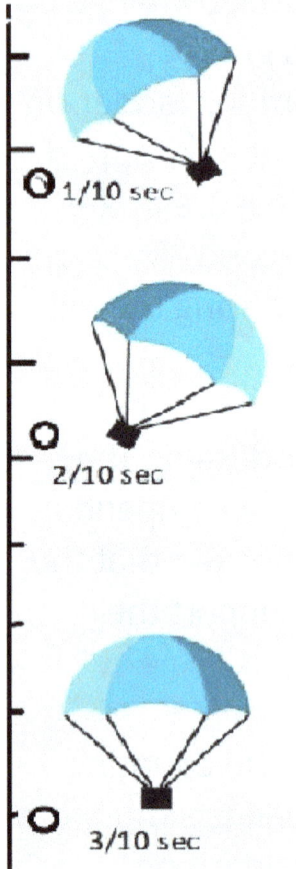

1/10 sec

2/10 sec

3/10 sec

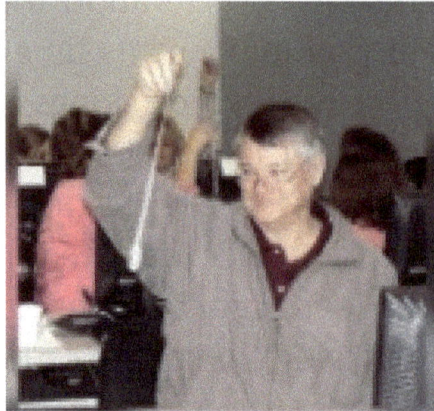 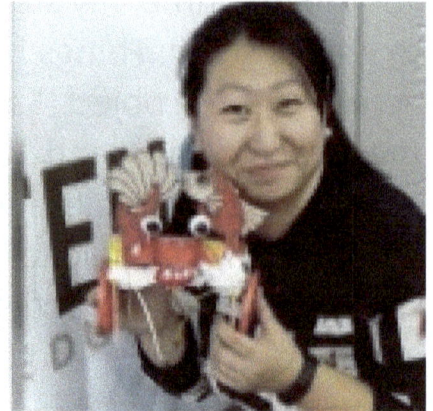

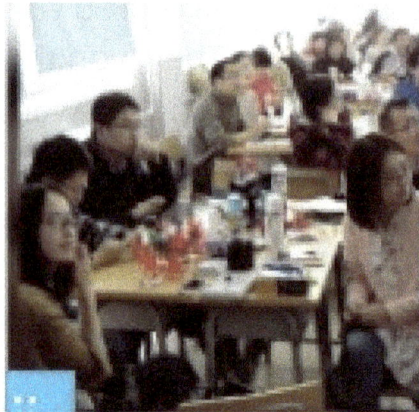 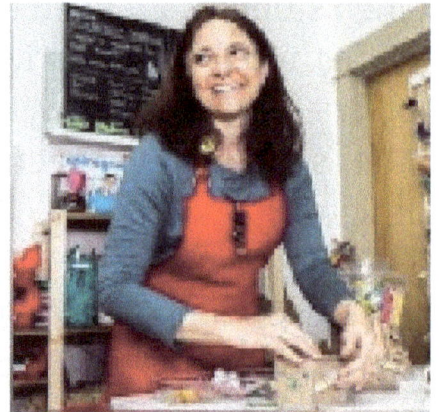

IV. 5 Simple Pieces
Foster Innovation in the Classroom

1. **Emphasize effort over talent**
    When giving feedback to your students, focus on their effort rather than their innate ability. Encourage them to embrace challenges and view mistakes as opportunities for growth.

2. **Teach the power of "yet".**
    When a student says, "I can't do this," remind them to add the word "yet" at the end. This simple addition changes the statement from a fixed mindset to a growth mindset and encourages students to keep working towards their goals.

3. **Use growth mindset language**
    Be mindful of the language you use when talking to your students. Avoid phrases like "you're so smart" or "you're a natural at this." Instead, use language that emphasizes effort and growth, such as "I can see you worked really hard on this" or "I'm proud of you for persevering through this challenge."

4. **Provide opportunities for growth**
    Give your students opportunities to challenge themselves and learn new things. Encourage them to take on projects that are outside their comfort zone and provide support and guidance as they work through the challenges

5. **Model a growth mindset**
    Finally, be a role model for your students by demonstrating a growth mindset in your own work. Share your own challenges and mistakes with your students and talk about how you overcame them through hard work and perseverance.

By developing a growth mindset in our STEM students, we can help them become confident, resilient learners who are ready to tackle any challenge that comes their way. STEM education is a term that has gained widespread popularity in recent years, and with good reason. It is an approach to teaching and learning that focuses on the integration of science, technology, engineering, and mathematics (STEM) in a way that promotes critical thinking, problem solving, and creativity. As educators, it is essential that we understand the basics of STEM so that we can effectively teach and inspire our students.

The first step in understanding STEM is to recognize that it is more than just a collection of subjects. STEM is an interdisciplinary approach that emphasizes the integration of knowledge from different fields. This means that instead of thinking of science, technology, engineering, and mathematics as separate subjects, we should teach them as interconnected and interdependent disciplines. While each field possesses fundamental knowledge which must be taught, this knowledge alone is inadequate for achieving success in any career path other than the theoretical.

How do these subjects intersect with one another?
Teaching the Basics with a STEM

Science is about real, tangible things that move, fly, explode, burn, haul loads, float, record images, stop diseases, and explore the universe. It includes all the interesting exciting "creations" of the times in which we live. Science and mathematics have a symbiotic relationship.

Mathematics provides the language and tools for expressing scientific concepts and theories quantitatively. It helps scientists analyze data, formulate hypotheses, create models, and make predictions. Conversely, science provides real-world contexts and applications that inspire and drive mathematical investigations. The empirical observations and experiments of science often require mathematical reasoning and analysis for interpretation and understanding.

Engineering and Technology share a close relationship as well. Technology encompasses the practical application of scientific knowledge and engineering principles to create useful products, processes, or systems. Engineers utilize technology to design, develop, and optimize solutions for real-world problems. Technology, in turn, informs and supports engineering practices by providing tools, materials, and techniques. Engineering focuses on problem-solving, applying scientific and mathematical principles to design and build structures, devices, and systems that meet specific needs and goals.

Mathematics plays a crucial role in engineering. Engineers use mathematical principles and calculations to analyze, model, and optimize designs. Mathematics provides the foundation for engineering concepts like calculus, differential equations, statistics, and linear algebra. Engineers rely on mathematical tools and models to quantify and predict system behavior, assess feasibility, and ensure safety and efficiency.

Science, mathematics, technology, and engineering are interconnected disciplines that leverage each other's strengths to advance knowledge, solve problems, and drive innovation. The integration of these disciplines through Many of us remember how separated the core subjects were from each other in the not too distant past. In 2004, less than 20 years ago, a team of presenters from my emerging professional development company traveled to a different rural school in GA each day to present model lessons.

We called the program Math2Go and it was all about having kids and teachers Newton's three laws. I received a call when this team was refused entry to the classroom because the teacher proclaimed that she did not need math lessons in her science classroom.

Teachers are not being asked to teach an additional subject in an already crowded curriculum. They are tasked with recognizing the interdisciplinary nature of STEM, incorporating it across the curriculum, emphasizing hands on learning, promoting problem-solving, and encouraging creativity. Together, educators in a grade level or a school can create a learning environment that embraces STEM literacy for all students.

Planning a Lesson - Just the Basics

Planning an effective learning experience, a lesson, is a skill all effective teachers master. It can seem daunting at first, especially for new teachers who are just starting out in their teaching career. However, with the right tools and strategies, it can be a rewarding and fulfilling experience for both the teacher and the student. In this chapter, we will explore some Lesson planning starts with identifying the learning objectives. What do you want your students to learn? What skills do you want them to develop? What is the expected outcome? How will the learned skill or objective generalize to broader understanding. Once you have identified the learning objectives and many districts or schools take this step for teachers, it is time to start to design your lesson plan.

The next step is to choose the right activities and resources. STEM education is all about applied and often, hands-on learning, so it is important to choose activities that will engage your students and allow them to explore and discover new concepts while practicing the core skills for which you are responsible as a grade level teacher. You can choose from a wide range of resources, including online simulations, interactive games, and physical materials like building blocks and circuit boards. When designing your lesson plan, take the opportunity to consider the different learning styles of your students.

While the effectiveness of tailoring instruction to specific learning styles is still a topic of debate, some research suggests that instructional approaches that incorporate a variety of modalities and cater to diverse learning preferences can benefit all learners.

STEM education also emphasizes the importance of problem-solving through data. Including data collection and analysis in a lesson is a simple step that can help teachers avoid the significant pitfall of many STEM programs, especially those for younger grades. Programs only address the S, the T, and the E; the math is considered optional. When STEM became a sellable commodity, many science lessons were suddenly labeled STEM. This was done by large and small developers and helped create many problems in implementation of effective STEM practices.

In several states over the past decade, when administrators at the state level or in the University system created STEM standards, they made arbitrary rules such as needing to include at least two or three of the STEM subjects in the lesson for it to qualify as STEM.

In one state, the Eastern half required two subjects and the Western half decided to require three to differentiate their research and grant platforms. This is not a useful or meaningful way to define STEM learning.

Another fundamental aspect of STEM education is the importance of Project Based Learning. STEM subjects are best taught through hands-on experiences that allow students to engage, explore, experiment, explain, and extend learning. Making data driven decisions and conclusions is an important part of this process because a poorly designed lesson can waste a lot of time with hands-on but not minds-on learning. Poor planning can miss a multitude of opportunities.

Imagine a scenario where a science teacher seamlessly integrates scale lessons and scientific notation into her curriculum, when covering a wide array of subjects such as cells, planets, elements, animals, and speed. Coinciding with this, the math teacher is delving into exponents and decimals. This synchronicity in teaching not only imparts valuable skills to students but also offers them a platform to apply those skills. By engaging in daily exercises, or bell ringers, in both classes that involve gauging the magnitude of various attributes like size, speed, weight, area, volume, and density, students establish a foundation for essential benchmarks. These benchmarks, in turn, equip them to make estimations and identify mathematically nonsensical outcomes with confidence, thus enhancing their comprehension within the realm of mathematics.

Well-designed projects can involve anything from building an autonomously driving vehicle from an off-the-shelf radio-controlled car to creating a functioning robot to designing experiments in a laboratory. Recently the International STEM League projects have evolved with the addition of Esports blending hands-on learning with gaming to teach a number of physics concepts.

By engaging in hands-on, project-based activities, evidence has shown that students are more likely to retain what they learn and develop a deeper understanding of the subject matter.

This is not a new idea and there is a large research base available. An early study in Canada provides a good summary of the positive outcomes of this kind of learning: The Impact of Hands-On-Approach on Student Academic Performance in Basic Science and Mathematics *(Cecilia O. Ekwueme1 , Esther E. Ekon1 & Dorothy C. Ezenwa-Nebife, 2015) and The Effect of Active Learning Techniques on Academic Performance and Learning Retention in Science Lesson: An Experimental Study, Aykan, A. ., & Dursun, F. (2022). Vol. 2 No. 1 (2022): The Journal of STEM Teacher Institutes)*

More updated research is available through sites like the Journal of STEM Teacher Institutes. One new study and strategic plan published in NC by EdNC, "A vision for STEM education over the next decade," highlights project-based learning and problem-based learning as two promising instructional strategies that develop these skills:

"Through project-based learning, a well-established practice, students gain knowledge and skills by working for an extended period to investigate and respond to complex questions, problems, or challenges relevant to students' experiences and communities. Students engage in the work with careful support and guidance from teachers. Students learn and practice such skills as calculating acceleration and writing persuasively within the context of a substantive six-to-eight weeks project."

Failure is a bump in the road to success! Get Creative!

In the realm of STEM education, one crucial aspect is the significance of creativity. Recently, a LinkedIn group was formed to explore whether teachers think students are more creative today.

My thought was that students have always been creative, but now schools are more accepting of learning styles that foster creativity rather than stifle it. STEM disciplines go beyond rigid rule-following; they inherently demand a spark of creativity and a spirit of innovation. Encouraging students to transcend boundaries and think beyond the conventional, STEM education fosters the cultivation of fresh perspectives and the pursuit of inventive solutions to challenges. It celebrates the power of thinking "outside the box," encouraging learners to embrace their creative potential in shaping a future fueled by imagination and ingenuity.

The four main learning styles are visual, auditory, reading/writing, and kinesthetic. Some students may learn better through visual aids, while others may prefer hands-on activities. One style really does not fit all. By incorporating a variety of teaching methods into your lesson plan and using multiple representations to introduce new concepts, you can ensure that all of your students are engaged and learning.

When I taught my first workshop in China, our team was not expecting to be critiqued by our adult students until the end of the workshop. At the end of the first day, at their request, our team met with their lead teachers to reflect on the day and get their feedback on how well we met their needs, any questions they noted, and suggestions we might incorporate the next day. It was an extremely helpful, if somewhat intimidating, interaction that our team learned from and uses today. This communication also led us to watch closely how they interacted with one another during activities.

Asian teachers are incredibly open and sharing within their groups. They would compare how one group introduces a concept, demonstrate it, invite critiques, and then compare it to how another group introduces the same topic. The critiques left them with multiple ways to represent a concept to their students and helped individuals identify misconceptions.

Teachers must strive to provide opportunities for students to work collaboratively. STEM education emphasizes teamwork and problem-solving, so it is important to create a classroom environment that fosters cooperation and communication. You can do this by assigning group projects or encouraging students to work together on individual assignments.

Finally, it is important to assess your students' learning throughout the lesson. This can be done through formative assessments, such as quizzes and group discussions, as well as summative assessments, such as exams and projects. For project assessments, having a rubric allows students to self-assess as they progress through the project. It is also a template for feedback and grades given to the students. By regularly assessing students' progress, you can ensure through data that they are mastering the concepts and skills that you are teaching.

K-12 STEM Education is an opportunity to help students begin to connect the conceptual dots learned in all the traditional subjects including art and the humanities. It should offer educators concrete and clear opportunities to collaborate and reinforce ideas across subjects.

The problems with which students are taught cannot be as messy as the ones solved in industry. Classroom problems should be small enough to be investigated with quantifiable outcomes. They often have opposing variables: if one condition improves, another declines. They are often about maximization and may not have a right or wrong answer but one that depends on the conditions in which the test is run. Students need to be encouraged to identify and control variables. This is the beginning of learning to solve problems that are real world messy.

Here is an example of how project-based hands-on learning might look.

Create a project in which students collect data while teams drive radio-controlled cars with different weights taped onto the cars during a class or after school. Students are attempting to determine at what weight their vehicle is getting maximum efficiency. It is a Goldilocks problem with a score based on weight and speed.

One such score is (weight times distance) / average speed. Students use technology to record weight, length of the track, and elapsed time of each run in a logbook along with notes about any data that seems to be an outlier. For instance, "Marcia was not used to driving and her time was affected by that factor more than the weight of the car."

During the week, the math class uses the data to teach graphing, best fit lines, or derive linear and quadratic equations. In elementary classes, the data can be used to practice graphing and computation such as averaging times from three timers.

The graphs and math models that can be generated from this kind of investigation can be grade leveled from third through twelve by ramping up the math analysis of the data collected.

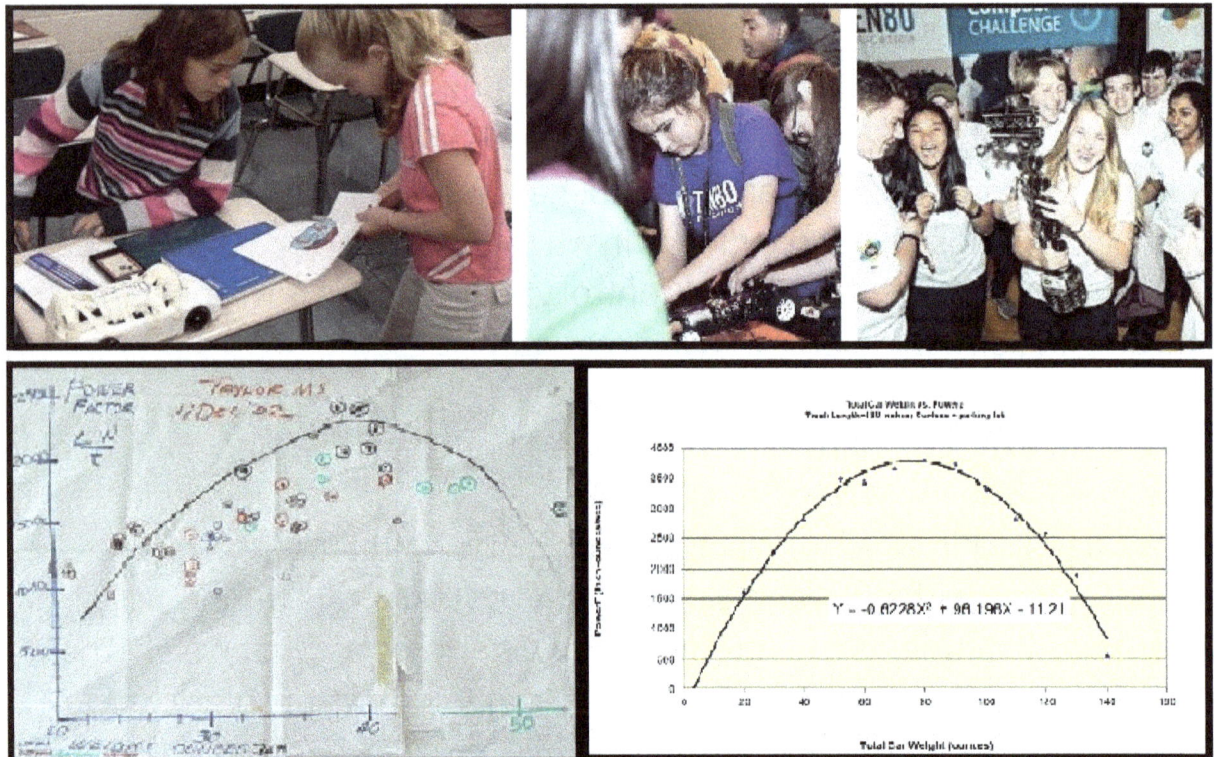

In science, the data lends itself to learning about mass and weight and Newton's laws of motion or thermodynamic, batteries, and energy depending on the objectives being taught at the time.

In CTE classes, carriers for placing weight on the car or ramps and bridges with adjustable heights for further investigation can be designed and built or online wind tunnels and CAD programs or Esports like iRacing can be used to show how digital or radio-controlled cars mimics what happens to actual vehicles. Data can also be downloaded from online iRacing for analysis.

History teachers can integrate the story of early developers of math, science, and technology used in automobiles into social studies lessons as appropriate.

The same decision-making process used in this lesson can be used to determine the maximum ticket price for a school concert. At what price point do the planners break even and at what point do student purchases begin to drop off? The process also generalizes to determining solutions in chemistry and to the concept of power and energy transfer in physics.

Though all this learning and practicing takes place, when asked what the kids did all day and all quarter, they will say they drove cars in math class every Fridays.

This example could have been about designing and prototyping a greenhouse for the school grounds. It could be about planning a garden with geometrically shaped flower beds that will attract butterflies and hummingbirds.

It is amazing how many teachers are doing great STEM lessons in the guise of projects and are simply unaware that their work is the true meaning of STEM. Others just need to think about their projects and make sure that they are tilting it toward STEM.

- Collect and Analyze Data! This is the first and simplest method for creating a STEM focus in a lesson for teachers beginning to integrate STEM into their planning. Use Good Investigative Practices (GIP). Incorporate an Engineering Design Cycle for prototypes.

- Use the Scientific Method to plan experiments. Integrate STEM into your classroom by looking at each lesson with an eye to what can be evaluated or investigated that lends itself to data collection. Any investigation uses the scientific process and any time you use data to predict how something will react or to improve its performance, you are engaging in very basic engineering design thinking.

Planning any lesson requires careful thought and preparation, but with the right tools, strategies, and mindset, it can be a rewarding and engaging experience for both you and your students.

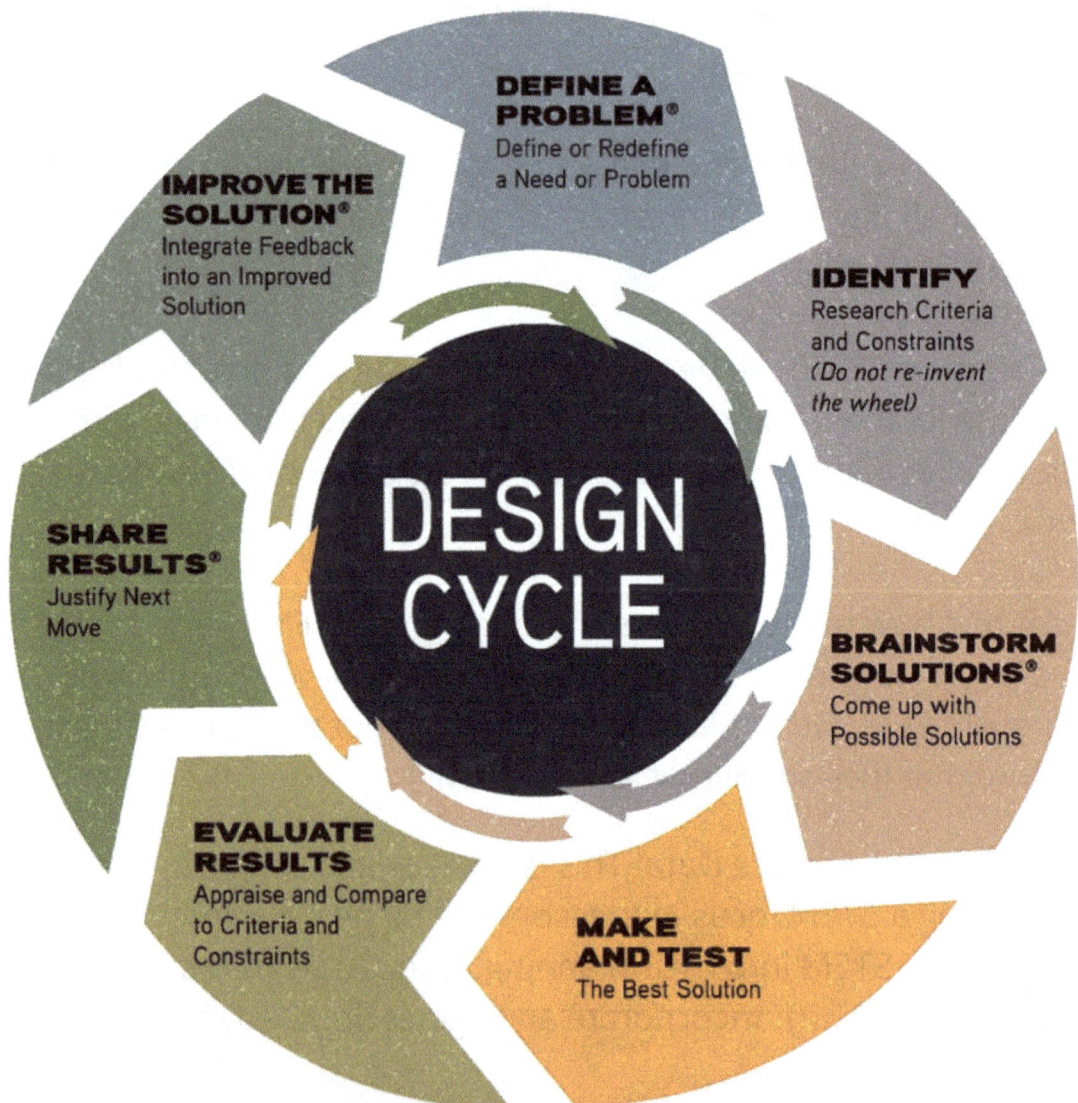

DESIGN CYCLE

DEFINE A PROBLEM®
Define or Redefine a Need or Problem

IDENTIFY
Research Criteria and Constraints (*Do not re-invent the wheel*)

BRAINSTORM SOLUTIONS®
Come up with Possible Solutions

MAKE AND TEST
The Best Solution

EVALUATE RESULTS
Appraise and Compare to Criteria and Constraints

SHARE RESULTS®
Justify Next Move

IMPROVE THE SOLUTION®
Integrate Feedback into an Improved Solution

Reflections: Pom Pom Catapults

By identifying learning objectives, choosing the right activities and resources, catering to different learning styles, promoting teamwork, and assessing student progress, you can create a dynamic and effective lesson that will inspire and empower your students. Integrating STEM can start with something as simple as looking up or collecting data to gain more insight into what you are studying. It can be as fun as shooting pom poms!

At the end of the book, you will find an index of several lessons that may help you think about how to plan your next STEM experience.

Pom Pom Catapults is one our team uses because students from K-6 can take part in the activity and the learning objectives can range from simple counting and measurement to controlling variables and finding patterns in collected data. My hope is that you will look at objectives you must teach and think about how you can customize this activity to help students practice skills as they solve a problem.

A copy of this lesson is included at the end of the book.

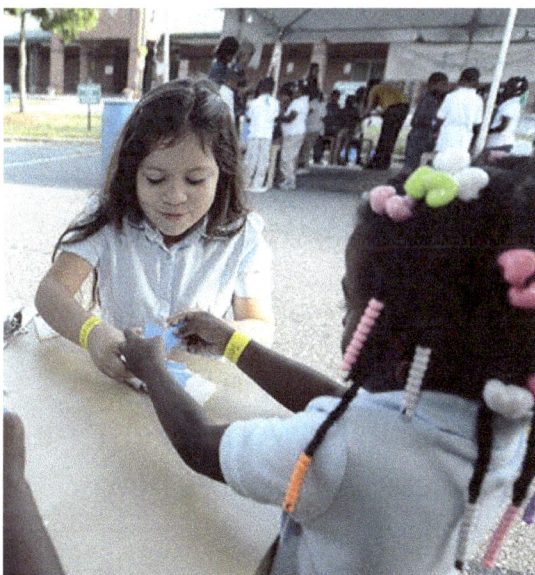

V: Creating a STEM-Friendly Classroom
Strategies for Making a STEM Focused Environment

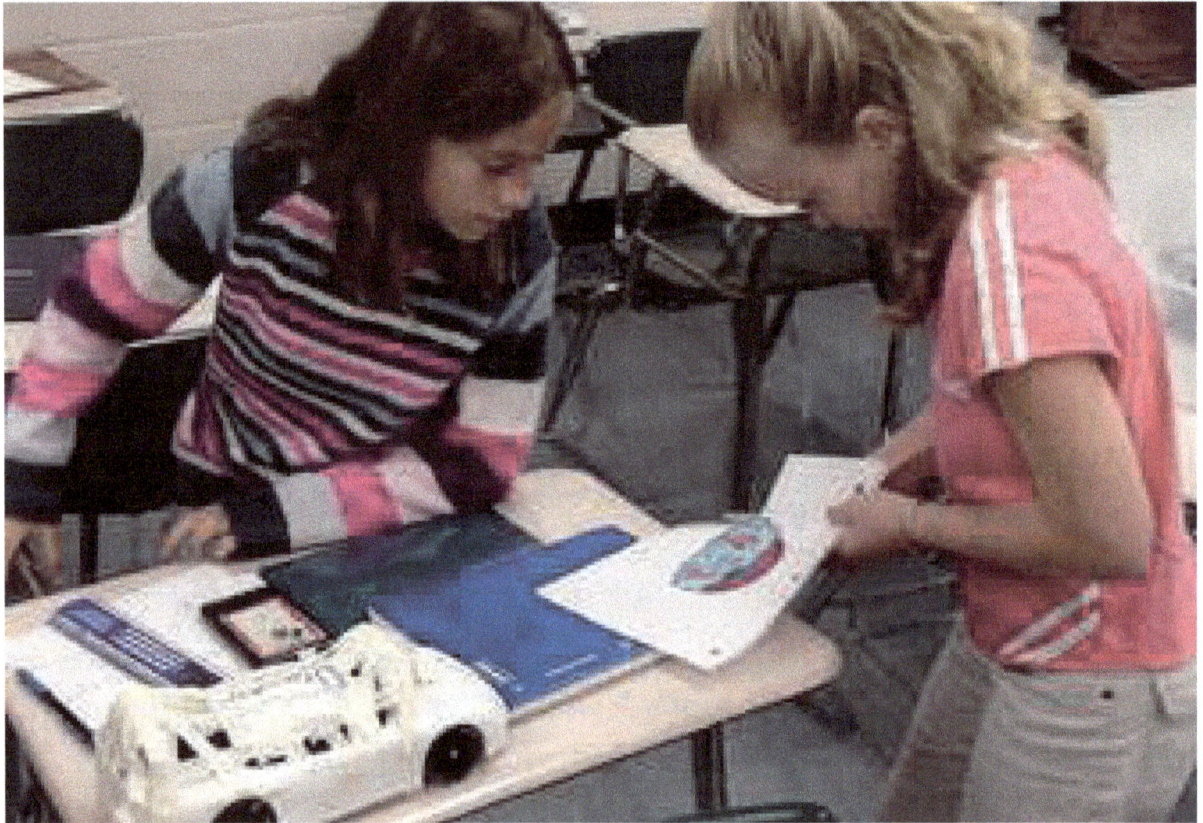

Creating a STEM-friendly classroom is essential to encourage students to develop a strong interest in the science, technology, engineering, and mathematics fields.

As a teacher in the STEM Education niche, you need to create an atmosphere that fosters creativity, innovation, and curiosity in your students. Here are some practical tips and strategies to help you create a STEM-friendly classroom:

Tables Encourage Collaboration: One of the essential skills in STEM education is collaboration. Encourage your students to work together in small groups to solve problems, brainstorm new ideas, and explore new concepts.

Provide Hands-on Materials and Tools: STEM subjects are best learned through hands-on experiences. Let them move, touch, and measure. Provide your students with tools such as scales, stopwatches, timers, multi- meters, and tape measures as well as opportunities to conduct experiments, build models, and work with technology. This will help to keep their interest levels high and engage them in the learning process.

Make Connections to Real-World Applications: Fostering connections to real-world applications is crucial for cultivating student engagement in STEM subjects. When students can directly witness the practical implications of science, technology, engineering, and mathematics, their enthusiasm and interest are more likely to be ignited. In my classroom, I found that designing programs centered around cars and racing captured students' attention effectively. Given that most individuals possess experience with cars or transportation, and the thrill of racing adds an element of excitement, this approach proved engaging.

It is imperative to demonstrate to students how STEM disciplines empower expert problem solvers to tackle complex real-world challenges, such as climate change. Just as budding professional baseball players start their journey by honing skills in T-Ball and Little League, novice and intermediate problem solvers must enthusiastically embrace the practice of STEM skills and participation in STEM competitions. This active involvement not only paves the way for skill development but also instills a profound appreciation for the practicality and impact of STEM knowledge.

Use Technology to Enhance Learning: Technology is an essential tool in STEM education. Use it to provide your students with access to online resources, virtual field trips, and simulations. This will help to enhance their learning experience and keep them engaged. Remember, technology is not always wired. It can be scales and calculators and calipers.

Celebrate Diversity: STEM fields are traditionally male dominated. As a teacher, you need to encourage diversity and inclusion in your classroom. Celebrate the achievements of women and minorities in STEM and provide your students with role models from diverse backgrounds.

Provide opportunities for self-directed learning: STEM subjects require a lot of independent study and self-directed learning. Provide students with resources such as textbooks, online tutorials, and educational games that they can use to explore the material on their own.

Incorporate interdisciplinary learning: STEM subjects are often interrelated, and incorporating interdisciplinary learning can help students see how different subjects connect. For example, a lesson on robotics could include elements of physics, engineering, and computer science.

Creating a STEM-friendly classroom requires a combination of practical strategies and a positive attitude. Encourage collaboration, provide hands- on learning opportunities, make connections to real-world applications, use technology to enhance learning, and celebrate diversity. By doing so, you will help to develop a love of STEM in your students and prepare them for success in the future.

Incorporating Technology in STEM Lessons

Incorporating technology in STEM lessons has become increasingly important in the current education landscape. Technology has revolutionized the way we teach STEM subjects, making it possible for teachers to engage their students in a more interactive and meaningful learning experience. Again, it is important to remember that not all technology is computer or network or cloud based. While computers and digital devices are commonly associated with technology, the scope of technology extends beyond just computers.

Technology refers to the application of scientific knowledge and tools to solve problems, improve efficiency, and enhance human life. It encompasses a wide range of tools, techniques, and systems that are designed to achieve specific objectives.

Tools are instruments or devices that are created to perform specific tasks or facilitate human activities. They can be manual, mechanical, or electronic in nature. Examples of non-computer-based technology include simple hand tools like hammers, wrenches, and screwdrivers, as well as more complex machinery, equipment, and appliances used in various industries.

Incorporating digital technology in STEM lessons can be accomplished using educational apps and software. There are numerous apps and software available specifically designed for STEM education, which can be used to supplement conventional teaching methods. For instance, there are apps that allow students to simulate scientific experiments, which can be especially helpful for teaching complex concepts that are difficult to demonstrate in a traditional classroom setting.

Another way of incorporating technology in STEM lessons is with multimedia resources. With my first experience using a headset and virtual reality, I took a trip to the moon in an Apollo capsule, and I stood beside a dinosaur later the same day. It was awe inspiring and made me begin to understand how many opportunities we can give our students.

Multimedia resources such as videos, animations, and interactive graphics can be used to illustrate complex concepts and make them easier to understand. Teachers can also use multimedia resources to create interactive quizzes and assessments to evaluate students' understanding of the subject matter.

Virtual field trips are another way of incorporating technology in STEM lessons. Virtual field trips allow students to explore different environments and ecosystems without leaving the classroom. There are many virtual field trip platforms available, which offer a wide range of subjects and topics to choose from. Teachers can use these platforms to supplement their teaching and provide students with a more immersive learning experience.

Incorporating technology in STEM lessons can also involve the use of social media and other online platforms. This method is subject to safety concerns at each location. Teachers can use social media platforms such as Twitter and Facebook to share resources and engage with their students.

Online platforms such as Google Classroom can also be used to facilitate collaboration and communication between teachers and students.
In today's rapidly evolving educational landscape, educators face the imperative of embracing and integrating new technologies within their classrooms. With the advent of AI, the role of technology in education has become even more significant. Students rely on their teachers to possess awareness and updated knowledge about the ways in which emerging technologies can enhance the learning experience. I can recall an instance where a business education teacher opted for retirement, citing an inability to adapt to new tools like "excel." This underscores the importance of teachers taking personal accountability for staying abreast of changes in the professional world, as it directly impacts the students' preparation for future success.

While not every teacher needs to be a coding expert, it is essential to comprehend the essence of coding and possess resources to support students in this area. Embracing the lifelong journey of learning may be time-intensive, yet it distinguishes effective educators and instills in students a sense of confidence inspired by their teachers' commitment to growth and adaptability.

As cloud computing and generative Ai and other technologies that are confusing to many who are not in IT fields, policy makers need to make sure teachers are offered workshops to keep them up on what these technologies are even if they are not expected to use them. We must think of these challenges to be lifelong learners as exciting rather than overwhelming.

Problem-Solving Prowess with Data-Driven PBL

Project-based learning is a teaching approach that has gained popularity in recent years, especially in the field of STEM education. It involves organizing classroom activities around projects that require students to solve real-world problems or create something new.

You may notice that many of the projects highlighted in the book have to do with cars. That is because my team learned that we could inspire and engage kids with the theater of racing in grades K-12. Where does your passion overlap with a topic that lends itself to engaging kids while offering ways to explore, investigate, prototype, and do on a classroom scale what experts do in the real world.

Project-based learning is a student-centered approach to teaching that promotes critical thinking, collaboration, communication, and creativity.

In this image, you see the progression of the same basic problem of maximizing performance of radio-controlled cars PreK to Grade 12. Lessons expand each year based on grade level math and science skills.

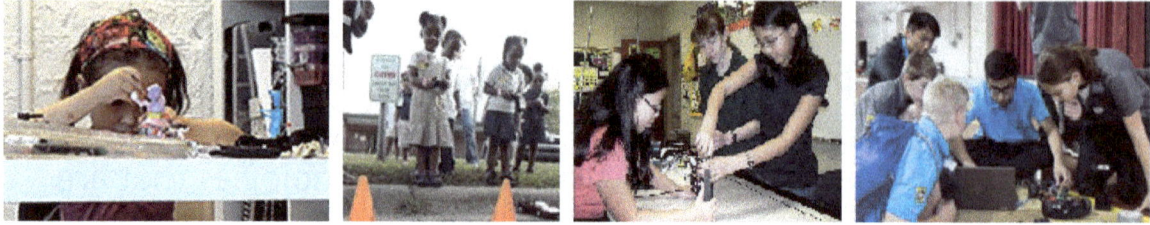

PBL also gives students the opportunity to work on projects that are interesting and challenging, which motivates them to learn more about STEM subjects. Post COVID-19, INSL projects evolved to focus on hands-on projects designed to accompany Esports gaming.

Here are some practical tips and strategies for implementing project-based learning in STEM education:

- Start with a clear learning objective.
  Before you begin a project, make sure you have a clear learning objective in mind. This will help you identify or design a project that is aligned with your learning goals and will enable students to achieve the desired outcomes.
- Create a rubric.
  Rubrics make explicit the way in which the team and the project itself will be evaluated. This makes sure that everyone is working toward the same goal and has the same expectations.
- Choose a relevant and engaging topic.
  Select a topic that is relevant to your students' interests and experience. This will help them engage with the project and stay motivated throughout the learning process.
- Provide guidance and support.
  While project-based learning is student-centered, it is essential to provide guidance and support to students throughout the project.
- Offer feedback and constructive criticism to help them improve their work and provide resources to help them overcome challenges.
- Encourage collaboration.
  Collaboration is an essential part of project-based learning. Encourage students to work together in groups to solve problems and create

innovative solutions. Have a list of "jobs" or "roles" that need to be filled so that each team member knows what is expected of them. This will help them develop teamwork skills that are critical for success in STEM careers.

- Celebrate success.
  When the project is complete, celebrate the students' success. Display their work in the classroom or have them present it to the school community.

Celebrating success will help students feel proud of their achievements and motivated to continue learning. Some groups are creating online portfolio galleries in Metaverse form using software that is free or relatively inexpensive for a school or youth organization.

Students enjoy a gamified atmosphere and respond well to earning points for their work as it is completed and awards or certificates for completion of the project.

Reflections on "interesting and relevant."

During my tenure as the developer of The Eagle Team, an Expanded Age Group Learning Experience, I had a transformative experience that underscores the effectiveness of project-based learning. This narrative serves as a testament to convince educators that this approach can effectively meet objectives while fostering student ownership of their work.

In my last three years as a science teacher, I was part of a four-member team instructing middle grades in a standard 800-student Georgia middle school. Our wing was granted the opportunity to experiment with a multi-age classroom concept, and we collectively taught 120 students: forty each from sixth, seventh, and eighth grades. Although those three years could fill a book on their own, it is pertinent to highlight a specific incident during the third year, which coincided with my nomination for an award.

Unexpectedly, an evaluation team from GA Tech and UGA visited my classroom. Gathered around a table as the bell rang, we observed thirty students entering the room. Instead of disruption, what unfolded was a testament to the efficacy of project-based learning. These students, selected at random apart from excluding "gifted" or "highly qualified" students, engaged in their self-chosen projects within multi-age groups. The environment was alive with quiet collaboration as they pursued their interests. One student even took charge of attendance by passing around a clipboard, a role performed seamlessly. Inquisitively, the evaluators inquired about the harmony they witnessed.

On that particular day:

One group deconstructed a donated motor, driven by their curiosity to comprehend its inner workings. What started as an exploration culminated in a comprehensive presentation analyzing various motor fuels and their global climate impacts, aligning with our earth science curriculum.

At a nearby table, another group crafted clay models of planets, complemented by a video illustrating the scale of planets when compared to our school acting as the sun scaled down to seventeen inches in diameter. This creative endeavor addressed multiple science and math objectives. Furthermore, they collaborated with our English teacher to delve into the evolution of optics and telescopes.

Meanwhile, a separate group engaged in crafting flower paper and ink for a calligraphy project, using plants cultivated in our school garden. The introduction of an adult volunteer enriched their experience. When they attended a calligrapher's assembly who designed pencils using a metal lathe, their interest pivoted towards learning calligraphy. Although not initially aligned with our objectives, they ingeniously justified its integration into our earth science curriculum.

This pattern extended across all eight projects, creating a hands-on learning environment that creatively aligned with state standards. In our outdoor garden, a living testament to three years of projects flourished. This group project setup liberated my time, enabling me to provide individualized attention, ensure completed readings, grade assignments, expand vocabulary, and foster math's relevance to each project. This integrated approach reverberated throughout their other classes, amplifying my lesson's impact. Ultimately, the garden emerged as our central hub for holistic integration.

The data showed significantly improved scores in math and science over three years and many students, as they left us to attend high school, tested in to the "gifted" category for the first time. Our standardized test scores were some of the highest in the state leading to our team's award as Team of the Year and to invitations to present our research with our University of Ga partners nationally.

This episode underscores how project-based learning transformed my classroom into a dynamic hub of exploration, learning, and innovation. It highlights the power of nurturing student interests to achieve learning objectives while organically fostering collaboration and critical thinking.

Inquiry-based Learning in STEM

Inquiry-based learning is an approach to teaching and learning that focuses on asking questions and seeking answers. In STEM education, inquiry-based learning is an effective way to engage students in the scientific process and help them develop critical thinking skills.

Benefits of Inquiry-Based Learning in STEM

Inquiry-based learning has several benefits for STEM education. First, it encourages students to take an active role in their learning. Instead of simply memorizing facts and formulas, students are encouraged to explore and discover information on their own. This can lead to a deeper understanding of the subject matter and a greater sense of ownership over the learning process.

Second, inquiry-based learning can help students develop critical thinking skills. By asking questions, students learn to analyze information, evaluate evidence, and draw conclusions. These skills are essential in STEM fields, where problem-solving is a key component of the work.

There are levels of inquiry from a novice problem solver to expert. This chart gives an overview of the basis of inquiry in a classroom project. Inquiry-based learning can help students develop a love of learning. When students are engaged in the learning process and feel like they are discovering new information, they are more likely to be motivated to continue learning and pursuing STEM subjects.

Levels of Inquiry

Problem Type	Problem Solving Level	Problem	Methodology	Solution
Tame	Novice	Given	Given	Given
Tame	Beginner	Given	Given	Unknown
Tame-Complex	Intermediate	Given	Unknown	Unknown
Wicked Messy	Expert	Unknown	Unknown	Unknown

Implementing Inquiry-Based Learning in Your Classroom:

Implementing inquiry-based learning in your classroom can be challenging, but there are several strategies you can use to make it more effective. Here are some practical tips for implementing inquiry-based learning in your STEM classroom:

Start with a question: Begin each lesson with a question that students will explore throughout the lesson. This will help focus their attention and give them a sense of purpose.

Provide guidance: While inquiry-based learning is student-driven, it is important to provide guidance and support along the way. Provide resources and scaffolding to help students explore the question and develop their understanding.

Encourage collaboration: Inquiry-based learning works best when students work together to explore the question. Encourage collaboration and discussion among students to deepen their understanding.

Celebrate the process: In inquiry-based learning, the process is just as important as the final product. Celebrate the process of learning and discovery, even if the students do not arrive at a definitive answer.

Inquiry-based learning is an effective approach to teaching and learning in STEM education. By encouraging students to ask questions and seek answers, inquiry-based learning can help students develop critical thinking skills, a love of learning, and a deeper understanding of STEM subjects. By implementing practical strategies in your classroom, you can make inquiry- based learning a success for your students.

Reflections on 5 Es:

Using the 5 E's with one of your Favorite Lessons.
This is my version of this model. Yours may differ. Here is a succinct breakdown of the 5E Model's five phases:

1. ENGAGE: The initial step revolves around the teacher assessing students' current knowledge and pinpointing gaps. Here, learners get their first glimpse of the new concept. This stage also aims to pique students' curiosity about upcoming topics. The instructor might ask students to pose questions or jot down their understanding of the subject. I like to use those wow experiments. Placing a cup of water on a board with ropes attached to the board. Swing the board in a circle as kids watch the cup of water go upside down without spilling or splashing them with water. That is a wow moment. Then teach centrifugal force.

2. EXPLORE: At this juncture, students delve into the topic actively through hands-on experiences. They might engage in the scientific process, collaborating with classmates to make observations. This offers a tactile approach to learning. In professional development workshops, we use this time to experience several stations. Students can also go through six or so stations in groups of 3-4. Stations can allow students to play with static electricity, handle magnets, plant seeds, mix chemicals or create paper airplanes.

3. EXPLAIN: In this instructor-guided stage, students consolidate their new knowledge and seek any necessary clarifications. An effective approach involves students recounting their discoveries from the 'Explore' stage, after which the teacher introduces detailed insights. Multimedia tools like videos or software might also be employed to enhance comprehension.

4. ELABORATE: This phase centers on allowing students to apply their newly acquired knowledge, facilitating a richer understanding. Educators might prompt students to craft presentations or embark on further explorations, ensuring the knowledge takes root. This might offer a setting in which a student's interest can guide how they pursue this topic.

5. EVALUATE: Evaluation within the 5E Model spans both informal and formal assessments. The evaluation can also encompass self-evaluations, peer reviews, written tasks, and tests.

VI: Assessing STEM Learning
Embrace the Rubric

Assessing student learning is an essential part of any teacher's job, and that holds true for STEM education as well. STEM education is unique in that it incorporates multiple subjects and skills, making it challenging to assess students' understanding comprehensively. However, there are different ways to assess STEM learning that can help teachers gauge their students' progress effectively. It does not always look like pencil and paper tests. This one has several forms depending on the age of students with ranges of points for each of the four parts of the rubric.

Project-based assessments: STEM education relies heavily on hands-on learning, and project-based assessments are ideal for assessing student understanding in this context. Teachers can assign projects that require students to apply their knowledge to real-world problems, and evaluate their performance based on the quality of their solutions.

Published Rubrics can help set goals and streamline evaluation. Rubrics give a range of points for the parts of a project that will be judged.

Collaboration assessments: Collaboration is an essential part of STEM education, and teachers can assess how well students work together by assigning group projects. Teachers can evaluate students based on a Rubric that sets out goals with respect to their ability to collaborate effectively, communicate their ideas, and problem-solve together.

Formative assessments: Formative assessments are an ongoing evaluation of students' understanding, and they can be used to identify areas where students need more support. Teachers can use quizzes, exit tickets, and other informal assessments to gauge students' understanding of a particular topic.

Performance assessments: Performance assessments involve students demonstrating their understanding of a particular concept or skill. For example, a teacher might ask students to design and build a simple machine, then evaluate their performance based on how well they meet specific criteria. Again, those criteria should be clearly set forth in a rubric.

Self-assessments: Self-assessments are a useful tool for promoting metacognition and encouraging students to take ownership of their learning. Teachers can ask students to reflect on their progress, identify areas where they need improvement, and set goals for the future.

The International STEM League publishes project rubrics. Students upload their project log books and presentations, then use an app to self-assess and award themselves points according to their adherence to the rubric. Judges provide feedback and allow for changes to be made by students prior to awarding final points to the projects.

It is possible to use apps to let students self-evaluate with the knowledge that their evaluation points may change when the teacher grades projects using the same rubric and awards final points. Self-evaluation can identify how a student may need additional clarification.

These methods are examples of authentic ways to assess STEM learning that can help teachers evaluate their students' understanding effectively. Project-based assessments, collaboration assessments, formative assessments, performance assessments, and self-assessments are all valuable tools that can help teachers gauge their students' progress and identify areas where they need more support. By using a variety of assessment methods, STEM teachers can ensure that they are meeting the needs of all their students and promoting their success in the classroom.

iNSL TEAMS

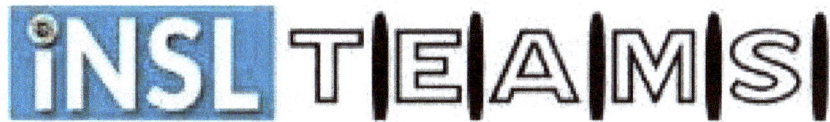

iNSL 5 Tool Stadium Project & Presentation Rubric

Category/Points	1	2	3	4
Is the scale model project accurate?	The project has some aspects that are correctly modeled, but most are not.	About half of the model is accurate.	The model is mostly accurate, but a few dimensions are slightly off.	The project is correctly modeled and the scale is consistent throughout.
Does the scale model project look like you put in a lot of effort?	The project was extremely simple, but one or two elements of detail were added to make it more complex. Some effort was put in to make the project good.	The project was somewhat complex, but no elements of detail were added. Some effort was put in to the project to make it look good.	The project was somewhat complex and elements of detail were added. A good amount of effort was put in to the project to make it look good.	The project was more complex or many details were added to make the project more complex. It is clear that a lot of time and effort were spent on making the project look good.
Did you complete the presentation including drawings?	The presentation is mostly complete and one drawing is attached.	The presentation is complete with drawings and graphics attached.	The presentation and model are complete including scale drawings & logbook.	The project is full realized and presented to the "press" including scale model & drawings.
Are the stadium areas clearly marked & present?	Areas are clearly marked but without graphic design.	Signage is present for all areas but sloppy or hastily completed.	Signs and markings are present through the stadium with clear graphics.	The stadium is has clear signage, finished graphics, and logos throughout.
Were you an effective presenter?	"Um" and "like" were said a lot throughout. You were nervous and unsure of what to say. No visual aids were used for the presentation.	There is evidence of some practice. While you might be nervous, you knew what you wanted to say and used an appropriate volume. Visual aids were used.		You were confident and did not use the words "um" or "like" frequently. You used an appropriate volume and used visual aids.

Using Technology to Assess STEM learning

Assessment is a vital component of any STEM education program. It is the process of gathering information about what students know and can do and using that information to make decisions about instruction and learning. Technology can play a significant role in facilitating assessment in STEM education.

One of the most popular ways of using technology to assess STEM learning is through online quizzes and assessments. These tools allow teachers to create and distribute quizzes and tests to students electronically.

Online quizzes and assessments are easy to administer and grade, and they provide instant feedback to students. Teachers can also use online quizzes and assessments to track student progress throughout the school year.

Virtual simulations and labs are another way in which technology can be used to assess STEM learning. These tools allow students to engage in hands-on activities and experiments in a virtual environment. Virtual simulations and labs are particularly useful in situations where access to physical equipment or materials is limited. Teachers can use virtual simulations and labs to assess students' understanding of scientific concepts and their ability to apply that understanding in a practical context.

Data analytics and visualization tools can help teachers to assess STEM learning by analyzing student performance data. These tools can provide insights into student strengths and weaknesses, as well as patterns of learning across the class. With data analytics and visualization tools, teachers can identify areas where students need additional support, and adjust their instruction accordingly.

Technology can be a valuable tool in assessing STEM learning. Online quizzes and assessments, virtual simulations and labs, and data analytics and visualization tools are just a few examples of how technology can be used to support assessment in STEM education. By leveraging the power of technology, teachers can gain deeper insights into student learning and provide more targeted instruction and support.

Strategies for Providing Feedback on STEM Projects

As a STEM teacher, providing feedback on student projects is an essential aspect of your job. Feedback is not assessment but a step in the engineering design process.

Feedback helps students understand their strengths and weaknesses, identifies areas of improvement, and encourages them to strive for excellence. However, delivering feedback can be a daunting task, especially if you are a new teacher.

To help you provide constructive feedback, here are some effective strategies that you can use in your classroom.

- **Start with positive feedback:** Begin by highlighting the strengths of the project. This approach helps students feel appreciated and motivates them to work harder. It also sets a positive tone for the rest of the feedback.
- **Be specific:** Vague feedback can be confusing for students. Be specific about what you like and what needs improvement. For example, instead of saying "good job," you can say "I liked your clear explanation of scientific concepts."
- **Provide Rubrics:** If rubrics were provided for presentations, logbooks, project plan, and lab reports, giving feedback is more targeted and effective.
- **Use the sandwich technique:** This technique involves starting and ending with positive feedback and placing constructive criticism in the middle. This approach helps students feel motivated to improve.
- **Avoid criticism:** Avoid using negative language that demotivates students. Instead, provide specific suggestions for improvement.
- **Focus on the process, not just the product:** It is essential to focus on the process of creating the project, not just the final product. Encourage the growth mindset. This approach helps students understand the importance of planning, research, and problem-solving skills.
- **Encourage self-reflection:** Encouraging students to reflect on their work and identify areas of improvement helps them take ownership

of their learning. It helps them become more self-aware and confident.

- **Provide opportunities for revision:** Giving students the opportunity to revise their work based on feedback helps them learn from their mistakes and improve their skills.

Data tells the story that matters. Assess before, during, and after a lesson or activity to be sure that students are learning what you are teaching. Adjust how and what you teach based on those assessments. Providing feedback on STEM projects is an integral part of teaching. By using these strategies, you can help your students understand their strengths and weaknesses, motivate them to improve, and encourage them to continue learning. Remember to focus on the process, be specific and constructive, and encourage self-reflection. By doing so, you will help your students become confident and successful STEM learners.

VII: Changing the sysSTEM
Addressing Common Misconceptions about STEM

STEM education has gained a lot of popularity in recent years because of its potential to equip students with the skills and knowledge required to thrive in the 21st-century workplace. However, despite its numerous benefits, there are still some misconceptions associated with STEM education. In this section, we will address some of these misconceptions and help teachers understand the true essence of STEM education.

Misconception 1: STEM education is only for high-achieving students.

One of the most common misconceptions associated with STEM education is that it is only suitable for high-achieving students. However, this is not true. STEM education is for all students, regardless of their academic abilities.

The goal of STEM education is to equip students with the skills and knowledge required to succeed in the 21st-century workplace. Therefore, it is essential to provide all students with access to STEM education and support them in developing the necessary skills.

Misconception 2: STEM education is only for students who want to pursue STEM careers.

Another misconception associated with STEM education is that it is only for students who want to pursue STEM careers. However, this is also not true. STEM education provides students with a diverse range of skills and knowledge that can be applied to various fields. For example, the critical thinking, problem-solving, and analytical skills developed through STEM education can be applied to fields such as finance, law, and healthcare.

Misconception 3: STEM education is only about memorizing facts and figures.

Another common misconception associated with STEM education is that it is only about memorizing facts and figures. However, this is not true. STEM education is about developing critical thinking, problem-solving, and analytical skills. These skills are developed through hands-on activities and projects that require students to apply their knowledge to real-world problems.

Misconception 4: STEM education is only for students who are good at math.

Another misconception associated with STEM education is that it is only for students who are good at math. However, this is certainly not true. STEM education requires students to have a diverse range of skills, including critical thinking, problem-solving, and analytical skills. While math is an essential component of STEM education, students who struggle with math can still excel in STEM education and technology offers help in this area.

STEM education is an essential component of modern education, and it is essential to address the misconceptions associated with it. By understanding the true essence of STEM education, teachers can provide all students with access to STEM education and support them in developing the necessary skills to succeed in the 21st-century workplace.

Dealing with Student Disengagement in STEM

Dealing with student disengagement in STEM is a common challenge that many teachers face. As a STEM educator, it is important to recognize that disengagement can be caused by various factors such as lack of interest, difficulty in understanding, and boredom.

However, there are several strategies that teachers can implement to re-engage students and promote a love for STEM. Post-COVID, the issue of engaging students has become a top priority. Too many students who had to learn at home in less than ideal settings have come to think of school as optional. One of the most effective ways to combat disengagement is to make STEM education relevant and relatable to students' lives. Teachers can do this by incorporating real-world examples and applications into their lessons.

For instance, if teaching math, teachers can relate equations to everyday scenarios such as calculating the distance a car travels or the cost of groceries. This helps students understand the importance of STEM in their daily lives and makes the subject more interesting.

Another strategy is to incorporate hands-on activities and projects that allow students to apply what they learn in real-life scenarios. This helps students see the practical application of STEM and promotes a deeper understanding of the subject. Teachers can also encourage collaboration among students by assigning group projects that require teamwork and communication skills.

It is also important to create a positive and supportive classroom environment. Teachers can do this by praising students' efforts and acknowledging their achievements. This helps build confidence and encourages students to take risks and ask questions. Teachers can also provide personalized feedback and support to students who are struggling, which can help them feel more engaged and motivated.

In addition, technology can be used to enhance STEM education and promote engagement. Teachers can incorporate interactive software and apps that allow students to explore STEM concepts in a fun and engaging way. This not only makes learning more enjoyable but also helps students retain information better.

In conclusion, dealing with student disengagement in STEM requires patience, creativity, and a willingness to adapt teaching strategies. By making STEM education relevant, hands-on, collaborative, and fun, teachers can help students see the value of STEM and promote a lifelong love for learning.

Supporting Struggling Learners in STEM

Supporting struggling learners in STEM can be a challenging task for any teacher.

However, with the right strategies and practical tips, you can help struggling learners to overcome their difficulties and achieve success in STEM subjects.

One of the first steps to supporting struggling learners in STEM is to identify the areas where they are struggling. This can be done through observation, assessment, and feedback from the students themselves. Once you identify the areas where the student is struggling, you can develop a plan to address those specific areas.

Having students collect data in a middle grades classroom and calculate a score from their data allowed a teacher to identify the one fundamental error in how a student treated mixed fractions. Once remediated, the student was offered additional ways to practice place value and estimation so that they could better identify an answer that was not reasonable.

In another classroom a high school engineering teacher who took part in a special event argued that her "highly capable" students should be allowed to use calculators to calculate their scores, but relented when the presenter insisted on paper and pencil for at least the first round of data collection. At the end of the lesson, the teacher and her colleagues had to regroup as they learned that students who were the top of their classes and planning to attend college in one year were unable to accurately read minutes and parts of a second on an analog stop watch, struggled to measure out a track length longer than the tape measure they were using and could not correctly average the times of all the timers for a run of the radio controlled car.

Over reliance on tools that do the work for you before you learn to do it for yourself is leaving huge gaps in what students learn. Hand-on activities offer one solution.

Mentors offer another effective support for struggling learners in STEM. Providing one-on-one support or tutoring sessions gives student the extra attention they may need. College chapters of national organizations such as the ASA (American Statistics Association) and NSBE (National Society of Black Engineers) are examples of kids willing to help as near peer mentors. The adults in these organizations often hold Saturday meetings with groups of students and foster STEM through academic competitions like the International STEM League or Vex Robotics. Daily exercises that build a sense of comfort with basic scale, computation, and measurement can help students grow in their comfort with mathematics.

Scaleville is a series of these daily activities that a teacher can use as bell ringers to grow a sense of number and estimation. After using such interventions, students can recognize an unreasonable answer because they have developed a sense of how much things weigh, how fast they move, how much area they cover and what powers of ten can do to help in estimation. These also help teachers build that same sense of scale. It was ignored in most teacher education paths. Therefore, it gets ignored when we teach. This is an example of a Scaleville daily activity that can be used over one day or a week. There are activity books for elementary, middle, and high school classes.

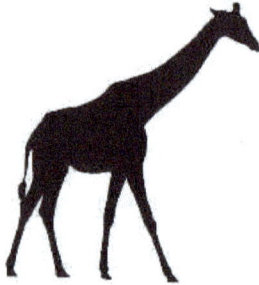

Distance and Speed
Activity 53

Step # 1
Remember our 14 to 18 feet-tall giraffe?
What is its top running speed?

Step # 2
Name something 10 times as fast.

Name something 1/10th as fast.

Step # 3
Convert the measurement from # 1 to metric,
or convert to standard if already in metric.

Step # 4
The measurement from #1 falls between what
two powers of ten?

10   and   10

Why would a giraffe need to run?
Who would chase a giraffe?

scaleville

53

Another strategy that can be used to support struggling learners in STEM is to adjust your teaching methods to better suit their learning style. For example, if a student is struggling with a concept that is presented verbally, you may want to provide visual aids or hands-on activities to help them better understand the material.

It can also be helpful to break down complex concepts into smaller, more manageable pieces. This can help struggling learners to better understand the material and build confidence as they see their progress. I usually lean into the data, but this is one instance in which I am not convinced that the studies can isolate the variables well enough to tell me this does not work, so I would try it because it seems like a reasonable strategy

.

Finally, it is important to encourage struggling learners in STEM to persevere and not give up. Reassure them that it is okay to make mistakes and that learning is a process. Provide positive feedback and celebrate their successes, no matter how small. Always remember the STEM Mindset includes the Growth Mindset. Supporting struggling learners in STEM can be a challenging task, but with the right strategies and support, you can help these students to achieve success and build confidence in their abilities.

Addressing the Gender Gap in STEM

STEM (Science, Technology, Engineering, and Mathematics) fields have traditionally been male dominated. The gender gap in STEM is a significant concern that needs to be addressed. According to the National Science Foundation, women earn only 20% of bachelor's degrees in engineering, 18% in computer science, and 43% in mathematics. This gap is not only unjust; it also limits the potential talent pool for these critical fields.

Teachers play a crucial role in closing the gender gap in STEM. Here are some practical tips and strategies that can help teachers address this issue:

Foster a welcoming and inclusive classroom environment: Teachers can create a welcoming classroom environment that is inclusive of all genders. They can encourage students to share their experiences and ideas without fear of judgment or ridicule. Teachers can also use examples and case studies that feature women in STEM to inspire and encourage female students.

Create a Who's-Who file box (virtual or real) organized by topics you teach in your main subject area and in STEM fields. Behind each one, place examples of people who we should know about, but may not. Do not be exclusive but inclusive. This makes it simple to give examples that include various genders and ethnicities and races when that teachable moment arrives.

Provide mentorship and role models: Female students in STEM often lack role models and mentors who can guide and inspire them. Teachers can help by connecting their female students with successful women in STEM fields and in their own communities. They can also serve as role models themselves by sharing their experiences and successes in STEM fields.

Use gender-neutral language: Teachers should avoid gender-specific language when teaching STEM in their lectures, assignments, and tests. This will help create a more inclusive learning environment and make female students feel more comfortable and welcome. It is enlightening when we learn how often we say "he."

Encourage collaboration: Teachers can encourage collaboration among their students, especially between male and female students. Collaborative projects and group work can help break down gender barriers and promote teamwork and inclusivity. Make sure that on hands on projects, male roles do not always have the males doing the "fun" part while the females calculate and write the lab reports.

Celebrate diversity: Finally, teachers should celebrate diversity in their classrooms. They can organize events and activities that celebrate the accomplishments of women and minorities in STEM fields.

Closing the gender gap in STEM is a critical goal that requires the support and commitment of all educators. By creating a welcoming and inclusive classroom environment, providing mentorship and role models, using gender-neutral language, encouraging collaboration, and celebrating diversity, teachers can help address this issue and inspire the next generation of female STEM professionals.

VIII: Professional Development and Resources

Yes, workshops can really feel as exciting as this one.

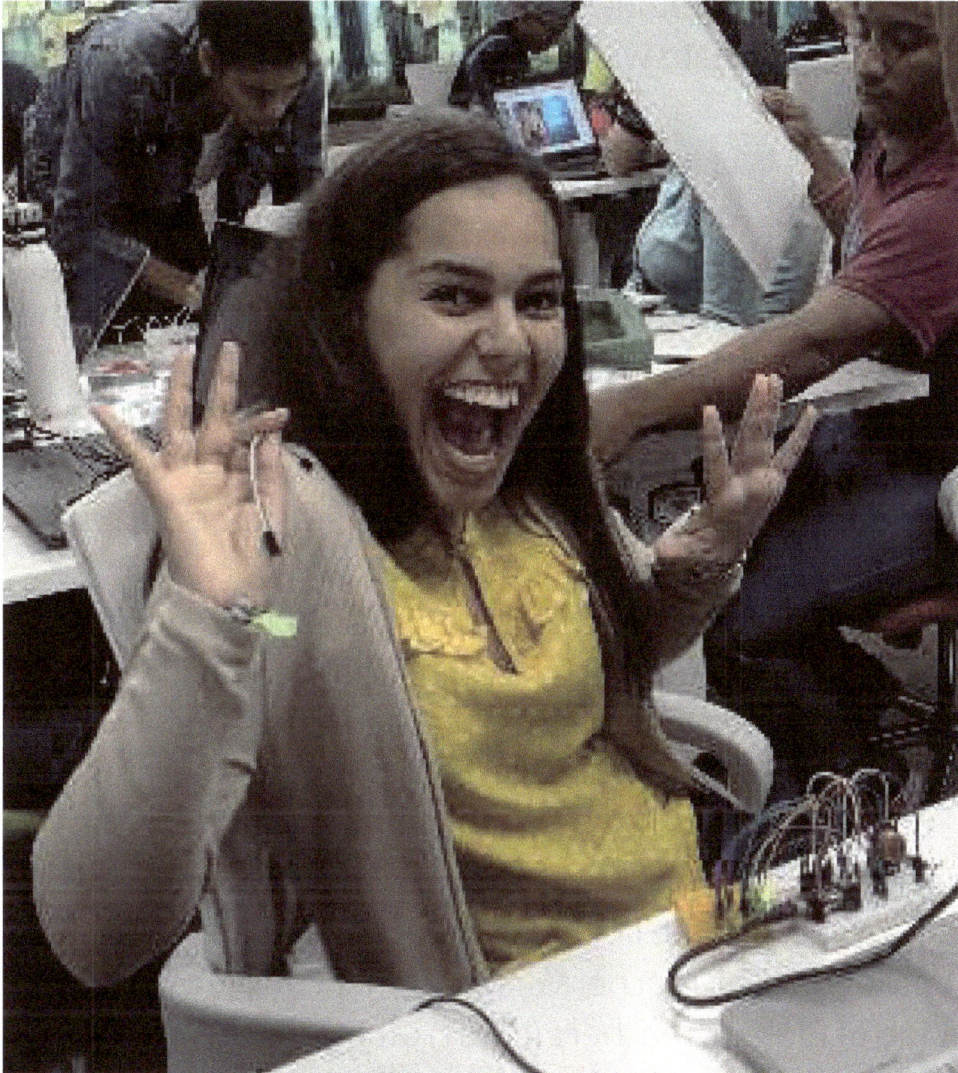

These teachers were new to the field and excited to be integrating science, computer science, and mathematics with an engineering program. In a one-week STEM Sprint, they experienced it as a student and learned to facilitate it as a teacher. They used an Esports game as the HOOK for their kids and their classrooms were exciting places this year.

STEM education is a rapidly evolving field. As a teacher, it is essential to stay updated on the latest developments and best practices in STEM education to ensure that your students receive the best education possible. Fortunately, there are many opportunities for professional development in STEM education that can help you improve your teaching skills and stay up to date with the latest trends.

Attend Conferences and Workshops
Conferences and workshops are an excellent way to learn from experts in the field and connect with other STEM educators. Many conferences and workshops offer hands-on learning opportunities, keynote speakers, and networking events that can help you stay current with the latest trends and best practices in STEM education.

Some popular conferences and workshops for STEM educators include the National Science Teachers Association (NSTA) Conference, the International Society for Technology in Education (ISTE) Conference, and the STEM Conference for Educators. You may find that your budget and needs are better served by attending more local and state level conferences.

Join Professional Organizations
Professional organizations like the National Science Teachers Association (NSTA), the National Council of Teachers of Mathematics (NCTM), and the National Association of Biology Teachers (NABT) offer a wealth of resources and opportunities for STEM educators. These organizations provide access to professional development resources, networking opportunities, and the latest research and best practices in STEM education.

Take Online Courses and Webinars
Online courses and webinars are convenient options for STEM educators who want to continue their professional development without leaving

their homes. Many online platforms, such as Coursera, Udemy, and edX, offer free or low-cost courses on a variety of STEM topics. Khan Academy can help you fill in your own gaps should that increase your confidence. It is a great refresher for math concepts.

Participate in Mentoring Programs

Mentoring programs are another excellent way for STEM educators to develop their skills and knowledge. Many schools and professional organizations offer mentoring programs that pair experienced teachers with novice educators.

Mentoring programs provide opportunities for new teachers to learn from experienced educators, receive feedback on their teaching, and gain valuable insights into the teaching profession.

Professional development is essential for STEM educators who want to stay current with the latest trends and best practices in the field. Attending conferences and workshops, joining professional organizations, taking online courses and webinars, and participating in mentoring programs are just a few of the many opportunities available for STEM educators to continue their professional growth and development. By taking advantage of these opportunities, you can improve your teaching skills, enhance your students' learning experience, and advance your career as a STEM educator.

STEM Resources for Teachers

STEM education is rapidly growing and is becoming an essential part of every student's academic journey. However, teaching STEM subjects can be challenging, especially for new teachers. And to help them with their teaching journey, here are some STEM resources for teachers that can aid them in delivering quality education and help students develop their STEM skills.

International STEM League- the iNSL is a 501c3 organization that provides a practice league for STEM careers. It has curriculum for K-12 project based learning and has recently created an Academic Esports Curriculum to use in conjunction with Gaming. iNSL runs an international STEM competition with an annual points race.
http://www.insl.org
Sprint workshops are available through the International STEM League now. https://www.insl.org/design-sprints

National Science Teaching Association - The National Science Teaching Association is a professional organization that supports science teachers in the United States. They provide resources such as lesson plans, professional development opportunities, and instructional materials for teachers.

Code.org - Code.org offers free, online coding courses for students of all ages. The website also provides teacher training and resources for teaching computer science.

NASA Education - NASA Education provides educators with resources, materials, and opportunities for professional development in STEM education. The website offers lesson plans and multimedia resources teachers to bring into classrooms.

PBS Learning Media - PBS Learning Media is an online library of K-12 educational resources, including STEM education materials. The website offers lesson plans, videos, and interactive activities that promote inquiry- based learning.

Art of STEM – Art of STEM brings blended learning to new heights with on site Art of STEM Festivals for elementary students and families. It has a suite of programs, classes, camps, and kits for remote and in person learning.

Ten80 Education – In its 17th year of national and international competition, this group offers effective STEM classes, camps, and curriculum as well as competitions

Teaching STEM subjects can be challenging, but with the right resources, teachers can deliver quality education and help students develop their STEM skills. These STEM resources for teachers can provide support, inspiration, and guidance to educators who are committed to promoting STEM education.

Building a STEM Teacher Network

As a STEM teacher, it is essential to build a network of like-minded educators who share a passion for science, technology, engineering, and math. Collaborating with other teachers can help you improve your teaching skills, stay current with the latest trends in STEM education, and create a supportive community of professionals.

Here are some tips for building a STEM teacher network:

Join Professional Organizations: Joining a professional organization is an excellent way to connect with other STEM teachers. You can attend conferences, workshops, and webinars, which provide opportunities to learn from experts in the field, network with other educators, and share your own experiences.

Connect on Social Media: Social media platforms like Twitter, LinkedIn, and Facebook are great places to connect with other STEM teachers. You can join groups and participate in discussions, share resources, and ask for help and advice.

Attend Local STEM Events: Attending local STEM events like science fairs, hackathons, and maker fairs can help you connect with other STEM teachers in your area. These events provide opportunities to learn about new teaching strategies, share ideas, and collaborate on projects.

Join Online Communities: Online communities like STEM Teaching Tools, Edmodo, and STEM Learning Communities offer a wealth of resources and support for STEM teachers. These communities provide a platform to ask questions, share teaching strategies, and collaborate with other educators.

Collaborate on Projects: Collaborating on STEM projects with other teachers can help you develop new teaching strategies, share resources, and create a supportive community of professionals. You can work together on projects like robotics competitions, coding challenges, and science experiments.

Building a network of STEM teachers is essential for professional development, staying current with the latest trends in STEM education, and creating a supportive community of professionals. Joining professional organizations, connecting on social media, attending local STEM events, joining online communities, and collaborating on projects are all great ways to build your network.

IX: Inspiring the Next Generation of Data Driven Global Problem Solvers

What characterizes a confident teacher?

- A confident teacher does not have all the answers, and is comfortable admitting that is the case.
- The confident teacher knows how to access resources to find answers or point students in the right direction for exploration
- The confident teacher knows how to experiment if that presents a better next step toward understanding.
- The confident teacher is an enthusiastic life-long learner who updates basic STEM skills to better serve students.

That is why professional development is so important. Having clarified this definition of teaching with confidence, why is it so important?

The students you teach are looking for guidance and knowledge from you. They need you to be confident in your abilities to teach them the skills and concepts that will help them succeed in their future careers. Additionally, a confident teacher can inspire confidence in their students, which can lead to greater engagement and better learning outcomes.

To teach with confidence, it is important to stay up to date with the latest research and developments in your field, as well as seeking out professional development opportunities to improve your own teaching skills.

When you have a deep understanding of the subject matter, you can answer questions and provide explanations with ease and can find reliable sources when you need to know more.

Your comfort with the subject matter and with the things you do not know will help build your students' confidence in the subject matter as well. You will also better identify the subject matter intersections between your primary subject and others.

Another way to teach with confidence is to be prepared. This means having lesson plans and materials ready in advance, and anticipating potential challenges or questions that may arise during your lesson. Being prepared also allows you to be flexible when those teachable moments happen.

Prepared does not mean adhering to the lesson plan when better teaching opportunities arise. By being well-prepared, you can focus more on teaching and engaging with your students, rather than worrying about logistics.

Additionally, it is important to foster a positive classroom culture that encourages experimentation and learning from mistakes. This can help students feel more comfortable taking risks and asking questions, which can lead to greater engagement and understanding of the subject matter.

Always remember that teaching with confidence is not about being perfect or knowing everything. It is about being comfortable with the subject matter and being willing to learn alongside your students. By modeling a growth mindset and a willingness to learn, you can inspire your students to do the same and create a classroom culture that values curiosity and rewards exploration.

X: Cultivate a Passion for STEM!

Being passionate about STEM as a teacher is a powerful force that ignites curiosity, sparks inspiration, and propels students on a lifelong journey of discovery. It is a genuine dedication to fostering a love for science, technology, engineering, and mathematics that goes beyond the classroom walls.

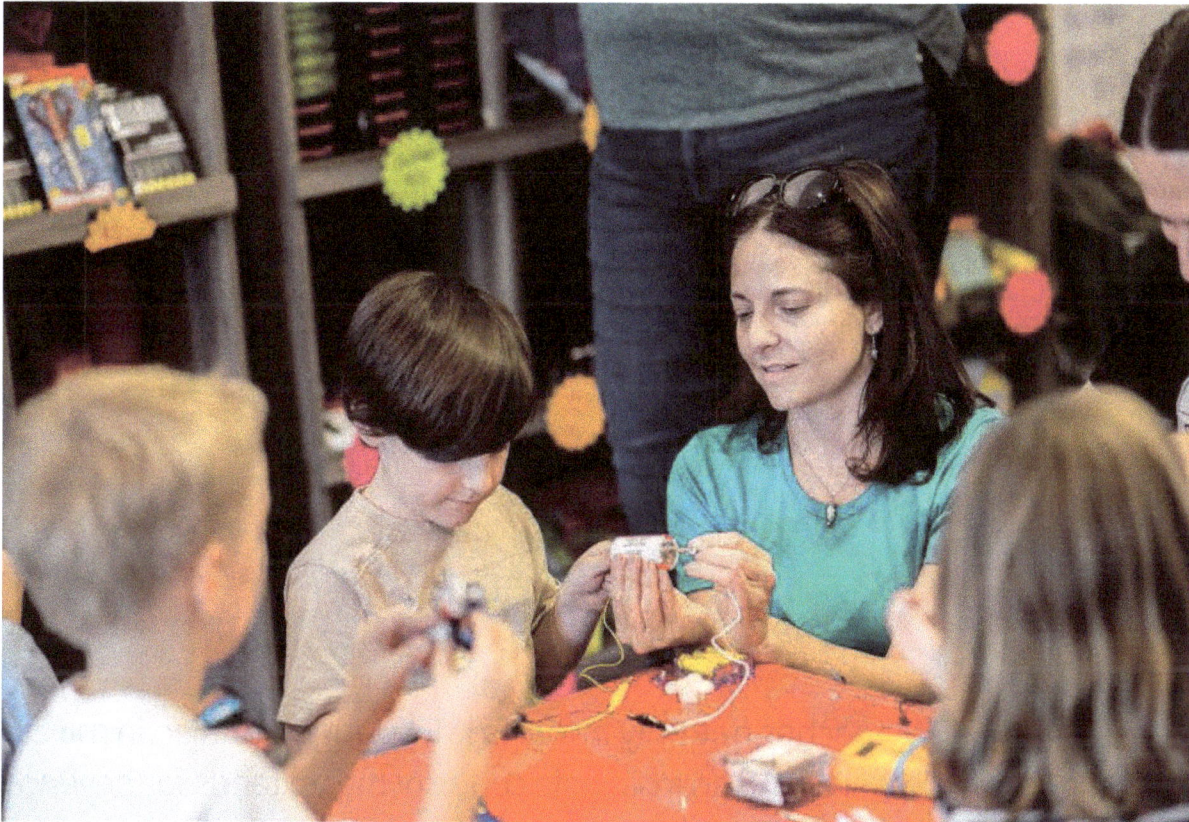

Passion for STEM is evident in a teacher's unwavering commitment to creating engaging learning experiences. It means designing hands-on experiments that captivate students' imaginations, encouraging them to ask questions, make connections, and explore the world around them. It is about infusing real-world context into lessons, enabling students to see the relevance and applicability of STEM in their everyday lives.

Passion for STEM shines through in a teacher's contagious enthusiasm and genuine excitement for the subject matter. It means staying current with the latest advancements, embracing new technologies and teaching methodologies, and constantly seeking out opportunities for professional growth.

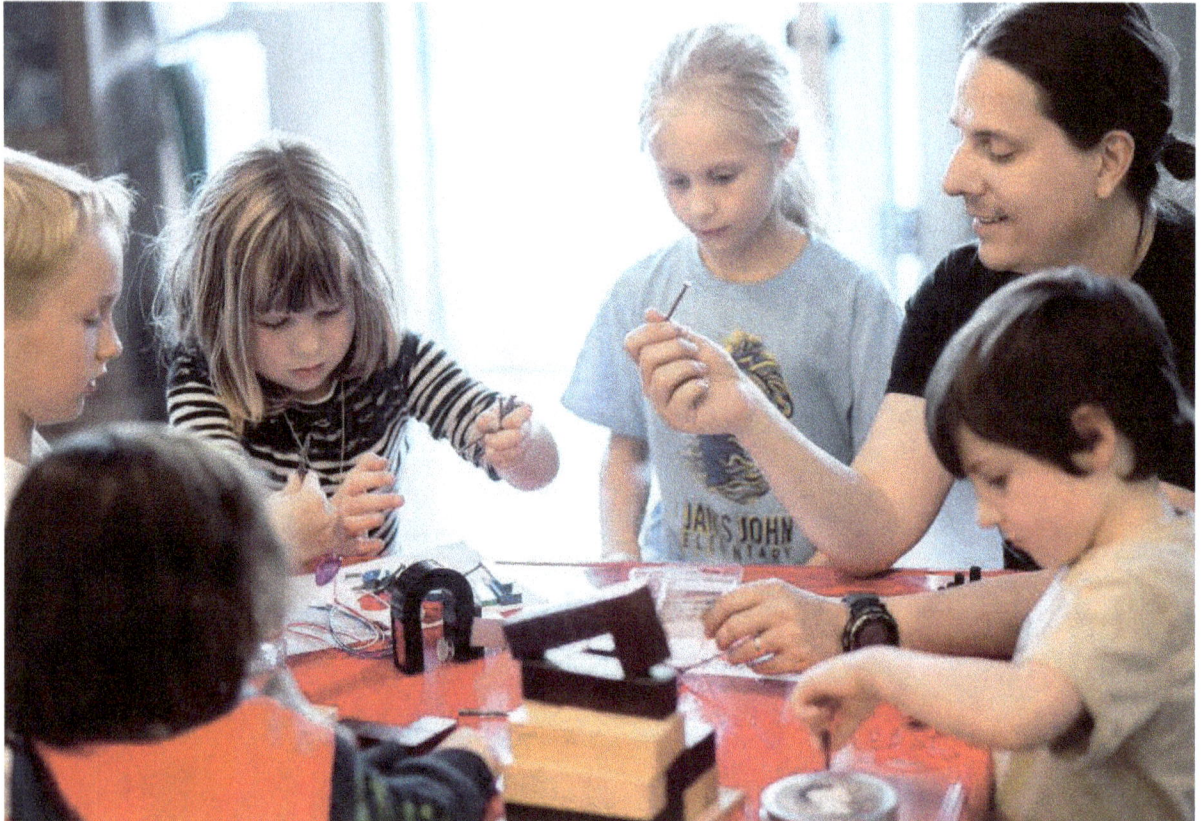

A passionate STEM teacher not only imparts knowledge but also inspires a lifelong love for learning and an insatiable curiosity that extends far beyond the classroom. Ultimately, being passionate about STEM as a teacher means being a catalyst for change, nurturing the next generation of innovators, problem-solvers, and critical thinkers who will shape our future.

A passionate STEM teacher is a relentless advocate for equity and inclusion, ensuring that all students, regardless of their background or gender, feel welcomed and empowered in the pursuit of their interests. They strive to break down barriers, challenge stereotypes, and foster a diverse and inclusive learning environment where everyone has the opportunity to thrive and succeed. It means instilling in students the belief that they have the power to make a difference and contribute to the world through their STEM knowledge and skills.

Passion for STEM is a transformative force that fuels the fire of learning, unlocks potential, and empowers students to reach new heights. It is this passion that lights the way, guiding students on a path of endless possibilities and inspiring them to embrace the wonders of STEM with open hearts and curious minds.

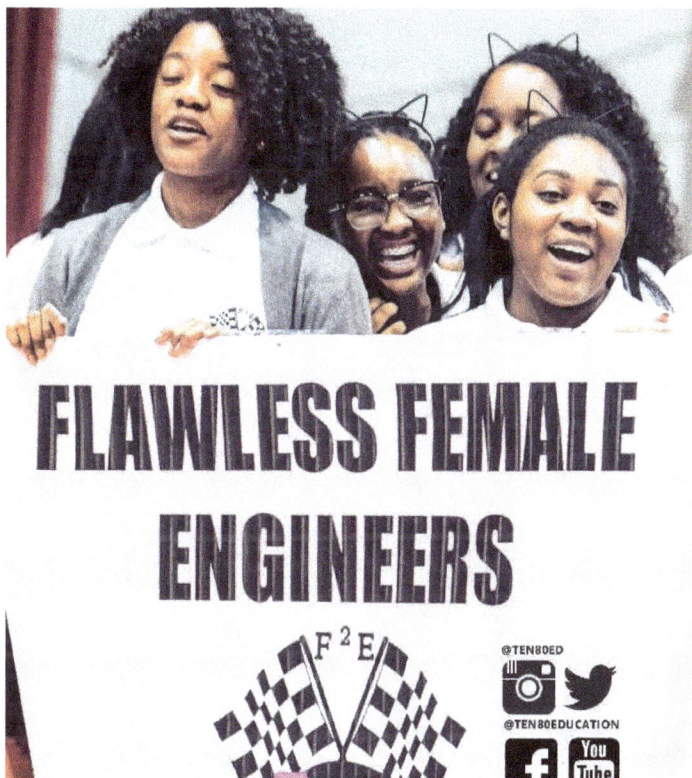

Sample Lessons

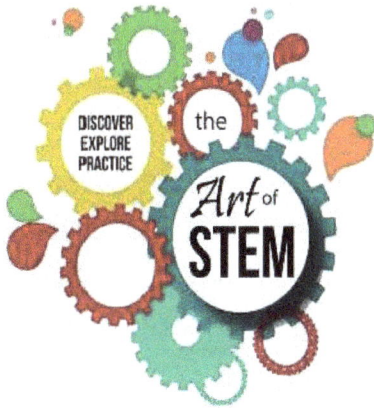

POM POM CATAPULTS

Materials:
5 craft sticks, 2 tongue depressors, 4 rubber bands, bottle cap, pom-poms, cardstock for bullseye, ruler, pencil, tape

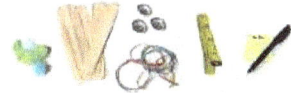

Description: Investigate lever and fulcrum (simple machines) with fuzzy pom poms and a pop stick catapult. The catapult is basically a lever. A lever is a simple machine with a beam on a fixed hinge, or fulcrum. A lever is rigid but can see-saw on its fulcrum. The catapult stores energy when its arm is pulled down over the fulcrum. Energy is released to launch the pom pom payload.
Where should you place the fulcrum to store the most energy and create the longest launch?

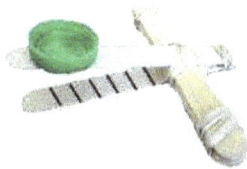

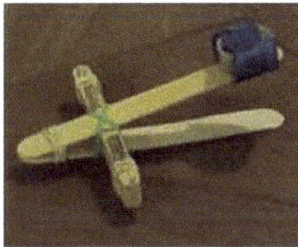

USE DATA TO FIND THE BEST PLACE FOR YOUR CATAPULT'S FULCRUM

START HERE

A catapult uses the sudden release of stored potential energy to launch its payload. Types of catapults have been used by the Greeks, Romans, and Chinese. Early catapults tried to increase the range and power of a crossbow. A Greek historian was the first to document a mechanical arrow firing catapult (called a Ballista) in 399 BC. Our catapult is a small scale machine that will launch fuzzy pom poms.

CONSTRUCT AND INVESTIGATE

1. Turn one of the tongue depressors into a ruler by marking centimeters or inches along the stick. This allows you to collect data on the best place to put your crossbar given the target's distance and height.
2. Stack and band together 5 pop sticks.
3. Band the tongue depressors at tip and criss-crossed over the crossbar.
4. Glue or tape the cap (experiment with attaching the cap as a variable).

COLLECT AND ANALYZE DATA

Put the projectile into the cap, hold down the top stick, release and watch the object fly. Practice aiming by setting up a target.
These numbers will help you decide the best launch setup for your catapult.

Create a chart to collect the distance travelled vs. fulcrum placement.
- Write the fulcrum measurement on the chart (Independent Variable).
- Measure the distance travelled by each pom pom (Dependent Variable).

X Fulcrum Where is the beam?	Y Landing How far did the pom pom travel?
2 cm	300 centimeters

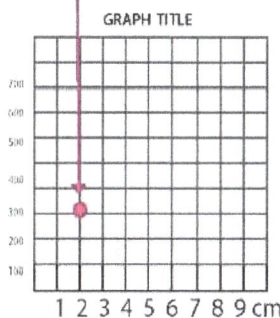

GRAPH TITLE

GRAPHS HELP DATA TELL STORIES

Move the chart data to a graph so the patterns in data are easy to read.
The X axis along the base is an independent variable that you control. You control the location of your fulcrum. Y axis is the dependent variable that changes as a result of your decisions like the distance a pom pom travels. Place a finger on the X axis number. Place a finger on the matching Y axis number. Bring your fingers together and place a dot.

REDESIGN

What other "variables" can you test to change the catapult's launch power? Examples: Test rubber bands. Test number of pop sticks in your fulcrum. Collect data. Read the data, and redesign your catapult using data!

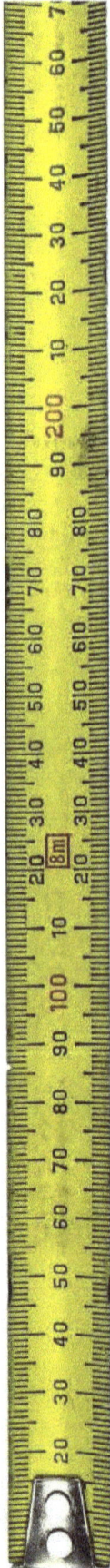

Driving STEM

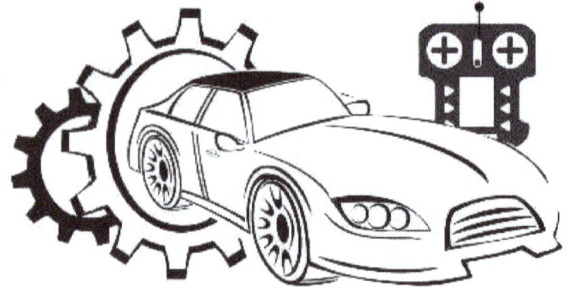

FORCES & MOTION
Energy Bounce

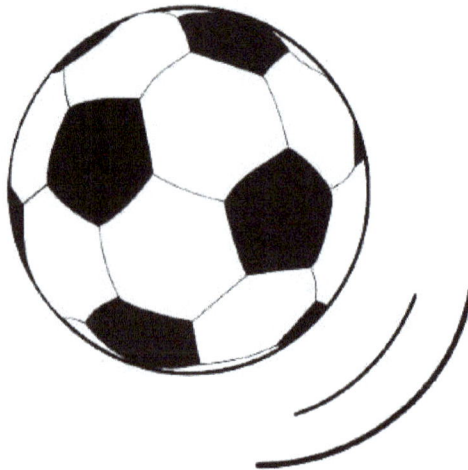

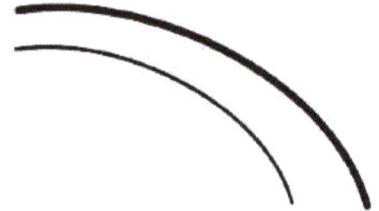

MATERIALS
4 different types of balls rubber
bands
tape measure handout
pencil

1

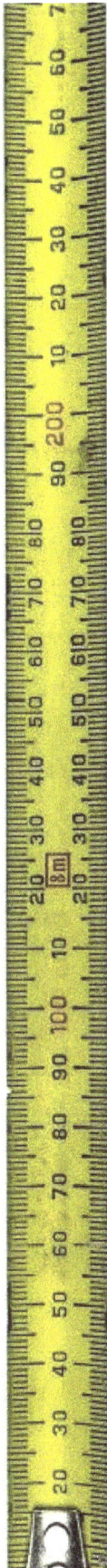

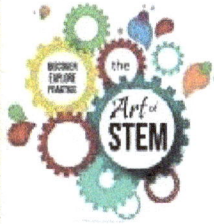

Forces & Motion
Energy Bounce

Energy Bounce
Procedures

Step 1
- Set the meter stick up vertically
- Hold the ball at the top of the meter stick and drop the ball. What force is acting on the ball?

- Does it bounce back the same distance it was dropped?

Step 2
- Measure and record how high the ball bounces when dropped from 4 ft...
- Drop 1 ___ Drop 2   Drop 3 _____
- Is the height of the first bounce the same each time?
- What is the average bounce of the ball?.

Step 3
Drop the ball from various heights, 1 foot, 2 feet, 3 feet
- Graph the highest recoil of the ball from each height.

Step 4
Repeat steps 3 and 4 for each different kind of ball and add to the group data chart and graph.

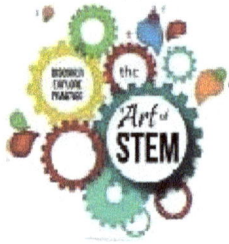

Forces & Motion
Energy Bounce

2

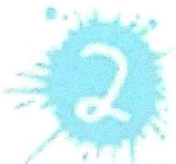

Energy Bounce

Energy cannot be created or destroyed but it can be changed in form.

Use 3 kinds of balls to determine if there is a pattern to the way balls bounce.

Essential Questions

- What is an elastic collision?
- What is stored energy?
- What is potential energy?
- What is kinetic energy?

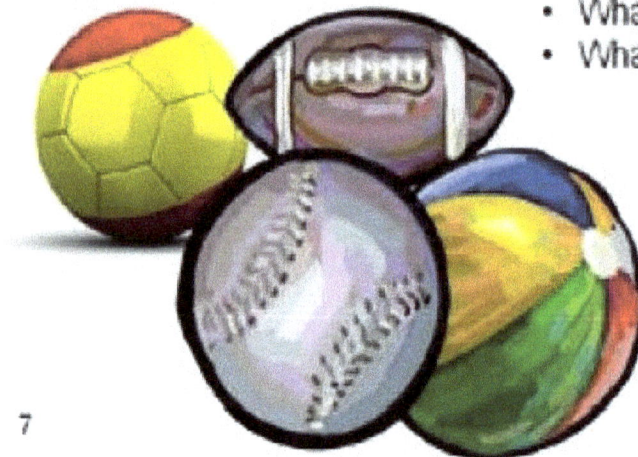

Materials
- Golf Ball
- Ping Pong Ball
- Wiffle Ball
- Graph
- Colored pencils

7

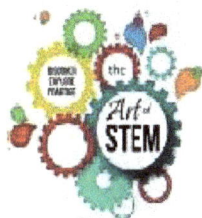

Forces & Motion
Energy Bounce

ENERGY BOUNCE DISCUSSION

Kinetic Energy describes the amount of energy an object has by virtue of it having some non-zero mass and traveling at some speed.
KE= 1/2 mv^2

Potential Energy describes the energy that could be gained by that object if it was not at that poten-tial. It is not really accurate to say that potential energy is energy at rest since it is very possible for moving objects to have potential energy.

A book sitting on a shelf has some gravitational energy. It's potential energy equals the amount of energy needed to put the book up there in the first place and the amount of energy which could be gained if the book falls down from the shelf. As the book is falling, before it hits the floor, the book has some fraction of its potential energy converted into kinetic, in other words it has both kinds of energy at the same time.

ENDURING UNDERSTANDING

1. Potential energy is energy that is stored in an object. If you stretch a rubber band, you will give it potential energy. As the rubber band is released, potential energy is changed to motion

2. Kinetic energy is energy of motion. A rubber band flying through the air has kinetic energy.

ESSENTIAL QUESTIONS

1.   What is the difference in kinetic and potential energy?
2.   What are some examples of energy transversions?

Look for Misconceptions

 Many students incorrectly assume that an object cannot have kinetic energy and potential energy at the same time.
  TRUTH: As objects convert PE to KE we can think of them as having both kinds of energy at the same time.

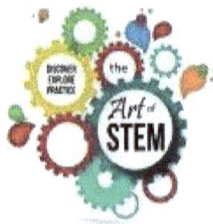

Forces & Motion
Energy Bounce

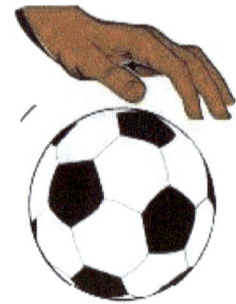

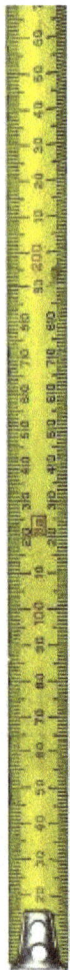

DIRECTIONS

Step 1: Set the meter stick up vertically, or hang a tape measure on the wall.
Hold the ball at the top of the meter stick and drop the ball.

What force is acting on the ball?

Does it bounce back the same distance it was dropped?

Step 2 : Measure and record how high the ball bounces when dropped from 4 ft.

Drop 1 ___Drop 2 _____ Drop 3 _____ Average:_____

Is the height of the first bounce the same each time?
What is the average first recoil bounce of the ball?.

Step 3: Drop the ball from various heights, 1 foot, 2 feet, 3 feet
Graph the first or highest recoil of the ball from each height.

Step 4: Repeat steps 3 and 4 for each different kind of ball.
Add data to the chart and graph

Initial Drop Height	4 feet	5 feet	6 feet	8 feet	Dig Deeper: What is the ratio of recoil to drop height?
Ball 1 recoil height					
Ball 2 recoil height					
Ball 3 recoil height					
Ball 4 recoil height					

Average recoil heights _____ _____ _____ _____

Real Reverse Engineering

Art of STEM for Ten80 Education

DISCOVER
EXPLORE
PRACTICE

the *Art* of
STEM

TEN80
EDUCATION

Lesson Plan & Notes

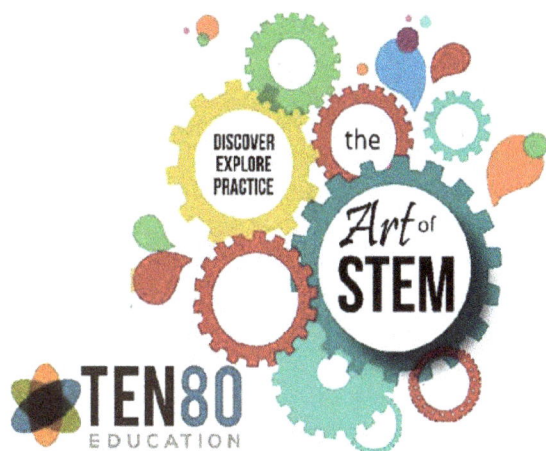

Objectives

Critically examine something mechanical that you see in everyday life, but may not think much about, then ask and answer the question, "How does it work?". Explain how it works so that others can understand how it works simply by watching your video, reading your description and/or looking at your illustrations.

Science and Engineering Correlations

HS.PS-FE.c. Evaluate natural and designed systems where there is an exchange of energy between objects and fields and characterize how the energy is exchanged.

HS-ETS-ED.b. Analyze input and output data and functioning of a human-built system to define opportunities to improve the system's performance so it better meets the needs of end users while taking into account constraints.

HS.PS-E.h. Design, build, and evaluate devices that convert one form of energy into another form of energy.

MS.ETS-ED.f. Communicate information about a proposed solution to a problem, including relevant scientific principles, how the design was developed, how it meets the criteria and constraints of the problem, and how it reduces the potential for negative consequences for society and the natural environment.

HS-ETS-ED.b. Analyze input and output data and functioning of a human-built system performance so it better meets the needs of end users while taking into account constraints (e.g., materials, costs, scientific principles).

ELA Correlations

RST.6-10.7. Integrate quantitative or technical information expressed in words in a text with a version of that information expressed visually.

SL.6-12.1. Engage effectively in a range of collaborative discussions (one-on-one, in groups, and teacher led) with diverse partners on grade appropriate topics, texts, and issues, building on others' ideas and expressing their own clearly.

GATHER MATERIALS

- Wind-up toy or pull-back vehicle
- Phillips Screwdriver (small)
- Needle-Nose Pliers (optional)
- Measuring tape or ruler
- Logbook
- Clear Tape
- *Tray to hold small parts*
- *Digital camera for documentation.*
  - *Take pictures as you go.*
  - *This is not part of the formal activity, but having images of each step helps with recall.*

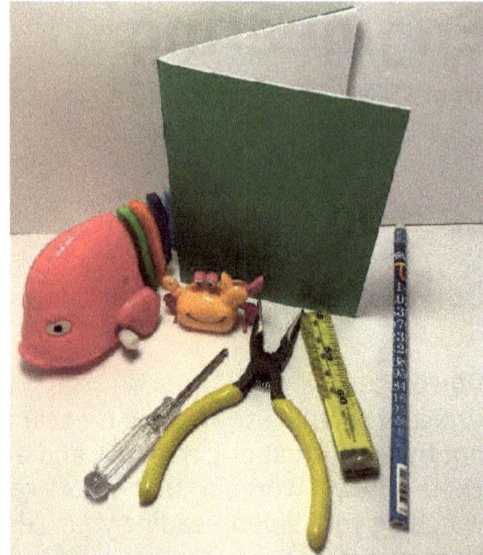

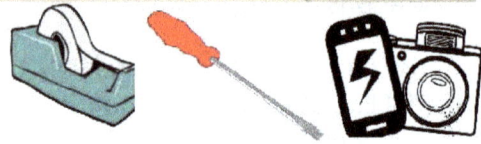

PREPARE WORKSPACES

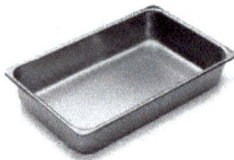

PURPOSE

The purpose of this activity:

- **Multiple representations** – Provide opportunities to explore and discuss gears, GIP, energy and engineering in a different context

- **Practice GIP** – focus on observations and DOCUMENTATION. Your goal is to understand how it works and be able to communicate that to others through your writing and figures (not just verbally).

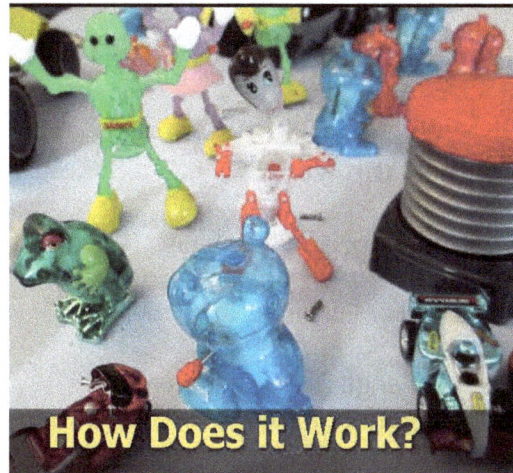

How Does it Work?

- **Reinforce lessons in energy** – your goal is to follow the energy from your hand through the mechanisms and movement. (Transformation of energy, kinetic, potential, etc.)

- **Foster Creativity** that often starts with sketches. Turn thoughts into tangible materials you can communicate to others.

Additional discussion on this idea.

Dream, Draw, Design

Dreams are often fueled by ideas, descriptions and pictures of places and things others have created, so without a base of knowledge and images to build upon, it is impossible for most of us to "dream up" things we don't already know about.

To convey your ideas to others, illustrations and sketches, are compelling tools. They are usually the first concrete step in making an idea you've created into a reality. Drawing and illustrating is a kind of language.

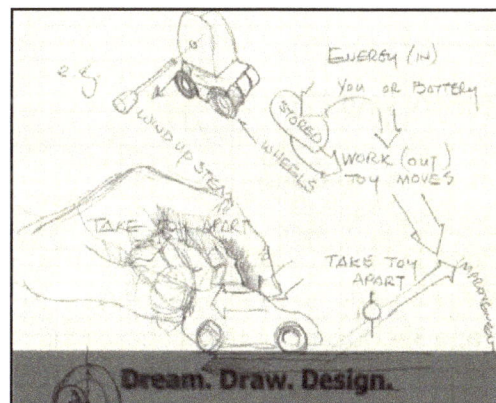

Dream. Draw. Design.

Design is the next step to transforming your dreams into something real. Taking a well defined idea and figuring out how to make it work is often a matter of choosing materials and defining manufacturing and testing processes through the application of scientific, mathematical and engineering analysis...but let's not go there yet.

Your first step to dreaming, drawing and designing truly new things, is building a mental library about how existing things work. Let's start building.

ENGAGE

The Challenge:

How Does this Work?

Wind, pull back, and demonstrate multiple toys to engage the audience. Issue the day's engineering "challenge."

"Your challenge is to reverse engineer something mechanical. Take apart a wind-up or 'rev' toy with the goal of understanding how it works and creatively (but accurately) communicating your new knowledge to others.

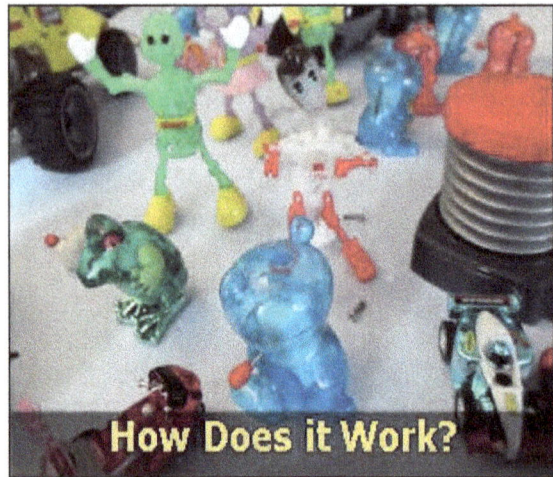

How Does it Work?

Your description should include the path of energy from your hand to ultimate movements of the toy. The path of energy will be stored and transformed in many ways. Use observations, reverse engineering, and detective work to explain that path."

EXPLAIN: Follow Good Documentation Practices = GIP

Prepare your logbook.

Enter a title and purpose.

Page 1 = Title, Purpose, Prediction
Page 2 = Add notes and diagrams.
Page 3 = Document final conclusions.
    Illustrate the energy transfer from
    windup to full stop.

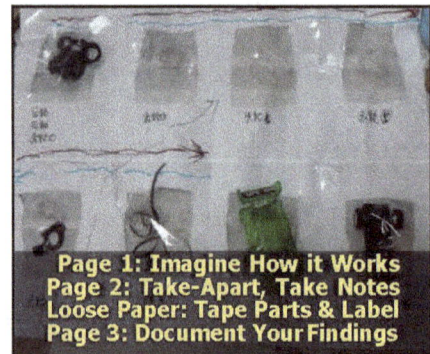

Page 1: Imagine How it Works
Page 2: Take-Apart, Take Notes
Loose Paper: Tape Parts & Label
Page 3: Document Your Findings

EXPLAIN: Injection Molded Toys

Before you start, look at a few common parts you'll find in the investigation.

This toy shown on the slide has the two main parts easily come apart with the removal of one screw on this toy. The blue body parts are simply 3 injection molded parts; front torso, back torso and legs.

Injection molding uses a hollow shaped mold and hot plastic (or other materials).

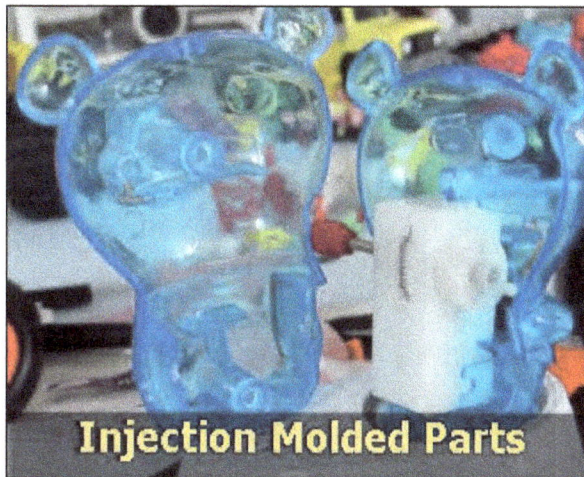

Injection Molded Parts

Read about injection molding with plastics <u>HERE</u>. https://www.thoughtco.com/what-is-injection-molding-820350
Learn about polymers used in injection molding <u>HERE</u>. https://www.thoughtco.com/definition-of-polymer-605912

What did you learn about injection molding and polymers?

EXPLORE – Preview the Project

Identify Parts

Draw what you see.

Tape parts to your notebook or paper

1. The Motor

The 'box' inside the toy is essentially its motor. Two pins can be seen opposite each other on the gear (colored red) on the outside of the motor.

When the motor turns, those pins turn and catch on the lever attached to the feet.

The little machine tilts enough to change its center of gravity. The wind up falls over.

Look for a motor box.

2. The Lever

What is a lever? This simple machine has a bar that moves on a fixed support, or fulcrum. Apply force by pushing **down** on one end of the lever to result in a force pushing **up** at the other end of the lever. Levers, like gears, can be used to increase the force available from a mechanical power source.

You May See: A Lever

What does your lever do?

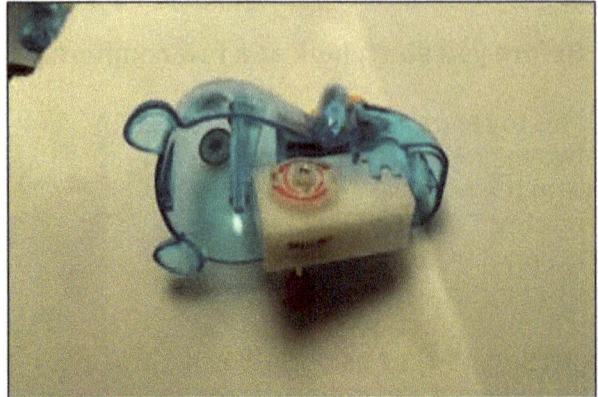

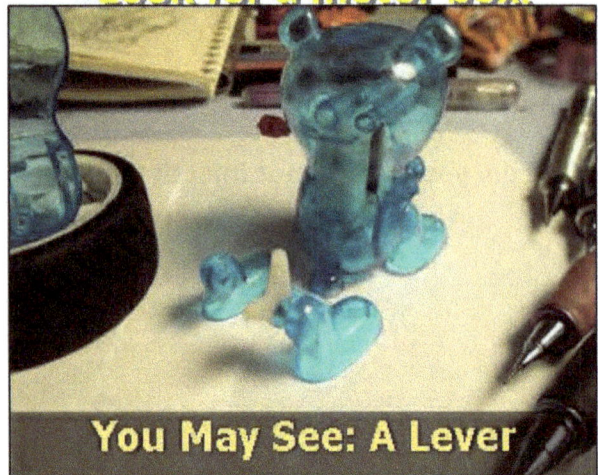

3. Springs

When the machine tilts over, the spring stretches. When the spring clears the legs lever, the spring snaps back and makes the toy stand upright.

This spring action doesn't just make it stand upright. It makes the toy flip over backwards.

Draw your lever.

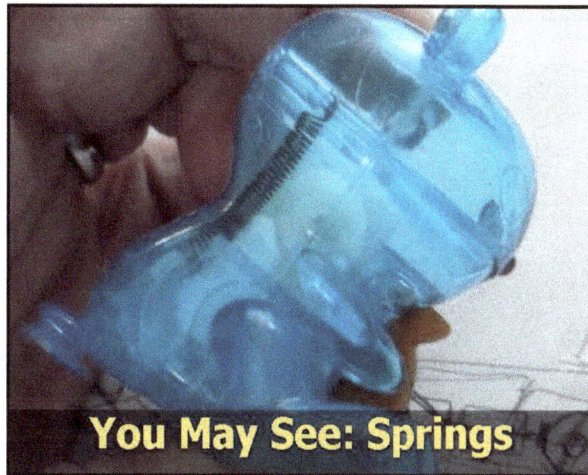

You May See: Springs

3b. Coiled spring in the Motor Box

Where does the energy to flip get stored when you wind up the toy?

There seems to be a split down the middle of the motor casing but no obvious way to open it. It is either glued together or a "forced fit". Place the box on a flat surface. Slide a screwdriver between the lines to split the box. Turn the tool into a lever as you GENTLY rock the tool back and forth to separate the two halves of the box.

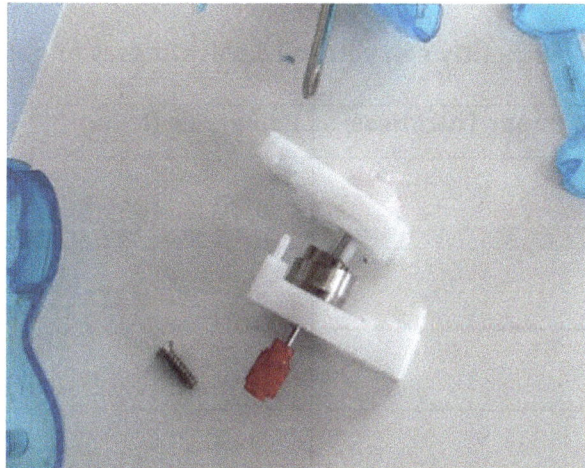

Once open, you can see that pins hold the box together in a forced fit. As the pins are pulled apart you can see a "coiled spring,"

Coiled springs get tighter and tighter as the handle is turned: this is the mechanism that causes a lot of action from a relatively few turns of the crank.

EXPLORE

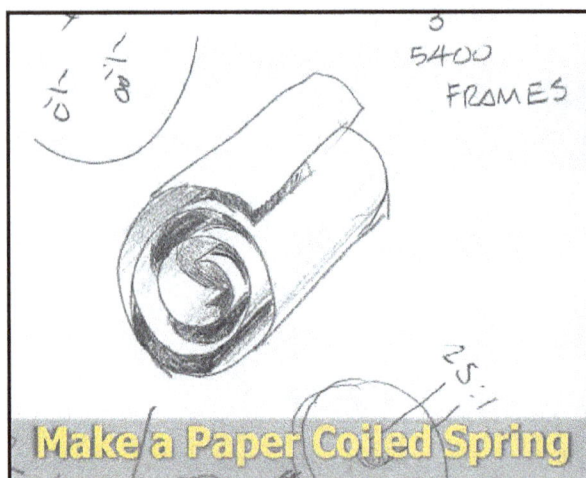

Make a Paper Coiled Spring

Mechanical advantage is a trade-off in force vs. distance. Each of the turns you make when winding up the toy provides more torque than is required to make the toy's motion (torque can be thought of as a rotational force). When winding, you input a lot of force over a little distance. The toy outputs a lot of distance that doesn't require a lot of torque.

To get a better idea of how coiled springs work, you might wind up a piece of paper – tightly – and let it go to see how the energy you put into the paper coil makes the paper spring out when released. This is the previously mysterious wind-up mechanism.

How tightly can you roll 3 thicknesses of paper?

*Paper Thickness	Paper size (l x w)	Roll Diameter	Observations
Ex: .05cm or .197cm	*letter paper* *215.9cm x 279.4cm* *8.5in x 11in*	*1cm* *or* *.394inch*	*Measures same when rolled from short or long side*

* To measure a single sheet of paper
  1. *Stack 20 sheets of paper.*
  2. *Measure the thickness of the stack.*
  3. *Divide thickness by # sheets of paper to find the thickness of 1 sheet.*
     Ex: 20 sheets measures 1cm
     1cm / 20 = .05cm per sheet of paper

How does this concept transfer to your toy?

EXPLORE: REVERSE ENGINEER A TOY

Prepare and Predict

- Give your project a Title.
- Explain the Purpose of this project.
- Observe the toy's motion. Talk about how you think it might operate. Once your ideas are formed, write down your prediction.
- Include observations that helped you make the prediction for your toy.

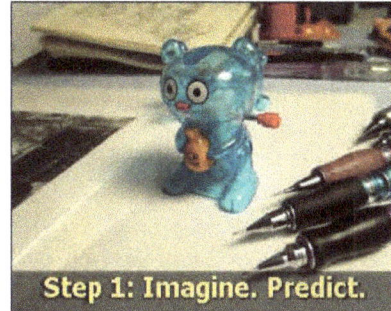
Step 1: Imagine. Predict.

Sample Prediction: How does the object store the energy you input as you turn the winder? I assume that because you wind it a little and it moves a lot, the toy must have some kind of coiled spring inside.

Take Apart
Take Notes
Collect Parts on a Paper

Now take the toy apart carefully.

- Take notes as you go.
- Also use your camera to take pictures. Though you cannot use them for your documentation, the images can be a good reminder of how it works.

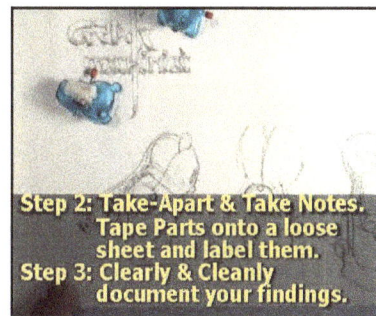
Step 2: Take-Apart & Take Notes. Tape Parts onto a loose sheet and label them.
Step 3: Clearly & Cleanly document your findings.

- Be very careful to open the toy so parts inside don't scatter or move inside the toy.
- Tape and label each part as you remove it. It is very easy to THINK you'll remember but it is also VERY easy to get confused. Tape and label AS YOU GO.
- When you think you understand how it works, and how the energy flows, document the process and clean up your sketches and flow-charts.

EXTEND

Present your findings to the group.

What can other groups add to the explanation?

Are there any constructive differences of opinion?

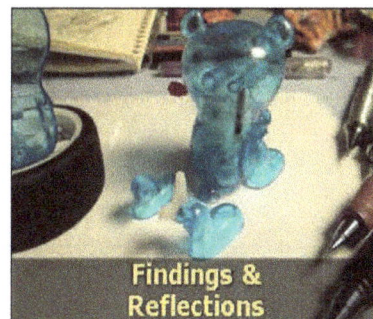
Findings & Reflections

Additional lessons can be found at the International STEM League website. www.insl.org

Additional lessons can be purchased from iNSL developer, Jeannie Ruiz, at her online store: Artofstemshop.com and Teacher Pay Teachers Art of STEM by Jeannie shop.

Please visit the book's website on Printing Futures website: www.printingfutures.com and send me an email with your thoughts and ideas for a more fleshed out version of the book due to publish later in the year.

Thank you for spending some of your valuable time with me as you read this book. I hope you will leave a review on my author's page on Amazon and on Goodreads. Reviews are important and I look forward to widening my network of amazing, dedicated, passionate and confident educators.

Perfect
Vision

Perfect Vision

The Original Bates Method Classic
Revised into Plain English

Michael Arnold, MD, L.Ac.

Mystery Dance Press
Monterey, California

Mystery Dance Press
1015 Cass St., #5
Monterey, CA 93940, USA
MysteryDancePress.com

Original work on which this derivative work is based:
"Perfect Eyesight Without Glasses,"
published by William H. Bates, MD, 1920.

The publisher's policy is to use paper manufactured from sustainable forests.

26 25 24 23 22 21 20 19 18   1 2 3 4 5 6 7 8 9

ISBN-13: 978-1-7321041-0-5

ILLUSTRATION CREDITS

All Figures are by Michael Arnold, MD, L.Ac. except the following:

Cover Photo   Melissa Lofton
Cover Design   Melissa Lofton
Figure 0.23   Dr. Bates Using the Retinoscope – Public Domain
Figure 0.24   The Snellen Test Chart – adapted from Public Domain
Figure 4.1   The Extraocular Muscles from Above –
                Adapted from "Treatise on Physiological Optics," Hermann von Helmholtz, 1851.
Figure 4.2   The Extraocular Muscles Labeled –
                Adapted from "Treatise on Physiological Optics," Hermann von Helmholtz, 1851.
Figure 4.3:   Lateral View of the Extraocular Muscles –
                Adapted from "A Textbook on Disease of the Eye," Henry D. Noyes, 1890.
Figure 4.4:   Extraocular Muscles, Lateral View, Labeled –
                Adapted from "A Textbook on Disease of the Eye," Henry D. Noyes, 1890.
Figure 4.5:   The Superior Obliques From Above –
                Adapted from "Treatise on Physiological Optics," Hermann von Helmholtz, 1851.
Figure 4.6:   Lateral View of the Oblique Muscles –
                Adapted from "A Textbook on Disease of the Eye," Henry D. Noyes, 1890.
Figure 11.1:   Cross section of the Fovea (19th Century Drawing) –
                Adapted from "Treatise on Physiological Optics," Hermann von Helmholtz, 1851.

Dedication

To Linda May Thornbrough,
with Great Love.

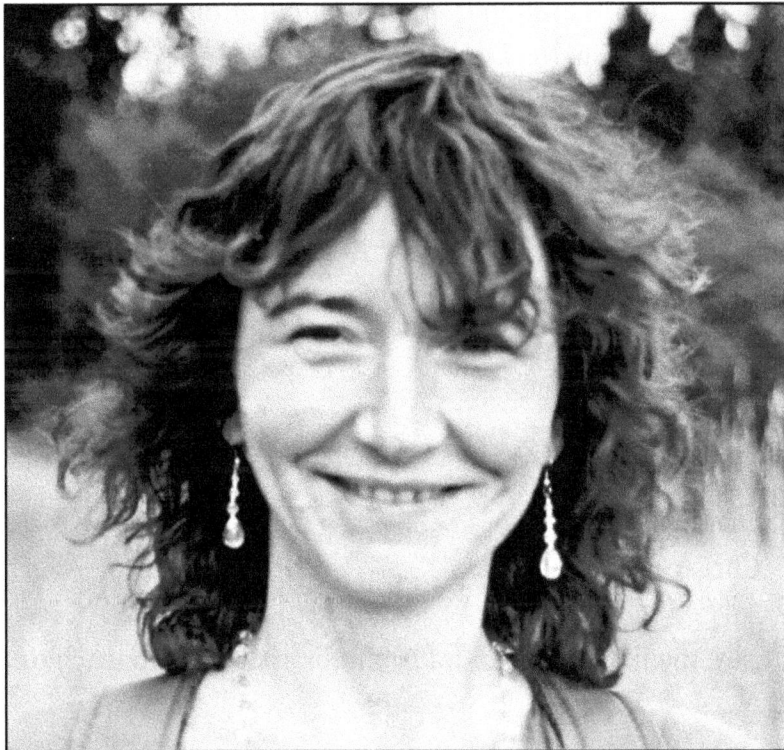

Acknowledgments

I have heard it takes a village to write a book. Thank you to everyone in the village of writing this book, named and unnamed.

Thank you Marlies Myoku Cocheret de la Morinière for your endless gentle encouragement.

Thank you Marilyn Power Scott for the copy editing par excellence and nonpareil.

Thank you Sandra Leader for your wondrously meticulous proofreading.

Thank you Patricia Hamilton (*parkplacepublications.com*), and Ginna and David Gordon, (*luckyvalleypress.com*) for all your technical expertise and patient encouragement.

Also, for all the encouragement and interest, thank you to:

    Sally Kempton
    Gloria Kalisher
    Barbara Rose
    Lisa Lee
    Steven Rothenberg
    Dr. Bill Little
    Dianne Burns
    Christopher Mankowski

And finally, thank you Alexandra Albin for asking me to teach on the subject.

Disclaimer

Many report great benefit from the Bates Eye Method. However, **this book is not a substitute for conventional Western medical care when needed.** Medical conditions such as high blood pressure, diabetes, or high pressure inside the eyeball (glaucoma) can cause a slow and preventable progression to blindness. Whether by alternative medical treatments or by conventional medicine, these kinds of conditions need to be cured or brought under control.

Sudden and severe symptoms are a red flag to seek conventional Western treatment immediately. These include (but are not limited to) severe pain in the eyes, double vision that lasts more than a minute or so, sudden loss of vision, and sudden occurrence of many new floaters. Seeking prompt conventional Western medical treatment in these circumstances could save not only your vision but your life.

This is all by way of saying, please use judgment and common sense. This book is for historic and informational purposes only. **The author, the publisher and the distributor can in no way be responsible for how you use the information in this book or any harm that may come to you as a result.**

TABLE OF CONTENTS

ILLUSTRATIONS

ILLUSTRATIONS (continued)

Preface
Michael Arnold, M.D.

About a century ago, an ophthalmologist named William Horatio Bates, MD, lived in New York City. In 1920 he published a book titled "Perfect Sight Without Glasses." In it he described his approach to healing the vision—an approach that we know today as The Bates Method.

In my own healing journey, I learned about many modern approaches to the Bates Method. Each teacher has developed his or her own unique perspective and emphasis, which is wonderful. However, I cannot say that I ever came across a systematic presentation of Dr. Bates's theories as to why his method is so effective.

Now, Dr. Bates himself would be the first to say that no theoretical understanding of vision and the eyes is necessary for his method to work. I myself, however, was never really able to benefit from the Bates Method until I went to the source and read what the originator wrote. Understanding his view as a physician gave me the insight and confidence to practice his method wholeheartedly. It also empowered me to adapt his method to my own personal needs and lifestyle.

"Perfect Sight Without Glasses" has long been in the public domain. You can find free downloads of it easily by searching the web. These versions are scans of the original book. They are difficult to read, especially if you have problems with your vision. The scans lose some of the resolution of the original; the layout is confusing. The photographs are neither sharp nor clear. After these obstacles comes the ornate prose style of an educated gentleman of 1920. Unravel the grammar in a marathon of run-on sentences, and you still find yourself mired in a jungle of ophthalmological terms that confounded me, despite my medical training. Penetrating to the meaning of all the technical terms, I still had to jump across the chasm between the conventional ophthalmological view and Dr. Bates's radically different view.

When I did persist, I found pure gold. It is my intention, by writing this book, to share that gold and spare you the obstacles.

My gift, I hope, is to explain a complex technical subject in an easily understandable and accessible way. I have gone through Dr. Bates's book chapter by chapter and have done my best to translate it into modern language that anyone can understand. I have mercilessly simplified the terminology. Occasionally, I have added comments, bracketed and tagged with my initials, when I felt what he was saying needed clarification. Finally, I trimmed away a few parts that I felt were entirely redundant.

I don't agree with everything Dr. Bates wrote, but my opinion is a matter for another time. The purpose of this present work is to make his point of view clear and accessible to today's readers. There is one exception: the issue of sun-gazing. After careful consideration, I included his teaching on the benefits of gazing directly at the sun, but only for purely historical purposes, and to honor the author of the original work. Please do not gaze directly at the sun. The wisdom of today is that doing so can blind you.

As you read Dr. Bates's book, recast into the language in use in 2018, please note that unless indicated otherwise, it is Dr. Bates speaking in the first person.

Michael Arnold, MD, L.Ac.
Monterey, CA
April 2018

Dr. Bates's Preface to the First Edition
(unedited)

This book aims to be a collection of facts and not of theories, and insofar as it is, I do not fear successful contradiction. When explanations have been offered it has been done with considerable trepidation, because I have never been able to formulate a theory that would withstand the test of the facts either in my possession at the time, or accumulated later. The same is true of the theories of every other man, for a theory is only a guess, and you cannot guess or imagine the truth. No one has ever satisfactorily answered the question, "Why ?" as most scientific men are well aware, and I did not feel that I could do better than others who had tried and failed. One cannot even draw conclusions safely from facts, because a conclusion is very much like a theory, and may be disproved or modified by facts accumulated later. In the science of ophthalmology, theories, often stated as facts, have served to obscure the truth and throttle investigation for more than a hundred years. The explanations of the phenomena of sight put forward by Young, von Graefe, Helmholtz and Donders have caused us to ignore or explain away a multitude of facts which otherwise would have led to the discovery of the truth about errors of refraction and the consequent prevention of an incalculable amount of human misery.

In presenting my experimental work to the public, I desire to acknowledge my indebtedness to Mrs. E. C. Lierman, whose co-operation during four years of arduous labor and prolonged failure made it possible to carry the work to a successful issue. I would be glad, further, to acknowledge my debt to others who aided me with suggestions, or more direct assistance, but am unable to do so, as they have requested me not to mention their names in this connection.

As there has been a considerable demand for the book from the laity, an effort has been made to present the subject in such a way as to be intelligible to persons unfamiliar with ophthalmology.

The Fundamental Principle

The fundamental principle in healing the vision is to relax.

If you have any difficult seeing, this principle is easy to demonstrate:

Close your eyes and rest them. Visualize pure black, or an extremely pleasant, restful scene. You could even gently cover the areas around your eyes with your palms if it helps you relax.

Keep your eyes closed until they feel rested or until any feeling of strain has been completely relieved. Now open them and look at something for a fraction of a second. If you have been able to relax, partially or completely, you will have a flash of improved or clear vision.

After opening the eyes for this fraction of a second, close them again quickly. Keep them closed until they again feel rested. Then again open them for a fraction of a second. Continue this alternate resting of the eyes and flashing of vision for a while. You may soon find that you can keep your eyes open longer than a fraction of a second without losing the improved vision.

In this way, you can demonstrate for yourself the fundamental principle of the cure of imperfect sight without glasses.

CHAPTER 0

Basics

It will probably be easier to read this book if you understand a few basic terms and concepts. The secret to reading about medicine is to understand the meaning of each word. Otherwise, things can get very vague, very fast.

I've done my best to keep technical jargon to an absolute minimum, but some medical words just have to be met. There is a glossary at the end of the book to refresh your memory.

In this chapter, I describe a few simple things about lenses, including the lenses we all have inside our eyes. I also show the three ways that eyes can go out of focus. And I show the three kinds of lenses used to correct that lack of focus. There is a brief section on the way eye doctors measure how well we see. And I introduce Dr. Bates's favorite instrument for examining eyes—the retinoscope.

Three Ways the Eye Loses Focus

First let me touch on the three basic ways the eye goes out of focus:

Nearsighted means being able to focus up close, but things far away are blurred.

Farsighted means being able to focus far away, but things up close are blurred.

Astigmatism means that the cornea is not the right shape, and it isn't possible to properly focus an image at any distance, near or far.

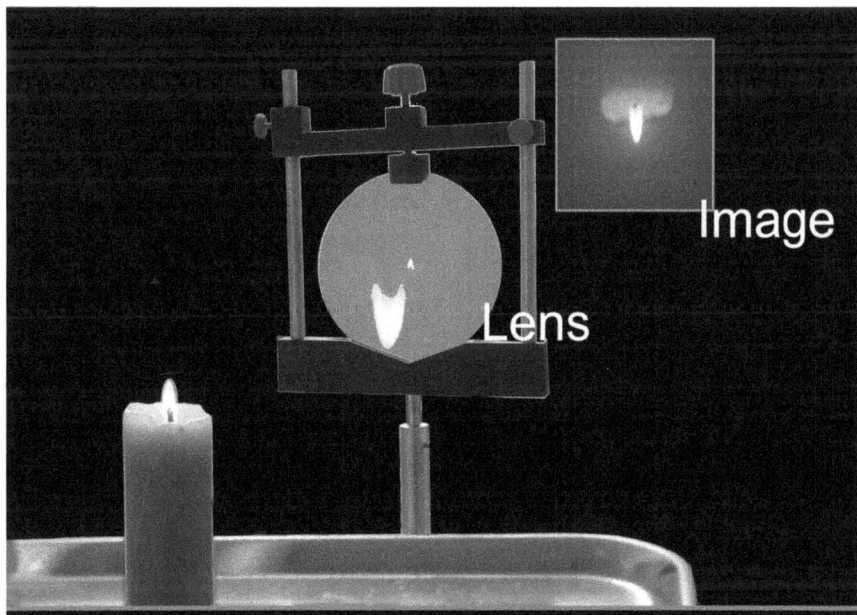

Figure 0.1: A Lens Can Project an Image

A Lens Forms An Image

A lens is a rounded clear substance that can project an image of what is in front of it onto a screen behind it. Because of the way light bends, the image will be upside down on the screen.

A clear image forms behind the lens only when the screen is a particular distance away from the lens. At any other distance, the image will be blurred. The distance from the lens to the clear image is called the **focal length**. The plane on which the image forms is called the **focal plane**—in this context, the physical screen.

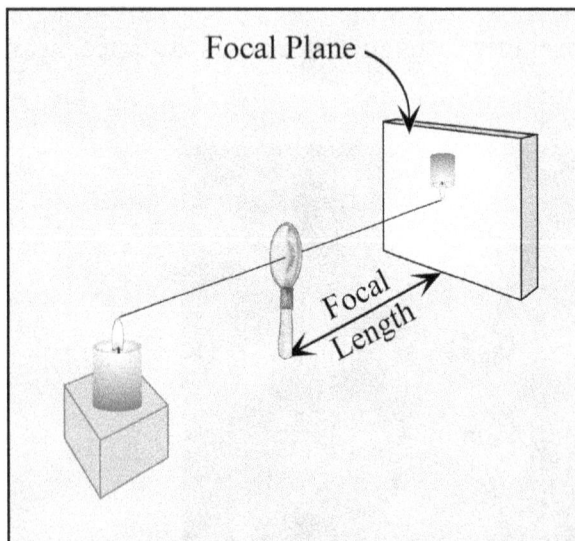

Figure 0.2:
Focal Length and Focal Plane

Focusing Up Close

When an object comes closer to a lens, the plane of focus moves back; the focal length increases (Figure 0.3).

To get a clear image of an object that is close to the lens, there are two choices (Figure 0.4):

1. Put in a stronger (i.e., thicker) lens, which would bring the plane of focus closer.

2. Move the screen back, farther away from the lens

Accommodation

The human eye changes when it has to focus on a close up object, and this change is called **accommodation**. Herein lies one of the key differences between Dr. Bates's theory and conventional theory. Conventional theory, then and now, believes firmly that the eye focuses for clear, close-up vision by making the lens in the eye thicker and thus stronger. Dr. Bates believed that the eye focuses for close-up clarity by using the muscles around the eye to make the eyeball longer (Figure 0.5).

Personally, I believe the eye probably does both. In general, that is how the body works. For example, you might think that it is just the heart that pumps blood through the body, but in fact the movement of many other muscles, as well as the action of breathing, also make important contributions to moving the blood. (This is one reason why people who never exercise are at higher risk for heart problems.)

light ray from afar

light ray from afar

focal plane
for far light

When light from a far away point
reaches the lens,
the light rays are more or less parallel.

focal plane
for near light

Plane of focus
moves back.

When light from a nearer point reaches the lens,
it comes in at a sharper angle.
This causes the plane of focus
to move back away from the lens.

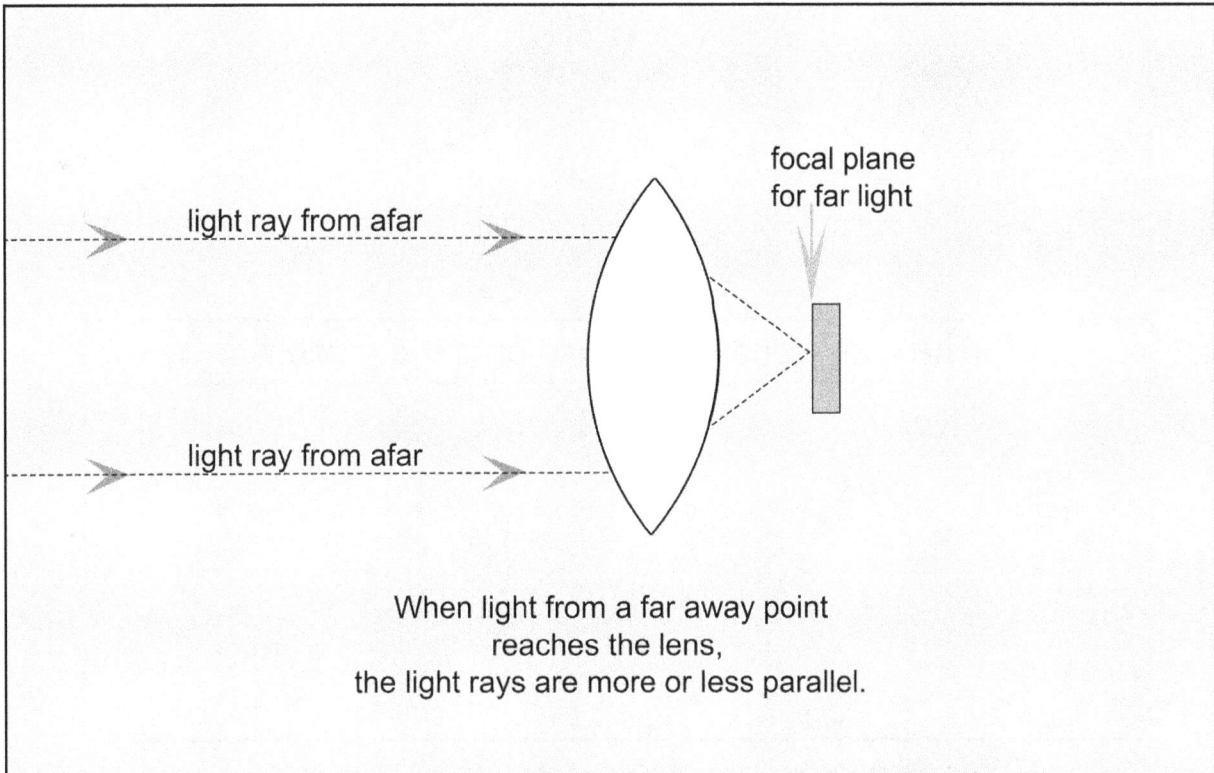

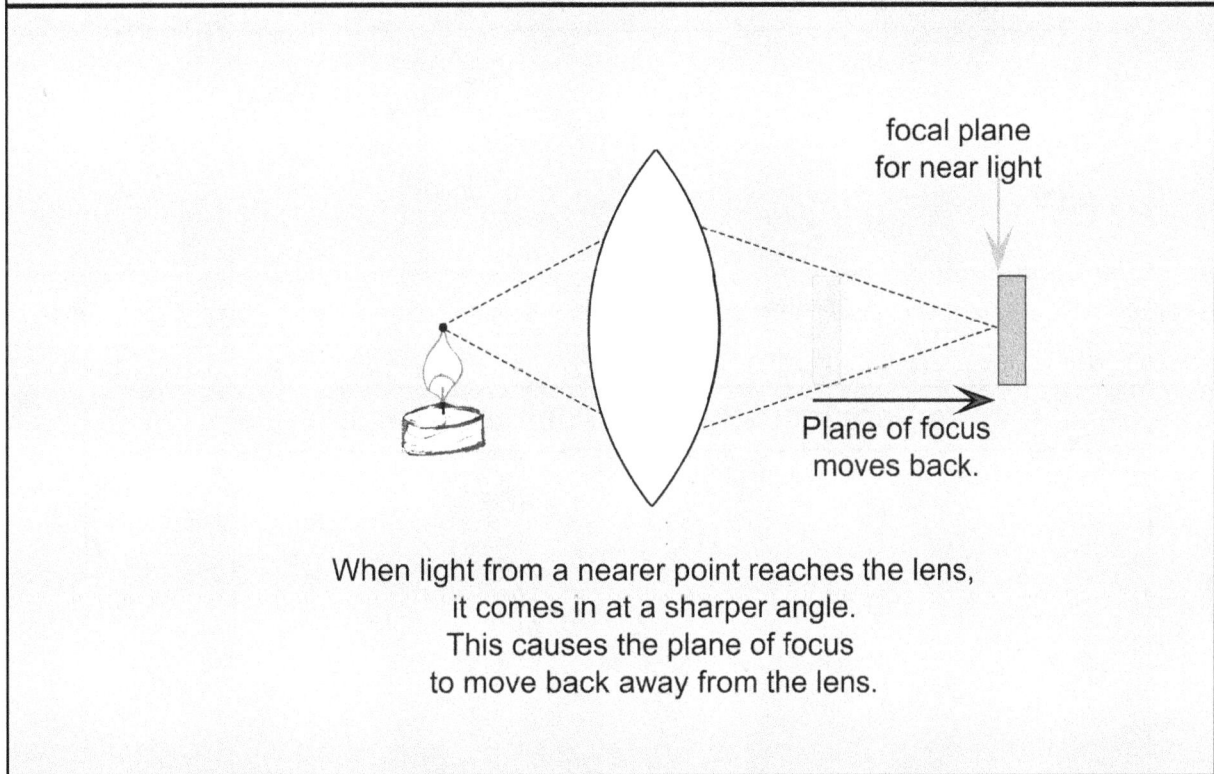

Figure 0.3: For Close Objects the Plane of Focus Moves Back

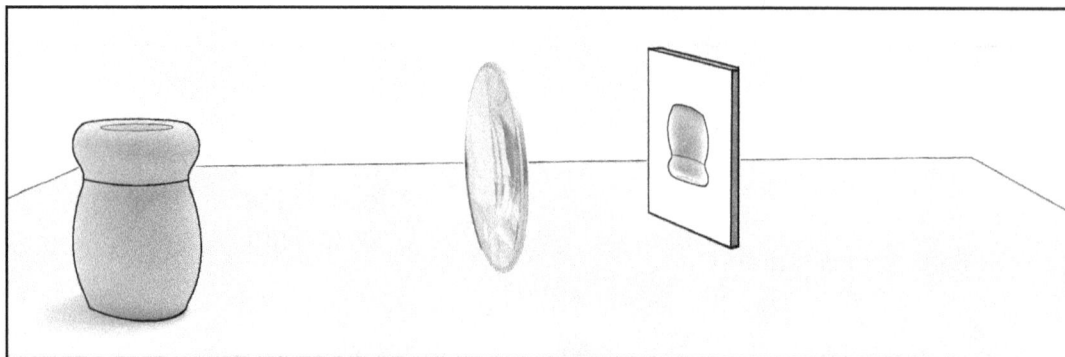

The lens focuses the vase onto the screen.

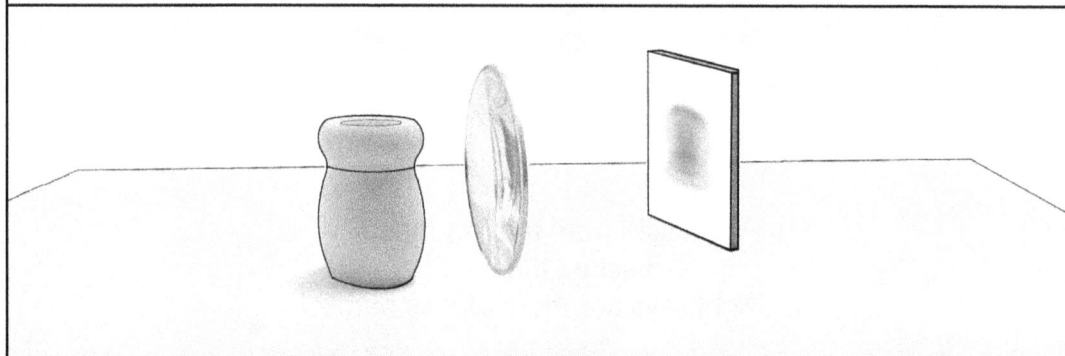

If the vase comes closer, the image is blurred.

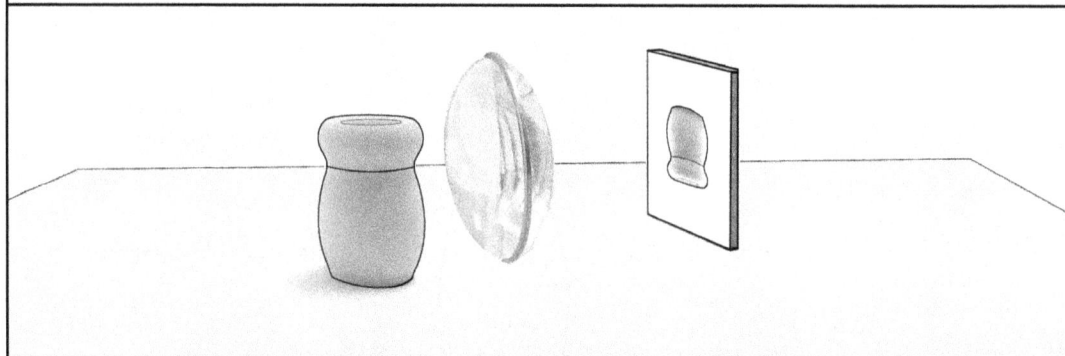

To restore focus, you can use a stronger lens...

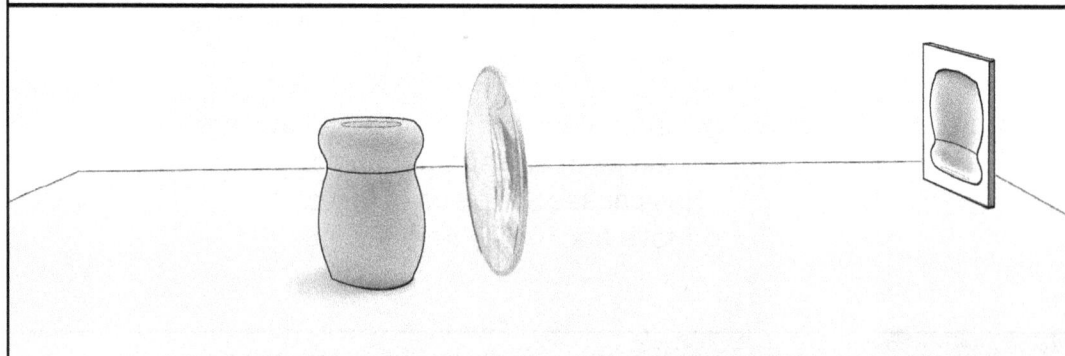

Or, just move the screen further back.

Figure 0.4: There Are Two Ways to Focus Close Up

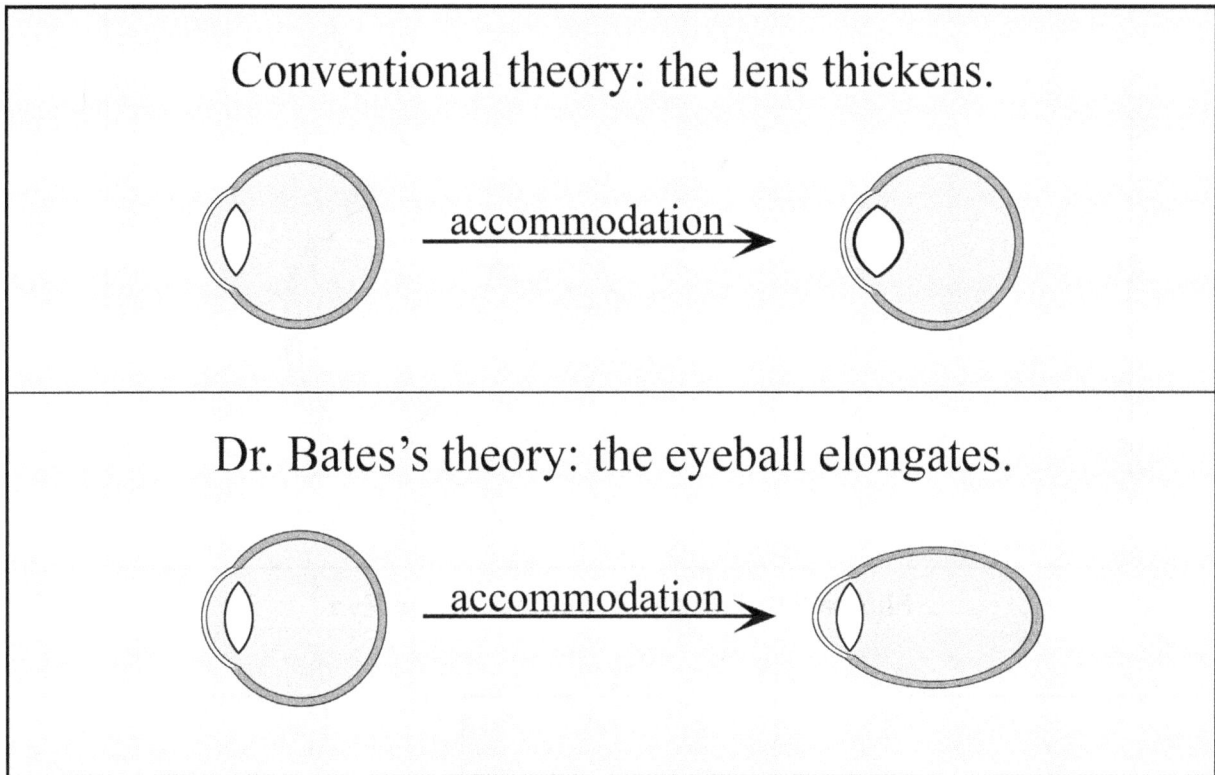

Figure 0.5: The Two Theories of Accommodation

The Optic System of the Eye

The optic system of the eye consists of two lenses, an iris, and an image receptor. Together, the lenses line up to project an image on the back of the inside of the eyeball, which called the retina. The retina is to the eye as film is to an old-fashioned camera or as a screen is to a projector (Figure 0.6).

The lenses are named the cornea and the crystalline lens.

The Cornea

The cornea is shaped like a hollowed-out bowl (Figure 0.7). The front surface of the cornea is exposed to the air and is covered by the eyelid when a person blinks or sleeps. People who wear contact lenses place them directly on the cornea and they fit perfectly. So if you want to know the shape of the cornea, just look at the shape of a contact lens (Figure 0.8).

The Crystalline Lens

The second lens sits behind the cornea. It's generally called the crystalline lens, or sometimes just "the lens." The crystalline lens acts pretty much like the lens in a strong magnifying glass. Anatomically, it bulges out a little more in back (Figure 1.9).

When lenses are mentioned, it can be confusing. Sometimes they refer to contact lenses or lenses in glasses. Sometimes they refer to the lenses inside our eyes. You usually have to tell which by context. It's the crystalline lens that can become cloudy in old age, causing cataracts. As you'll read later in the book, Dr. Bates says cataracts are reversible.

5

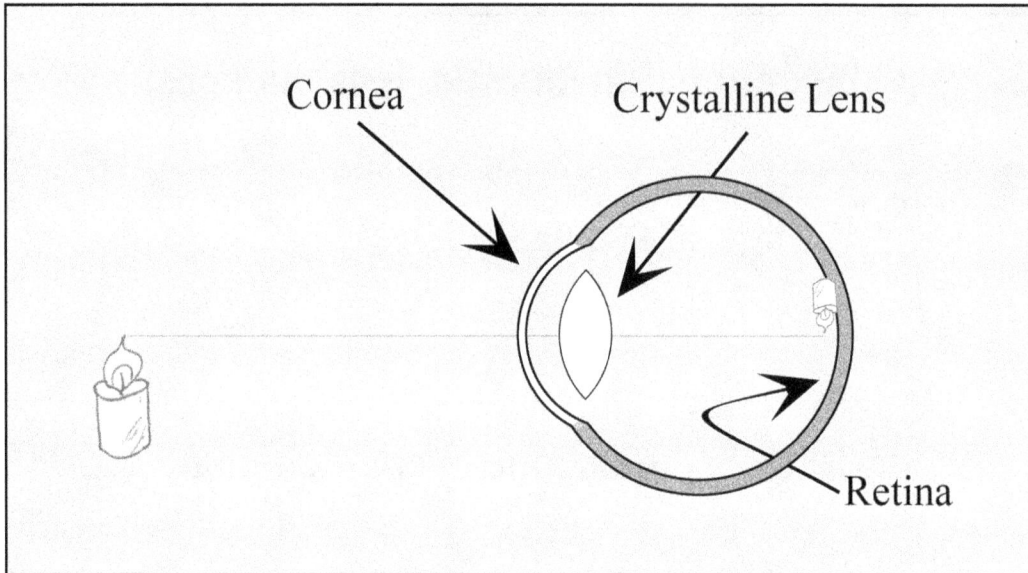
Figure 0.6: The Optic System of the Eye

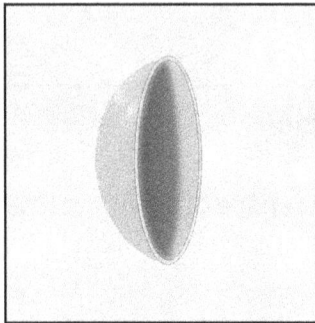
**Figure 0.7
The Cornea**

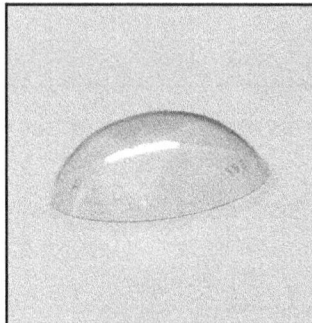
**Figure 0.8
A Contact Lens**

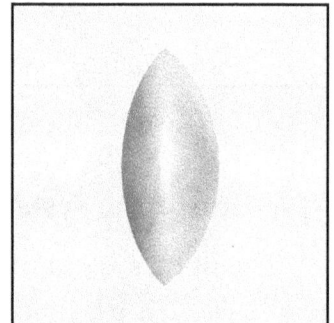
**Figure 0.9
The Crystalline Lens**

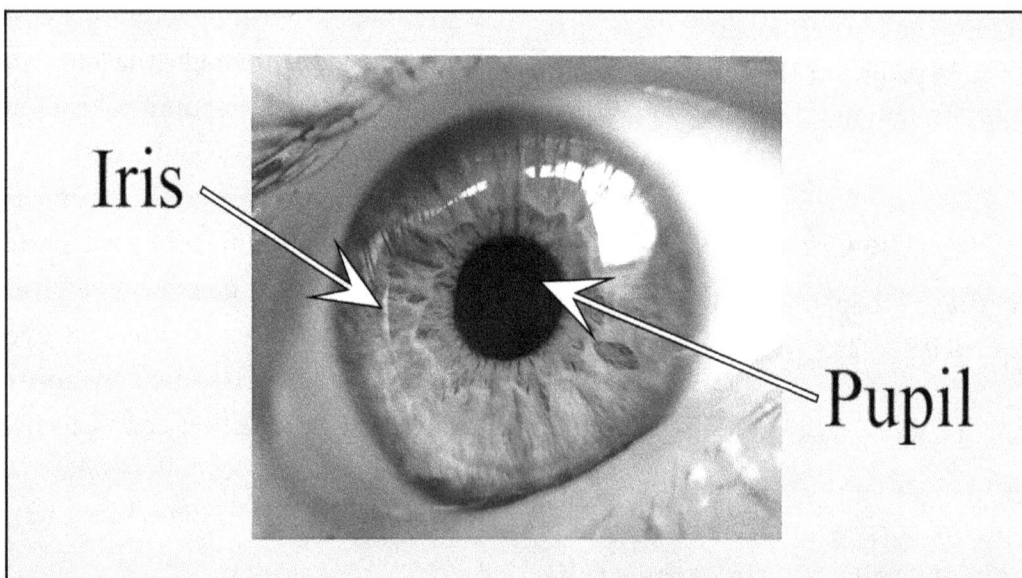
Figure 0.10: Iris and Pupil

The Iris

The iris controls how much light gets into the eye. The iris gives our eyes their color. The pupil is the opening at the center of the iris that gets larger and smaller

The iris is shaped like a flat disc with a round opening at the center, so from the side it doesn't look like much (Figure 0.10).

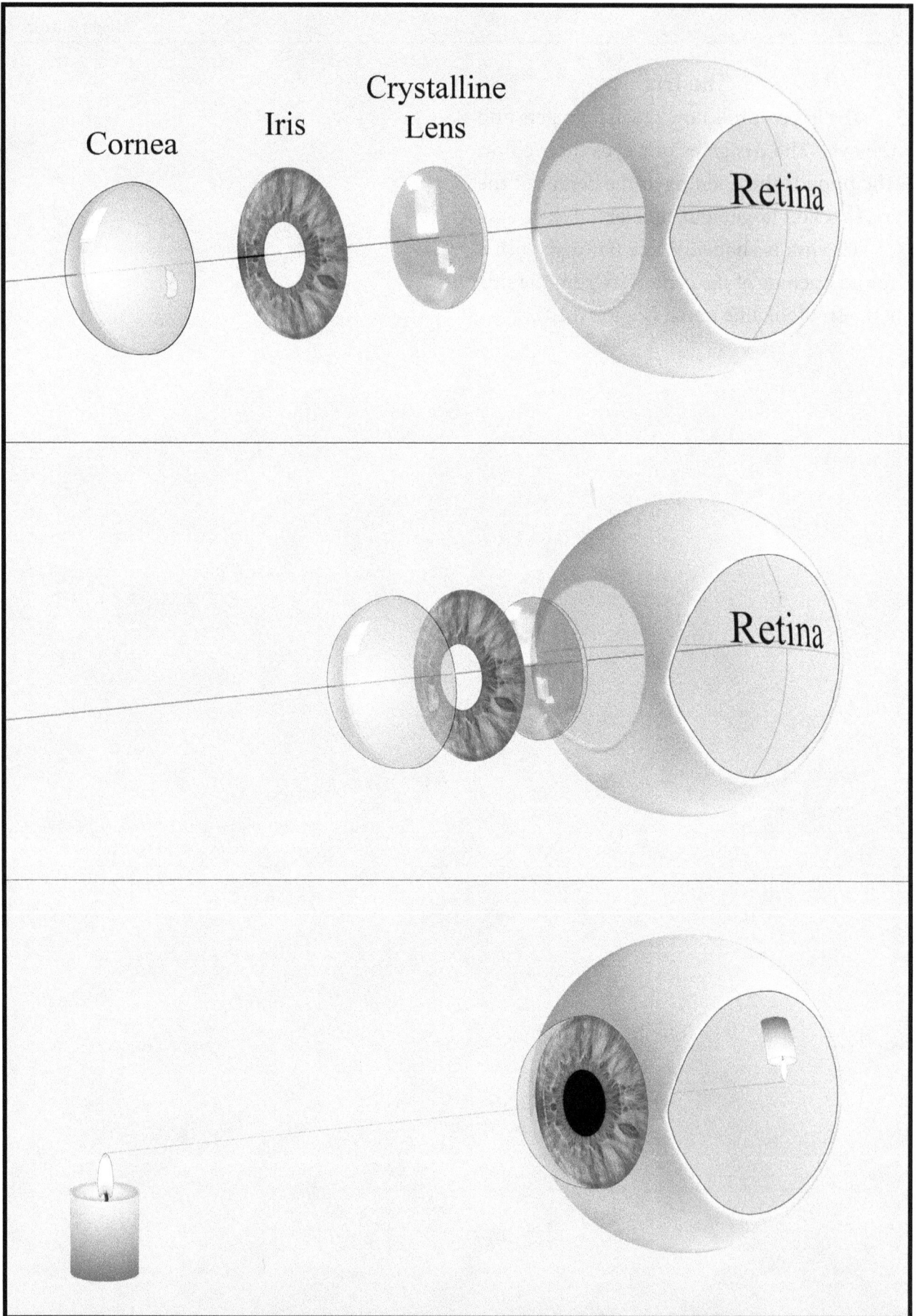

Figure 0.11: Expanded Views of the Optic System of the Eye

Three Basic Ways
The Eye Can Go Out of Focus

Nearsightedness

When the plane of focus falls in front of the retina, this causes nearsightedness (Figure 0.14, top).

Since the plane of focus moves back as an object comes closer, near-sighted people can see things clearly close up but not far away. The conventional view is that nearsightedness occurs because the eyeball is too long.

Farsightedness

When the plane of focus falls behind the retina, this causes farsightedness (Figure 0.14, middle).

Farsighted people may be able to compensate by squinting. This artificially brings the plane of focus forward and refocuses the image onto the retina. However, they still cannot clearly see close objects. Since they are always exerting effort to

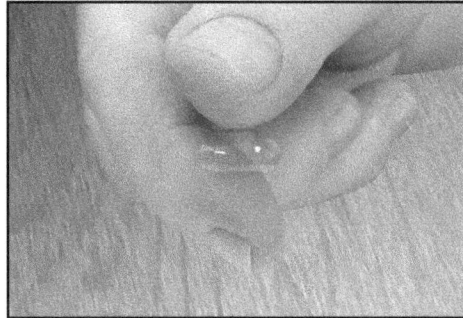

**Figure 0.12
The Astigmatic Cornea
is Shaped Like a
Compressed Contact Lens**

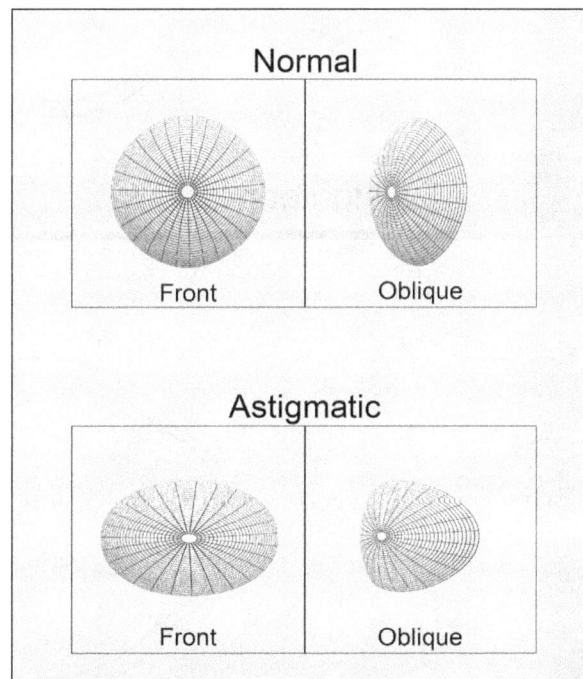

**Figure 0.13
Cornea Contour Lines**

focus as if everything were very close, they are subject to eye strain and eye pain.

Astigmatism

A lens creates an image because its surface is perfectly curved, like a slice off of a ball. That is why they are called spherical lenses. But very often, the cornea is not properly curved. It gets squashed shorter in one dimension and longer in another. In this situation there is no single plane of focus, near or far, on which a clear image can form (Figure 0.14, bottom). This deformity is called **astigmatism**.

The shape of the astigmatic cornea is like a gently compressed contact lens. It is no longer perfectly rounded (Figure 0.12).

Figure 0.13 shows the contours of a normal and an astigmatic cornea, as if on a topographic map.

9

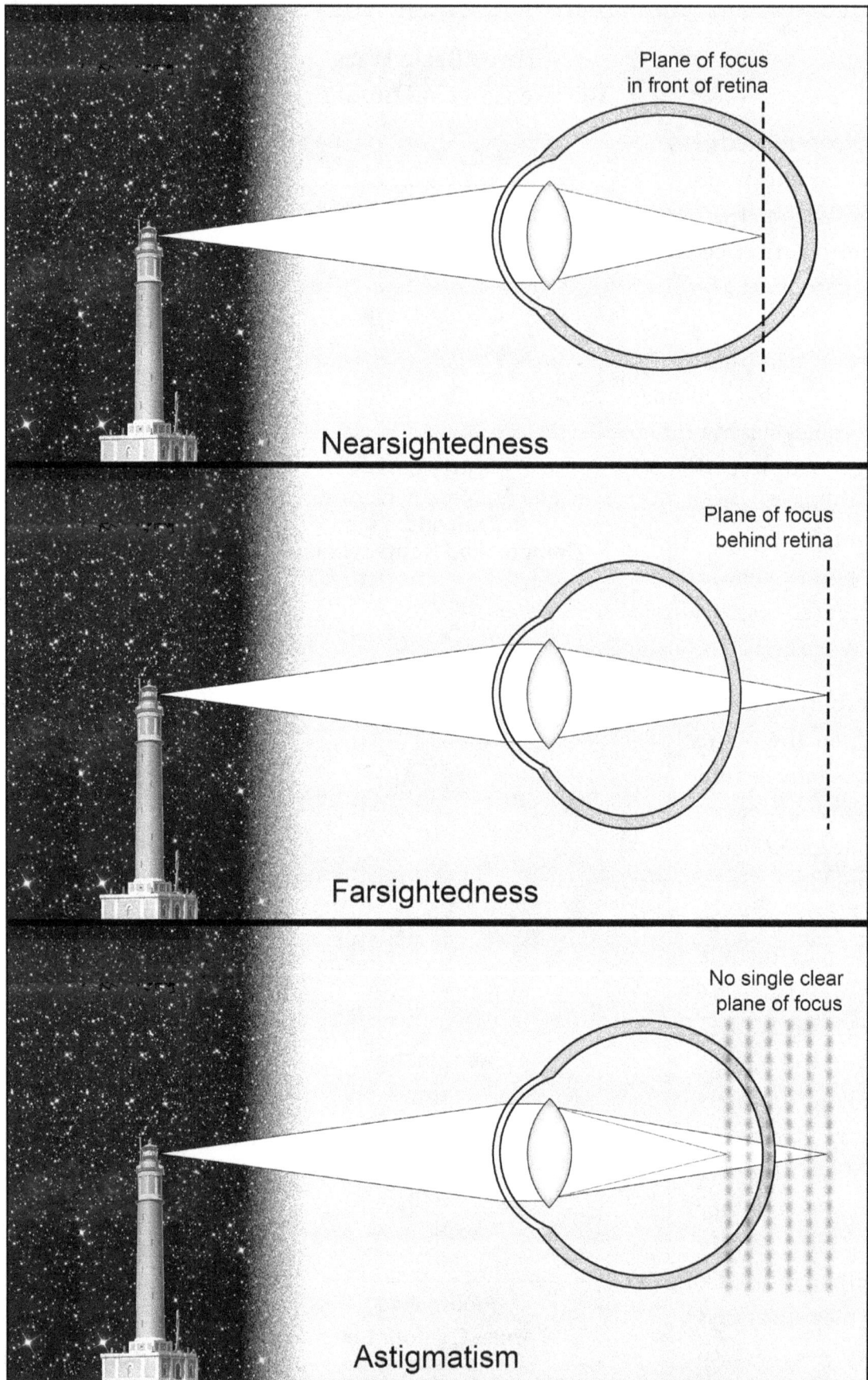

Figure 0.14: Three Ways the Eye Can Go Out of Focus

Demystifying the Diopter

People who work with optics use a unit of measurement, called a **Diopter**, to describe the strength of a lens. All prescriptions for glasses and contact lenses are written in Diopters.

The Diopter strength of a lens is defined very simply. Diopters are the inverse of the focal length (in meters) of a lens. This means that the higher the Diopters, the stronger the lens and the shorter the focal length. If, for example, a lens has a focal length of 2 meters, then that is a 1/2 Diopter lens (Expressed as "0.5 D") (Figure 0.15).

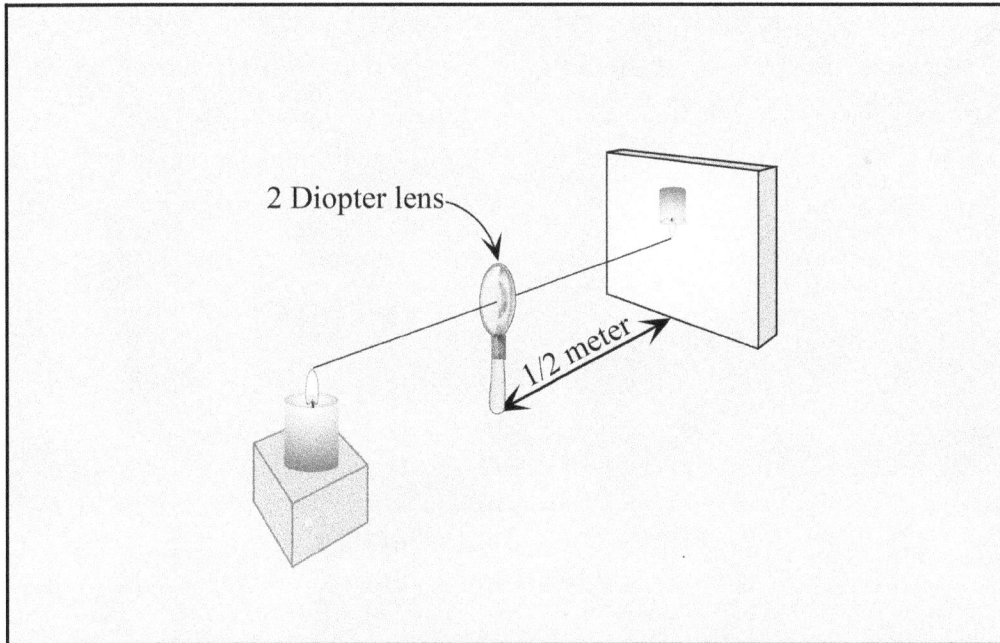

Figure 0.15: Diopters are the Inverse of Focal Length in Meters

Three Kinds of Corrective Lenses

If the lenses in our eyes cannot create a clear image on the retina by themselves, the image can be made clear by putting lenses in front of them. Since there are three basic ways the eyes go out of focus, it follows that there are three different types of lenses that can restore focus.

crystalline lens are both convex lenses. A hand-held magnifying glass is also a convex lens.

When a person is farsighted, the plane of focus falls behind the retina. So adding a convex lens in front of the eye pulls the plane of focus forward onto the retina.

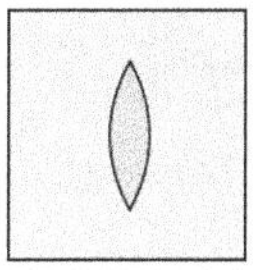

Convex Lenses

For farsightedness, the plane of focus is brought closer with a convex lens.

Convex means that the surface of the lens bulges outward. The cornea and the

Figure 0.16: Cross- Section of Convex Lens

11

Concave Lenses

For a nearsighted person, the plane of focus falls before the retina. Adding a concave lens in front of the eye pushes the plane of focus back onto the retina (Figure 0.20).

A concave lens curves inward (Figure 0.17). So instead of focusing all the rays of light to a point, it spreads them out. This effectively weakens the strength of the lens system to which it is added. For this reason, the strength of concave lenses is expressed in negative Diopters.

Cylinder Lenses

In astigmatism, the cornea is not perfectly rounded. The problem is not that the plane of focus comes before or after the retina, the problem is that there is no single clear plane of focus at all.

For this situation, a cylinder lens is needed. It's called a cylinder lens because it is shaped as if you shaved a piece off of a clear cylinder (Figure 0.18).

The cylinder lens balances out the lack of roundness of the cornea.

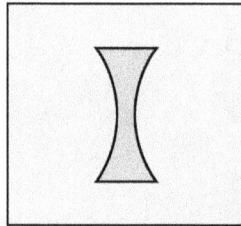

Figure 0.17: Cross-Section of a Concave Lens

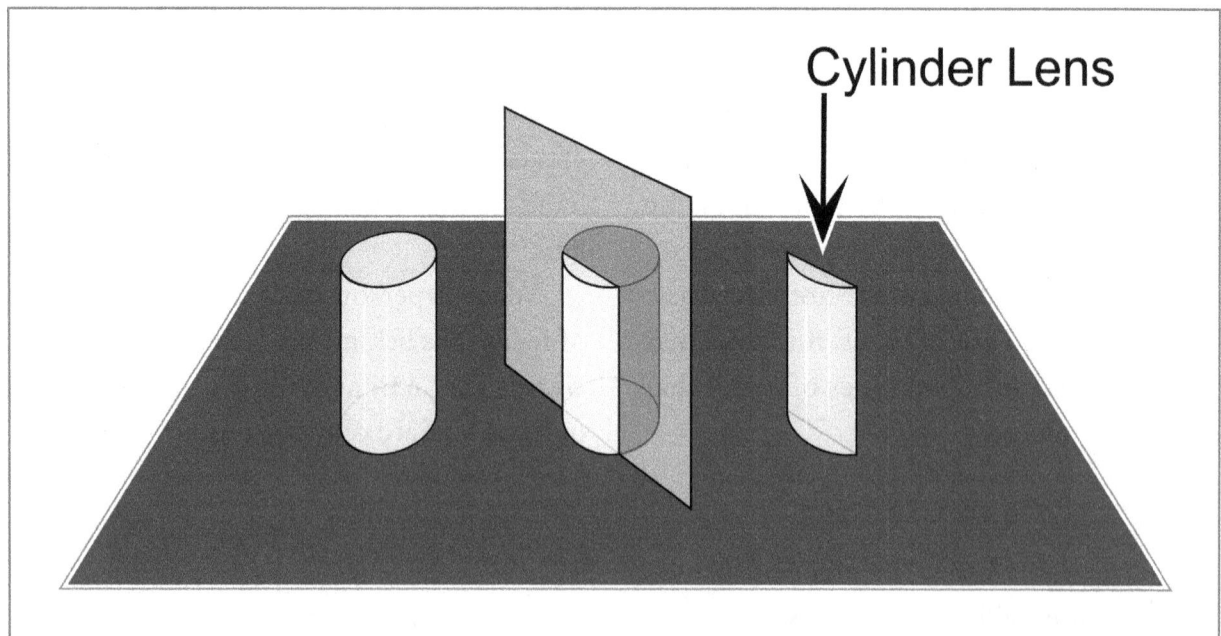

Figure 0.18: A Cylinder Lens is Cut from a Cylinder

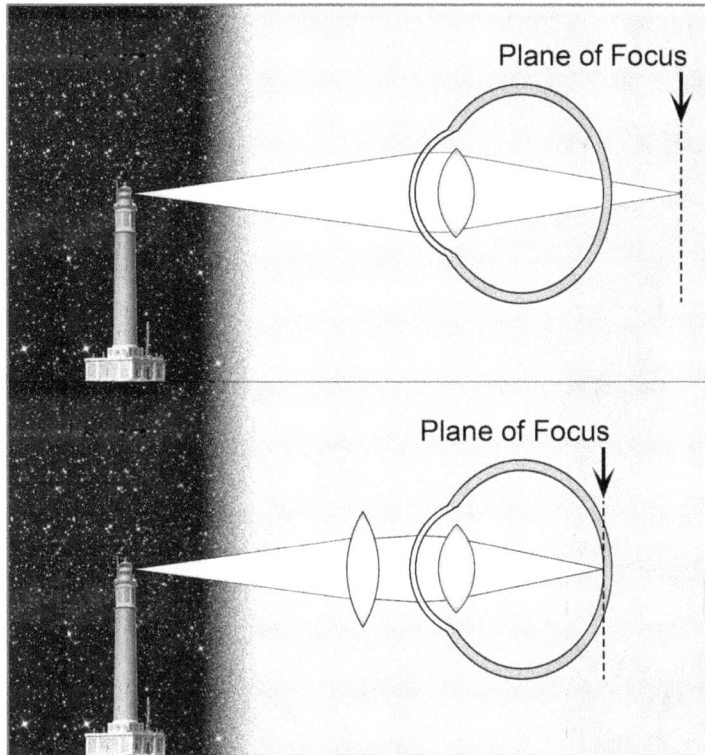

Figure 0.19:
A Convex Lens Corrects Farsightedness

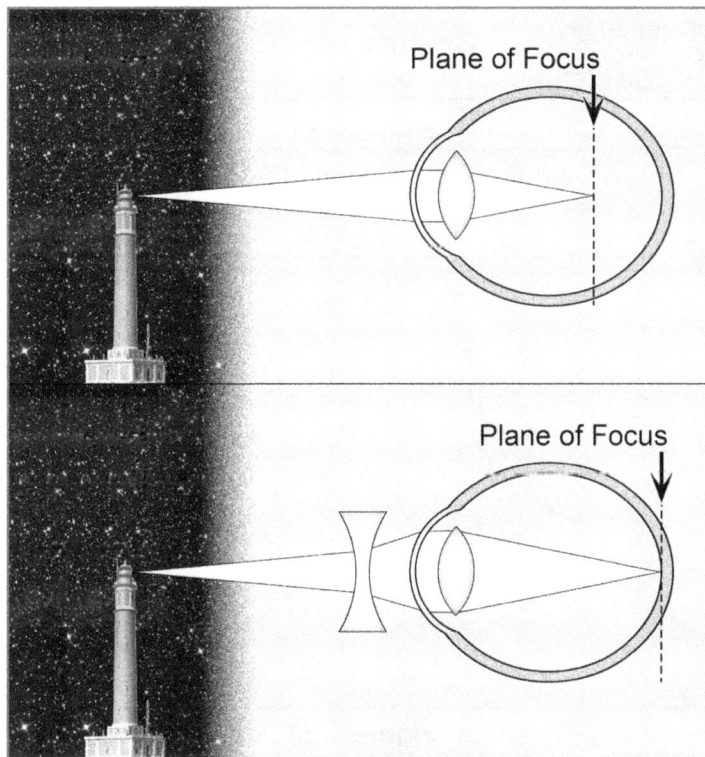

Figure 0.20
A Concave Lens Corrects Nearsightedness

13

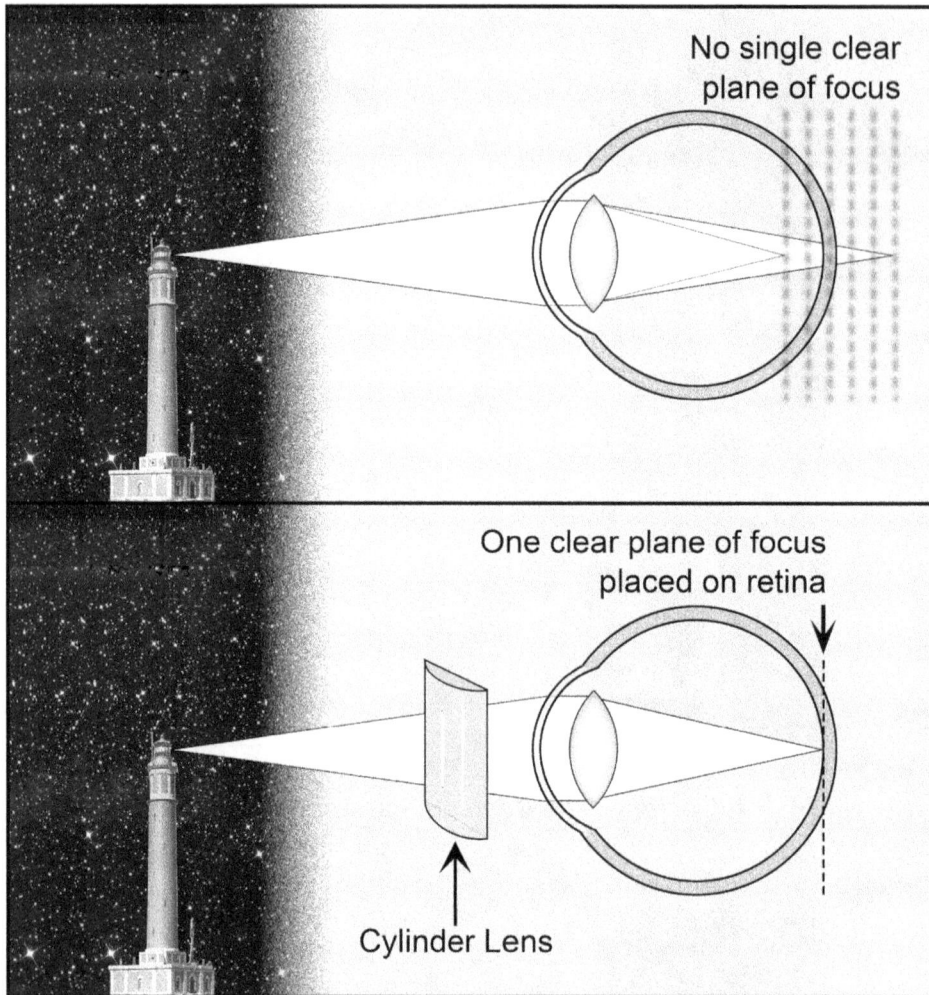

Figure 0.21
A Cylinder Lens Corrects Astigmatism

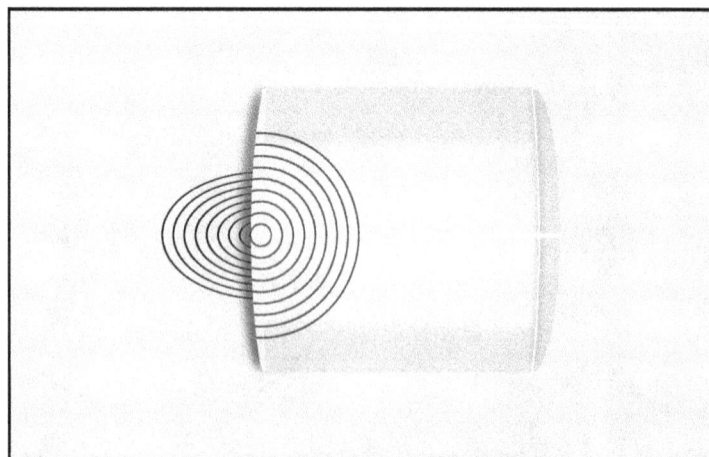

Figure 0.22
A Cylinder Lens Corrects for
the Cornea's Lack of Roundness

Why Don't My Corrective Lenses Look Like That?

It's true, the drawings and diagrams of lenses in this book don't look like the lenses in your glasses. I have shown the simple, exaggerated versions of the lenses for clarity of understanding.

Lens makers use special materials to keep the lenses as thin as possible. They have advanced plastics and special coatings. Also, they use more complex curves in the lenses, because in real life these are easier on the eyes. Through all the subtleties, however, the basic optical principles remain the same.

Visual Acuity

Visual acuity is a measure of how well a person sees. An eye chart is generally used to test this. You're probably familiar with them. Each line has smaller and smaller letters. This chart is named after Herman Snellen, a Dutch ophthalmologist who designed it in 1862.

Each line is given a number, which in Figure 1.23 you can see off to the right. The top line is referred to as "the one line." So if an eye doctor says, "He could read the ten line," the tenth line from the top is the one meant.

Visual acuity is expressed as two numbers that compare how well a person sees with how well a person with what's been deemed normal vision sees. The first number is how well the person being tested sees. The second number is the norm. So just remember, "Me first!" The first number is about your vision.

For example, if you have 20/20 vision, it means that you can see at twenty feet what a person with normal vision can see at twenty feet. That is normal vision.

If you have 20/40 vision, it means that you have to come up to twenty feet in order to see what a person with normal vision can see from forty feet away.

A combined number of 20/200 describes severe nearsightedness. A person with 20/200 vision needs to be twenty feet away from an object to see it as well as a person with normal vision sees it from two hundred feet away.

On the other hand, if you have 20/10 vision, it means you can see from twenty feet away what a person with normal vision needs to move up to ten feet away to see. That is really good vision!

For reference, in California in 2016, to get a driver's license, people have to be able to see, with both eyes, at least 20/40. In other words, with or without glasses, they have to be able to see at twenty feet what a normally sighted person can see at forty feet.

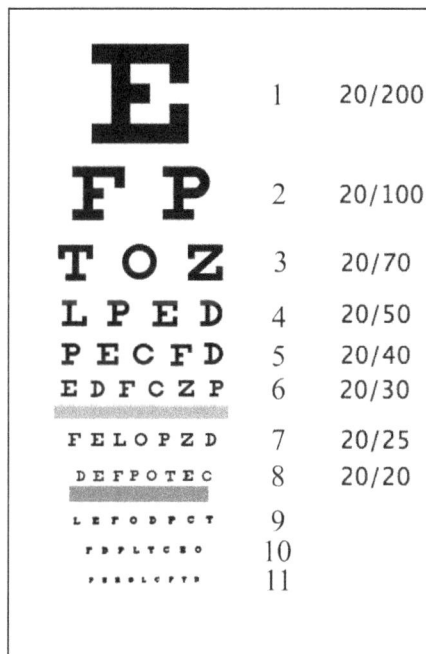

Line	Acuity
1	20/200
2	20/100
3	20/70
4	20/50
5	20/40
6	20/30
7	20/25
8	20/20
9	
10	
11	

Figure 0.23:
The Snellen Test Chart

The Retinoscope

Dr. Bates used an instrument called a retinoscope (Figure 0.24) to determine a person's error of refraction simply by shining a slit or streak of light into their eyes. The way that streak of light moves across the back of the eye tells how nearsighted or farsighted the person is or what kind of astigmatism they might have.

The advantage of the retinoscope is that it can be used on the eyes of any being, whether they can or cannot communicate. This includes infants, animals, people who have had strokes and cannot speak, and those in comas. It can even be used on a corpse. A further advantage is that using it only takes a few moments, while testing a person's vision with a chart takes some time. The final advantage for Dr. Bates was that he considered the retinoscope in his hands to be more accurate than visual acuity testing with the Snellen test chart.

The disadvantage is that it is incredibly difficult to master. Dr. Bates was a legendary virtuoso of the art. Indeed, he took his use of the retinoscope to a whole new level, which he named simultaneous retinoscopy. By this he meant that he could tell how a person's vision changed moment to moment by observing them through the retinoscope as they went about various activities.

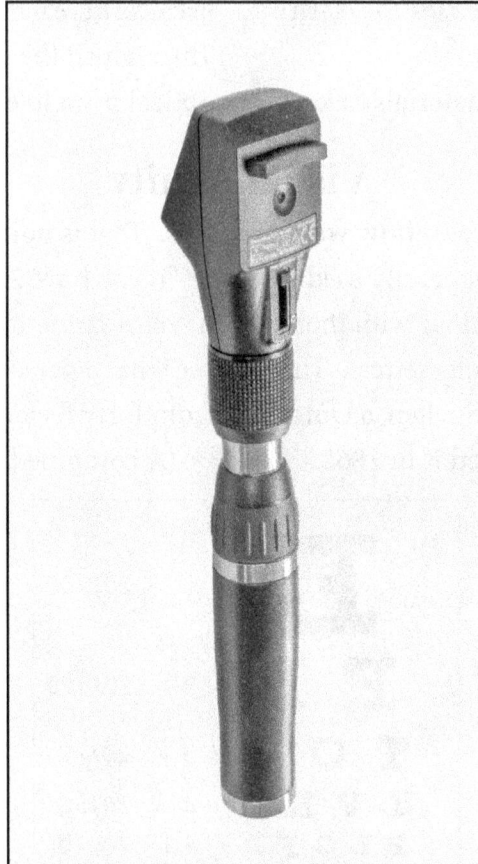

Figure 0.24: The Retinoscope

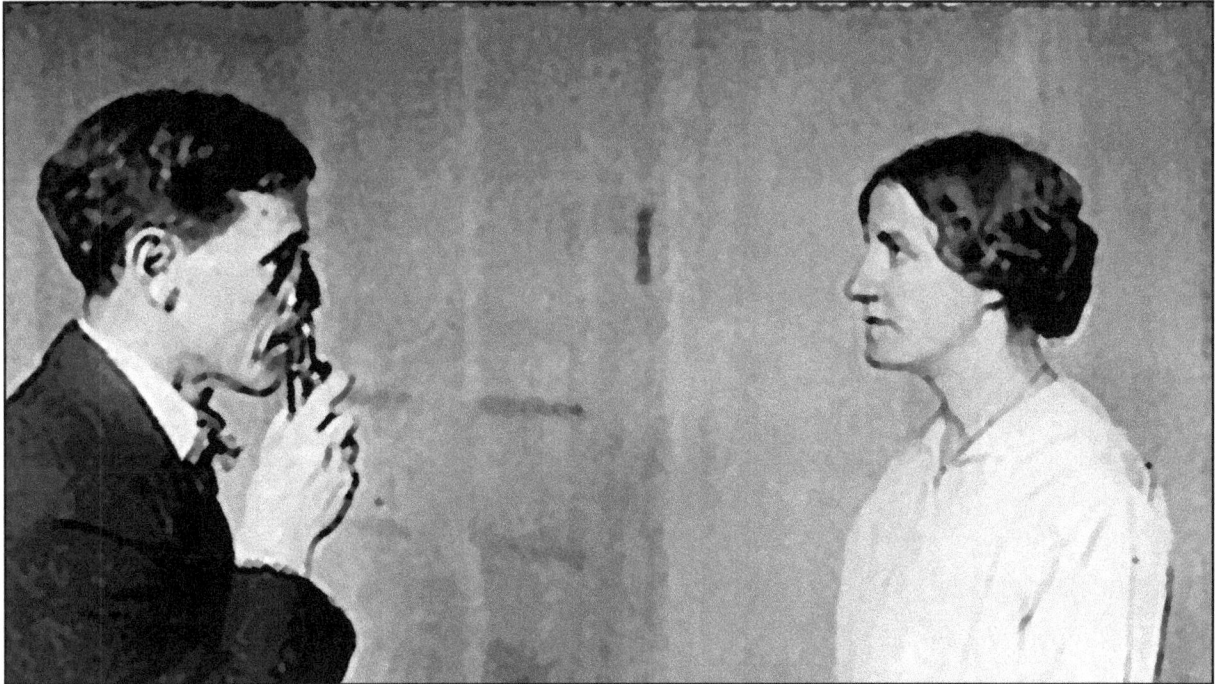

Figure 0.25: Dr. Bates Doing Retinoscopy

Congratulations!

This concludes Chapter Zero. You now have a basic knowledge of optics to prepare you for Dr. Bates . As I worked on this book, I found that the more I read of what Dr. Bates said, the better my vision got. I hope you find the same is true for you.

CHAPTER 1

Eyesight Can Change

These days, ophthalmologists think they have the final word on vision problems. Unfortunately, the final word is a rather depressing one. Practically everyone these days is nearsighted or farsighted. Poor vision is inconvenient and distressing. Often poor vision is even outright dangerous. Yet we are told there is no prevention, no treatment and no cure except for the crutch of glasses.

Certainly the human body seems to come with some design defects. But nowhere is Nature supposed to have blundered so badly as in the construction of the eye. With one voice, we blame the demands of modern life, especially the increased demand for close vision.

The healthy eye, when completely relaxed, is set to focus into the distance. For the eye to see up close, muscles in the eye must contract. This change in focus in order to see up close is called accommodation. The eyes accommodate to focus on something up close.

The accepted theory goes that indigenous people were usually looking far away, so their eyes were relaxed. By contrast, modern people are usually looking at things up close, and this puts a huge strain on the muscles that accommodate for close vision. This constant strain leads to poor eyesight.

The fact that indigenous women were seamstresses, embroiderers, weavers and artists in all sorts of fine and beautiful work appears to have been generally forgotten. Yet women living under indigenous conditions have just as good eyesight as men living under those same conditions.

A few hundred years ago, even princes were not taught to read and write. Now we compel everyone to go to school. A generation or so ago, books were scarce and expensive. Today they have been brought within the reach of practically everyone. The tallow candle has been but lately displaced by electric lights. We continue to use our vision into the dark hours of the night. Within the past couple of decades, the moving picture has come to complete the supposedly destructive process.

It is the accepted belief of ophthalmology today *[in 1920. And this is still the belief today.* **MA]** that the eyes simply cannot stand up to the demands of modern civilization. Certainly many facts support this view. Primitive people appear to have suffered little from defects of vision. By contrast, among those over the age of twenty-one living in civilized conditions, nine out of ten have imperfect sight. Among those over forty years of age, it is almost impossible to find a person free from visual defects.

Vision Requirements for Military Service

There are volumes of statistics to support the fact that modern people have poor vision. Just the visual standards of the modern army *[in 1920* **MA***]* show all the evidence required. A combat soldier ideally has perfect vision. Glasses can fall off or crack. They can get wet or dusty or scratched. A combat zone is no place for corrective lenses. Yet in Germany, Austria, France and Italy, you can be accepted into the military with vision so nearsighted that you cannot see anything clearly if it is more than six inches from your naked eye! In technical terms, these armies allow nearsightedness of up to six Diopters, which is severe nearsightedness indeed.

The German army requirement for vision during *[World War I* **MA***]* was that with glasses, the person had to be able to see 20/40 from at least one eye. In other words, the German soldier was considered fit for military service if the vision of one eye could be brought up to one-half of normal with glasses. In the German reserve army, they would even accept people who were blind in one eye.

In the armies of Great Britain, the recruits formerly were not allowed to wear glasses for their vision test. The requirement was they see at least 20/80 with their unaided right eye. The right eye is the eye used to aim a rifle. But this standard did not allow them to get enough soldiers. They had to loosen the requirement more or less to 20/40 in the right eye with glasses. In other words, the new standard was half of normal vision with the right eye.

Until 1908, the United States required normal vision in recruits for its military service. Then they had to loosen the requirement to 20/40 in the right eye, again because they could not get enough recruits. However, glasses were still not allowed.

In the first wave of recruiting in the U.S. for World War I, even these low standards did not allow for enough men to enter the military. Twenty-two percent of rejections for enlistment were due to inadequate vision. The standards were, therefore, interpreted very freely in the recruiting centers.

Later, the recruiters began to allow men who wore glasses if their corrected vision in the right eye was 20/40 or better. Yet poor vision was still among the top three causes for the rejection of potential recruits.

For more than a hundred years, the medical profession has been seeking some method of checking the supposed ravages of civilization on the human eye. Many approaches have been tried in the schools for young children. Nothing is working, as these military standards for vision show.

[FYI: In 2015, these are the current standards for US Military enlistment: A person may enlist if, with corrective lenses, their vision is as good or better than one of the following:

1. *20/40 in one eye and 20/70 in the other eye,*

2. *20/30 in one eye and 20/100 in the other eye,*

3. *20/20 in one eye and 20/400 in the other eye.* **MA***]*

Failure of Previous Methods

As for the prevailing method of treatment by corrective lenses, they are like crutches, which allow a lame man to walk. They help, but they do not heal. Some argue that they slow the decline of vision, but current experience does not support this.

A physician at the University of Zürich, Dr. Huguenin, published a study of thousands of cases. In these cases, patients practiced various methods to prevent decline in vision from nearsightedness and farsightedness. Dr. Huguenin states that all these methods failed, in spite of the fact that the patients followed his instructions for years "with the greatest energy and pertinacity." Sometimes they even changed their professions to do so.

I have been studying nearsightedness, farsightedness and astigmatism for more than thirty years. My observations confirm the uselessness of all the methods heretofore employed for the prevention and treatment of these conditions. I was very early led to suspect, however, that the problem was by no means unsolvable.

Trying to Explain the Variability of Refraction

Now, every ophthalmologist of any experience knows that errors of refraction are not always permanent and incurable. Some people recover normal vision spontaneously. Others go from nearsighted to farsighted or vice versa. It has long been the custom either to ignore these troublesome facts or to explain them away.

The usual explanation for the inconsistencies between ophthalmological theory and clinical experience is malfunction of the crystalline lens. According to accepted theory, the eye changes its focus for vision at different distances by altering the shape of the lens inside the eye. The assumption is that the shape of the eyeball does not change at all. Thus the healthy eye at rest is "set" to gaze into the distance. When the eye changes focus to see something up close, the theory is that the lens becomes more rounded to accomplish this.

How does the lens become more rounded? The accepted theory is that the lens is elastic and can change shape. In the resting state, the lens is suspended in the eye by fibers around its edge. This arrangement is similar to the way in which springs around the edge of a trampoline hold the mat on which we jump in place. These fibers pull on the lens even in the resting state, when the eye is looking far away. When we focus up close, the theory is that muscles around these fibers contract and the fibers loosen. The lens, which at rest is stretched flatter by the tension of the fibers, is now no longer pulled flat. It bunches up and becomes more rounded. When it becomes more rounded, it becomes a thicker, more powerful lens, and thus close objects are brought into focus.

The muscles around the lens of the eye that cause the fibers to loosen so the lens can get more curved are called the ciliary muscles.

People usually think that farsightedness means a person can see well far away but not close up. Actually, a farsighted person does not see into the distance that well but sees even worse up close. The conventional explanation is that the eyeball is too short from front to back. When the eye is at rest, all rays of light, from objects both near and far, are focused behind the retina instead of on it *[see Figure 0.14, page 10]*.

However, if the error is not too bad, the lens can increase its curvature and compensate, at least enough for the person to see far away.

In nearsightedness, the theory is that the eyeball is too long. While the divergent rays from near objects come to a point on the retina, the parallel ones from distant objects converge before reaching the retina *[See Figure 0.3, page 3]*.

Trying to Explain
How Prescriptions Change

Both of these conditions are supposed to be permanent. Yet any ophthalmologist will tell you that people's prescriptions change. But when the prescription does change, the doctors do not allow themselves to think that the shape of the eyeball has changed. They have to fall back on the idea that the behavior of the crystalline lens is causing the change in the prescription.

Consider the case when someone becomes less farsighted or even goes from being farsighted to having normal vision. Conventional ophthalmologists have to say that the entire time that the person was farsighted, the ciliary muscles in the eye were constantly exerting themselves to bring things more into focus, whether those things were near or far away. If farsightedness then improves, they theorize that the ability of the ciliary muscles to live in a continuous state of contraction to compensate for the error of

refraction has somehow improved.

If nearsightedness improves or goes away, they have to say that the nearsightedness was always due to a constant, pathological exertion of the ciliary muscle that caused the eye to focus up close. This would keep the crystalline lens in a continuously flattened state of near focus. Then they say, somehow that constant exertion has stopped and the eye can now see normally.

In this theory, if nearsightedness is caused by continuous contraction of the ciliary muscles, they call it apparent nearsightedness. This means that the eye only seems to be nearsighted because the ciliary muscle can't relax.

The purpose of refracting a patient is to determine the true focus of the eye in the absence of any contraction on the part of the ciliary muscles. This is why ophthalmologists like to put drops that paralyze the ciliary muscles into the front of the eye. These drops also make the pupils smaller. For this purpose, ophthalmologists use atropine eye drops, which also cause the pupils to dilate so the doctor can get a better look inside the eye.

The lens of the eye is really a mechanism for very fine tuning of focus. Most of the bending of light is done by the cornea. Doctors believe that after the age of about forty-five the lens slowly hardens and eventually cannot change the focus of the eye at all. This is why we start to need reading glasses for "old vision" (presby-opia). So for big changes in vision or changes after the age at which the lens hardens, no plausible explanation has ever been devised.

Disappearance of or changes in

astigmatism present an even more baffling problem. Astigmatism is due in most cases to irregularities in the shape of the cornea. Light does not focus uniformly onto any one plane, so regular lenses are of no help. The eye has no way to compensate. Yet astigmatism comes and goes with as much facility as do other errors of refraction. It is well known, too, that astigmatism can be produced voluntarily. Some people can produce as much as 3 Diopters of astigmatism. I myself can produce 1.5 Diopters of astigmatism at will.

No Error of Refraction is Ever Constant

Examining thirty thousand pairs of eyes a year at the New York Eye and Ear Infirmary and other institutions, I observed many cases in which errors of refraction either recovered spontaneously or changed their form. I was unable to ignore them. Furthermore, I was unable to satisfy myself with the orthodox explanations, even where such explanations were available.

In the course of time, I discovered that nearsightedness and farsightedness, like astigmatism, could be produced at will. I found that nearsightedness was not, as we have so long believed, associated with straining to see up close. The truth is quite the opposite: nearsightedness results from straining to see objects far away. Conversely, farsightedness results from straining to see objects up close.

I found that no error of refraction is ever a constant condition. Furthermore, I found that mild to moderate near- and farsightedness can be cured, while severe near- and farsightedness can be improved.

In seeking for light on these problems, I examined tens of thousands of eyes. The more facts I accumulated, the more difficult it became to reconcile them with the accepted views. Finally, about six years ago, I undertook a series of observations on the eyes of humans and animals with astonishing results.

I found that the crystalline lens is not a factor in focusing the eye. The eye focuses by changing its length, just as a camera does. How does the eye change its length? By the action of the muscles outside the eye—the extraocular muscles.

I further found that nearsightedness, farsightedness and astigmatism are not due to an improperly shaped eyeball or a malfunction of the lens in the eye. They are instead caused by a curable lack of proper function in the action of the extraocular muscles on the eyeball.

In making these statements, I am well aware that I am going against the almost undisputed teaching of ophthalmological science for the better part of a century. I have been driven to do so by the facts. The changes in my views came so slowly that I am now surprised at my own blindness.

CHAPTER 2

Simultaneous Retinoscopy

I have learned a great deal about the eyes from simultaneous retinoscopy. The retinoscope is just what it sounds like ("retina" and "scope"). It is a device for looking into the eye at the retina. The retinoscope shines light into the eye and has a lens through which the doctor looks to see what that light illuminates.

The retina is the inner coating of the back of the eyeball. It senses the image when light falls on it and sends information about what it senses to the brain.

Because of the optics of the eye, the retinoscope has a further virtue that has been key in my investigations. It can tell how much the eye is bending light. In other words, it can determine the eye's refraction. Furthermore, it can tell the refraction from moment to moment as the focus of the eye changes. This is why I call it "simultaneous retinoscopy."

How the Retinoscope Works

Here how it works: If the eye is not looking directly at the retinoscope, the edge of the pupil casts a shadow on the retina. The behavior of this shadow when the retinoscope is moved in various directions reveals how much nearsightedness, farsightedness or astigmatism there is in any given moment.

For accurate results, the retinoscope, or "scope," must be used from at least six feet away. Why? Because, as it turns out, the eye constantly changes its shape and focus in response to the environment. If you get closer than six feet to the patient or animal, they may become anxious. This immediately makes the eye become nearsighted. Unless the patient or animal trusts you completely, you cannot get an accurate reading from closer than six feet.

Now, if you see the shadow of the pupil on the retina and you move the retinoscope, the shadow might either stay still, move in the same direction you moved the retinoscope, or move opposite to the direction you moved the retinoscope.

If the shadow moves slightly in the same direction as the retinoscope, the patient has normal vision. Long experience brings the skill to know how much movement occurs in the normal eye.

If the shadow moves quite a bit in the same direction as the scope, the patient is farsighted.

If the shadow moves opposite to the direction in which the scope is moving, then the patient is nearsighted.

In the case of astigmatism, the movement of the shadow varies according to the meridian in which the movement occurs. What do I mean by meridian? Let's say you move the light up and down. We call that the 90-degree meridian. If you move the light back and forth, that is the 180-degree meridian. It's just like the meridians on a map of the world that are used to determine longitude.

It is usually necessary to put a mirror in front of the patient's eye if accuracy is desired. Usually I use a flat mirror. If the mirror is concave instead of flat, the movements described will be reversed.

The Shortcomings of Refracting with the Snellen Test Chart and Trial Lenses

The retinoscope is an exceedingly useful instrument. It has possibilities that have not been generally realized by the medical profession. Most ophthalmologists depend on the Snellen test chart and trial lenses to test the vision. *[Trial lenses are the test lenses the optometrist puts in front of the eyes while testing a person's vision with the Snellen test chart.* **MA]** This is a slow, awkward and unreliable method. This method cannot be used on young children, animals, or any adult who cannot or will not communicate.

The test chart and trial lenses can be used only under certain favorable conditions, but the retinoscope can be used anywhere. It is a little easier to use in a dim light than in a bright one, but it may be used in any light. It can even be used with the strong light of the sun shining directly into the eye. The retinoscope may also be used under many other unfavorable conditions.

It takes a considerable time, varying from minutes to hours, to measure the refraction with the Snellen test chart and trial lenses. With the retinoscope, however, refraction can be determined in a fraction of a second. With the Snellen test chart and trial lenses, it

would be impossible, for instance, to get any information about the refraction of a baseball player at the moment he swings for the ball, at the moment he strikes it, and at the moment after he strikes it. But with the retinoscope it is quite easy.

With the Snellen test chart and trial lenses, conclusions must be drawn from the patient's statements as to what is seen. The problem is that patients often becomes so worried and confused during the examination that they do not know what is seen. It becomes unclear whether the trial lenses are making the vision better or worse.

Moreover, visual acuity does not reliably reflect the state of refraction. I have had two patients, both of whom were mildly nearsighted at 2 Diopters, according to the retinoscope. When tested on the Snellen test chart, one of them had twice the visual acuity of the other.

The evidence of the test chart is, in fact, entirely subjective. That of the retinoscope is entirely objective and depends in no way on the statements of the patient.

In short, testing refraction with the Snellen test chart and trial lenses requires considerable time, can only be done under certain artificial conditions, and gives unreliable results.

Why the Retinoscope is the Best Way to Refract a Patient

By contrast, the retinoscope can be used under all sorts of normal and abnormal conditions. It can be used on the eyes of both humans and animals. When it is used properly, the results, can always be depended on. However, as mentioned earlier, the retinoscope must not be brought nearer to the eye than six feet. If it is brought closer, the subject may become nervous. When the subject becomes nervous the refraction changes and no reliable observations are possible. In the case of animals, it is often necessary to use it at a much greater distance than six feet.

Thirty Years of Practice with the Retinoscope

For thirty years I have been using the retinoscope to study the refraction of the eye. With it I have examined the eyes of tens of thousands of school children, hundreds of infants, and thousands of animals, including cats, dogs, rabbits, horses, cows, birds, turtles, reptiles and fish. I have used it when the subjects were at rest and when they were in motion. I have used it when I myself was in motion. I have used it when the subjects were asleep and when they were awake. I have even used it when the subject was under anesthesia.

I have used the retinoscope in the daytime and at night. I have examined subjects with it when they were comfortable and when they were excited. I have examined them when they were straining to see and when they were not; when they were lying and when they were telling the truth. I have performed this simultaneous retinoscopy when the eyelids were partly closed, shutting off part of the area of the pupil. I have performed it when the pupil was dilated and also when it was contracted to a pinpoint, when the eye was oscillating from side to side, from above downward and in other directions.

By this extensive use of simultaneous

retinoscopy, I discovered many facts that had not previously been known and that I was quite unable to reconcile with the orthodox teachings on the subject. This led me to undertake the series of experiments already mentioned. The results were in complete harmony with my previous observations and left me no choice but to reject the entire body of orthodox teaching about how the eye focuses and how people develop nearsightedness, farsightedness and astigmatism.

But before describing my experiments, I ask your patience. First let me present an overview of the evidence for the accepted view of how the eye focuses.

CHAPTER 3

Evidence for the Accepted Theory of How the Eye Focuses

The power of the eye to change its focus for vision at different distances is called accommodation. Accommodation has puzzled the scientific mind for centuries.

The Various Theories of Accommodation

In the early 17th century there lived a brilliant mathematician and scientist called Johannes Kepler. He expanded on the work of Copernicus about the orbits of the planets around the sun. He laid the groundwork for Newton to discover the Law of Gravity.

Kepler tried to explain accommodation by supposing a change in the position (rather than the shape) of the crystalline lens.

Later in history, every imaginable hypothesis was advanced to account for accommodation. Kepler's idea had many supporters. The idea that the eye changes focus by lengthening and shortening the eyeball also had many supporters.

Have you noticed that you can sometimes see better if you squint with your eyelids very close to being closed? This is because when light passes near an edge, it bends somewhat.

On this basis, some people believed that the narrowing of the pupil was sufficient to account for the eye changing focus. This theory was discredited when it was discovered that the eye focuses quite well even when the pupil is absent.

Some, dissatisfied with all these theories, discarded them across the board. They then boldly asserted that no change of focus took place. This view was conclusively disproven when the invention of the ophthalmoscope made it possible to see the interior of the eye.

The currently prevailing idea is that the change of focus might be brought about by a change in the form of the lens. This theory appears to have been first advanced in Austria by a Jesuit named Christoph Scheiner in 1619. In 1637, Descartes stated his agreement.

In the late 19th century in Germany, there lived an anatomist named Maximilian Langenbeck. He took an ingenious approach to proving the theory that the eye changes focus by changing the shape of its lens. This approach is based on looking at reflections of lights off the surface of the lens in the eye.

If a small bright light, usually a candle, is held in the right position near the eye, we can see three reflections of that light within the eye. One reflection is bright and upright. Another is large, less bright, and also upright. The third is small, bright, and inverted.

The first reflection comes from the front surface of the cornea. The second comes from the front surface of the crystalline lens, and the third from the back of the crystalline lens.

The Images of Purkinje

These three images were first described by an anatomist in Breslau in the early 19th century. His name was Johann Evangelist Purkinje. They are therefore known as the Images of Purkinje (See Figure 3.1, page 31).

So what? Any image reflected from a convex curved surface is diminished in proportion to the convexity of the reflecting surface.

One of these reflected images is from the front of the lens. If the lens changes shape, then the reflected image should change as well.

To focus on something close up, the lens must bend light more. To do that, the conventional theory is that the lens must become thicker. If the lens becomes thicker, its surface will become more curved, more convex. If the surface becomes more convex, the image should become smaller.

Therefore, if the conventional theory is correct, the size of the middle image, reflected from the front of the lens, should become smaller as the eye changes focus from far away to close up.

Those Who Followed After Purkinje

Langenbeck examined these images with the naked eye and concluded that the image reflected from the front of the lens does indeed become smaller as the eye changes focus from far to near.

In the latter part of the 19th century, in Holland, there lived another of the founders of modern ophthalmology—Dr. Franciscus Donders. He invented a way to measure the pressure inside the eye and was the first to

devise lenses for astigmatism.

Dr. Donders repeated the experiments of Langenbeck but was unable to make any satisfactory observations. He predicted, however, that if the images were examined with a magnifier, they would "show with certainty" whether the form of the lens changed during accommodation.

Dr. Antonie C. Cramer was another Dutch ophthalmologist of the time. Acting on Dr. Donder's suggestion, he examined the Purkinje images magnified from ten to twenty times, and thus convinced himself that the one reflected from the front of the lens became considerably smaller during accommodation.

Dr. Hermann Helmholtz was another 19th century physician who lived in Germany. He was also a physicist. Dr. Helmholtz confirmed these observations with a different method. His Handbook of Physiological Optics, published around the middle of the 19th century, is considered the cornerstone of early ophthalmology. In this book, he describes the Purkinje images as being "usually so blurred that the form of the flame cannot be definitely distinguished." So he placed two lights behind a screen with two little openings. In this way, two sets of Purkinje images were reflected from within the eye.

It seemed to Dr. Helmholtz that during accommodation, the two images on the front of the lens became smaller and approached each other. On the return of the eye to a state of rest, the images appear to grow larger again and separate. This change, he said, could be seen "easily and distinctly."

The Images of Purkinje

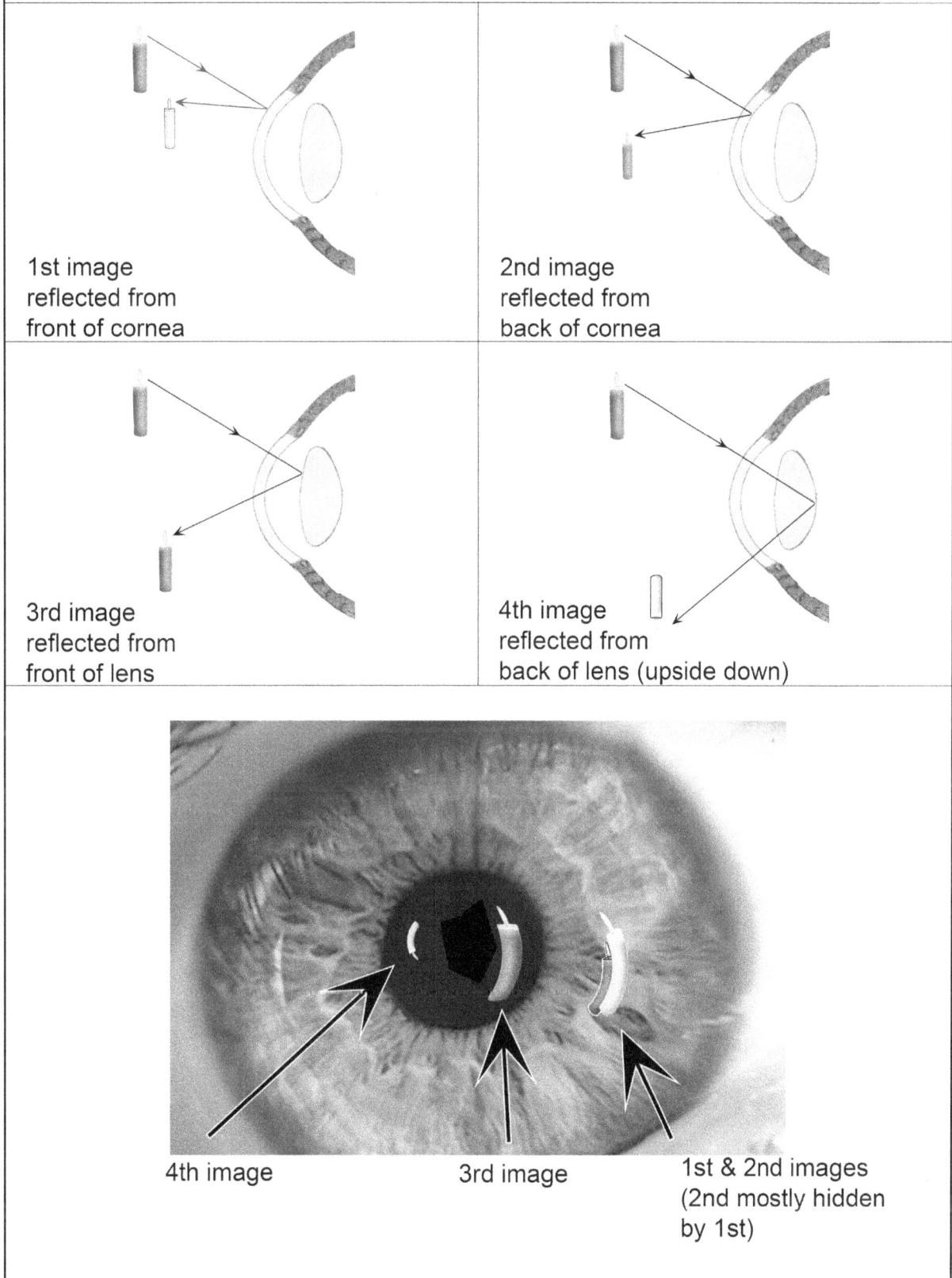

1st image
reflected from
front of cornea

2nd image
reflected from
back of cornea

3rd image
reflected from
front of lens

4th image
reflected from
back of lens (upside down)

4th image

3rd image

1st & 2nd images
(2nd mostly hidden
by 1st)

Figure 3.1: The Images of Purkinje

Helmholtz's Theory Accepted as Fact

Dr. Helmholtz's observations were soon accepted as facts. Ever since then, they have been presented as facts in every textbook dealing with the subject.

"We may say," writes Edmund Landolt in the late 1800s, "that the discovery of the part played by the crystalline lens in the act of accommodation is one of the finest achievements of medical physiology, and the theory of its working is certainly one of the most firmly established. Not only have knowledgeable men furnished lucid and mathematical proofs of its correctness, but all other theories which have been advanced as explaining accommodation have been easily and entirely overthrown... The fact that the eye is accommodated for near vision by an increase in the curvature of its crystalline lens, is, then, incontestably proven."

Yet when I myself examined the evidence for the theory that the lens is responsible for changing focus in the eye, I am not convinced. I can only wonder at the scientific credulity that could base the entire field of ophthalmology on such a mass of contradictions.

Dr. Helmholtz himself felt unable to speak with certainty of the means by which the supposed change in the shape of the lens was effected. Strangely enough, at present [1920 **MA**] the question is still being debated.

Dr. Helmholtz stated that he could find "absolutely nothing but the ciliary muscle to which accommodation could be attributed." He therefore concluded that the changes that he thought he had observed in the curvature of the lens must be caused by the action of the ciliary muscle. However, he was unable to offer any satisfactory theory to explain the way the ciliary muscle causes the lens to grow thicker.

Dr. Helmholtz explicitly stated that the mechanism he suggested was only a probability. Some of his disciples proclaimed as certain what Dr. Helmholtz himself, with much reserve, explained as probable.

No one except myself, so far as I am aware, has ventured to question that the ciliary muscle focuses the eye. As to exactly how the ciliary muscle works, there is generally felt to be much need for more clarity. My view is that since the lens is not a factor in accommodation, it is not strange that no one is able to find out how it changes its curvature. It is strange, however, that these difficulties have not in any way disturbed the universal belief that the lens does change shape and focus the eye.

With age, the lens can become milky and opaque. This is called a cataract. The treatment is to remove the lens. *[By 2017, an artificial plastic lens is inserted in place of the original crystalline lens in cataract surgery.* **MA**]

When the lens has been removed because of a cataract, patients usually appear to lose the power of accommodation. They have to wear one set of glasses to replace the lost lens and a stronger set of glasses for reading.

In a few of these cases, however, they can see perfectly well after surgery at the near point without any change in their glasses. *[The near point is the closest point at which one can focus.* **MA**]. This comes about after a period of time in which they become accustomed to the absence of the lens in their eyes.

The most common scenario of needing reading glasses after cataract surgery supports the theory that the lens focuses the eye. But the cases where people can still focus their eyes up close after cataract surgery are hard to explain away, and they are not going away. Every ophthalmologist of any experience has seen cases of this kind, and many of them have been reported in the scientific literature.

These cases have been the cause of great embarrassment to those who feel called on to reconcile them with the accepted theory.

The simple fact is that with the retinoscope, the lens-less eye can be seen to accommodate.

Astigmatism

Some people can voluntarily produce astigmatism. Why is this important? Astigmatism involves a change of shape in the cornea, which could only be produced by a change in the shape of the eyeball. This proves that the accepted theory that the eyeball cannot change shape is wrong. If the eyeball changes shape, simple physics dictates that the focus changes as well.

CHAPTER 4

The Truth About Accommodation

as Demonstrated by Experiments

[Note: In this chapter, Dr. Bates explains in detail the surgical and manual manipulation of the eye muscles of cadavers and live animals that he undertook in his research. **MA***]*

As mentioned in Chapter 3, prior to Dr. Helmholtz, some people believed that the external muscles of the eye, also called the extraocular or extrinsic muscles, help the eye to change focus. This belief almost vanished after Helmholtz's lens theory of focusing was accepted.

As Dr. Donders (mentioned in Chapter 2) noted, there were many cases of people whose extraocular muscles were paralyzed but whose ability to change focus was intact. He also described cases where the ability to change focus was lost but the movement of the eyes by the extraocular muscles was entirely intact. He concluded that the theory that extraocular muscles are involved in changing focus in the eye "scarcely needs refutation."

If Dr. Donders had not considered the question settled, he might have inquired more carefully into these cases. If he had inquired more carefully, he might have been less dogmatic in his statements. As was pointed out earlier, there are plenty of indications that the extraocular muscles do help focus the eye.

My own experiments on the remains of animals show conclusively that accommodation depends wholly on the action of the extrinsic muscles and not at all on the action of the crystalline lens. By the manipulation of these extraocular muscles, I was able to produce or prevent accommodation at will. I was able to produce or prevent nearsightedness, farsightedness and astigmatism. Let me describe the anatomy of these extraocular muscles so that my findings will make sense.

The Anatomy of the Extraocular Muscles

There are six extraocular muscles attached to the outside of the eyeball. Four are known as the "rectus" muscles and two as the "oblique" muscles. *["Rectus," just means "straight" in Latin.* **MA***]* The other ends of these muscles attach at various points at the back of the bony eye socket.

The four rectus muscles attach at cardinal points around the eyeball: top, bottom, inside and outside. In the language of anatomy, inside is "medial" and outside is "lateral;" top is "superior" and bottom is "inferior."

So the individual names of these four muscles on the outside the eye are simple: medial rectus, lateral rectus, superior rectus, and inferior rectus.

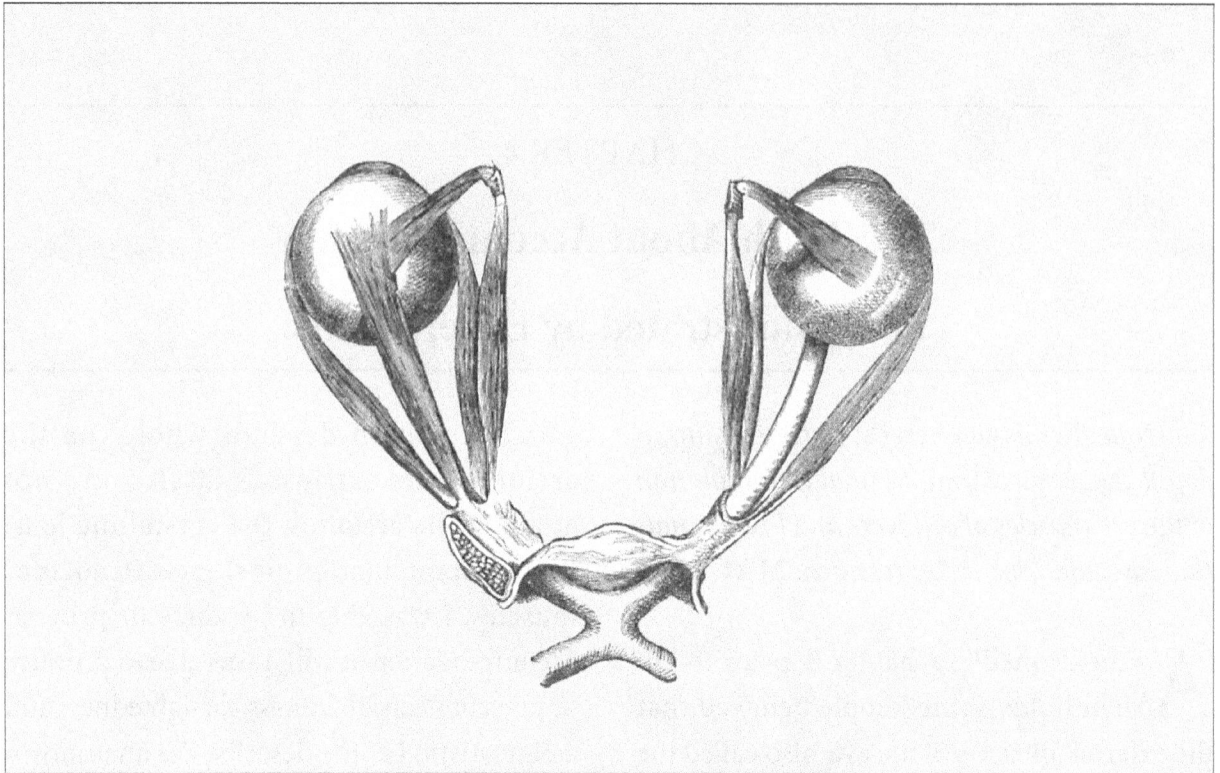

Figure 4.1 The Extraocular Muscles from Above

   We are looking down on the eyes and their surrounding muscles. The muscles that go directly from the eyeball to the back are the rectus muscles. The muscle that goes from the eyes to the midline and then back is the superior rectus muscle. The inferior rectus muscle is not shown.

   On the right side, the top rectus muscle is cut away to show the optic nerve below.

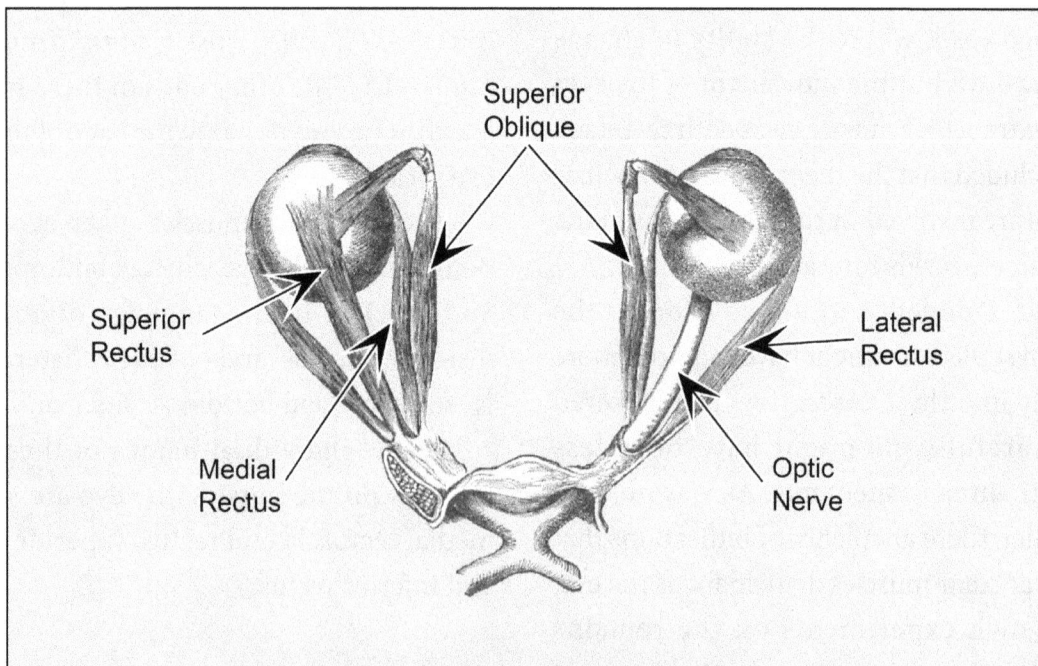

Figure 4.2 The Extraocular Muscles Labeled

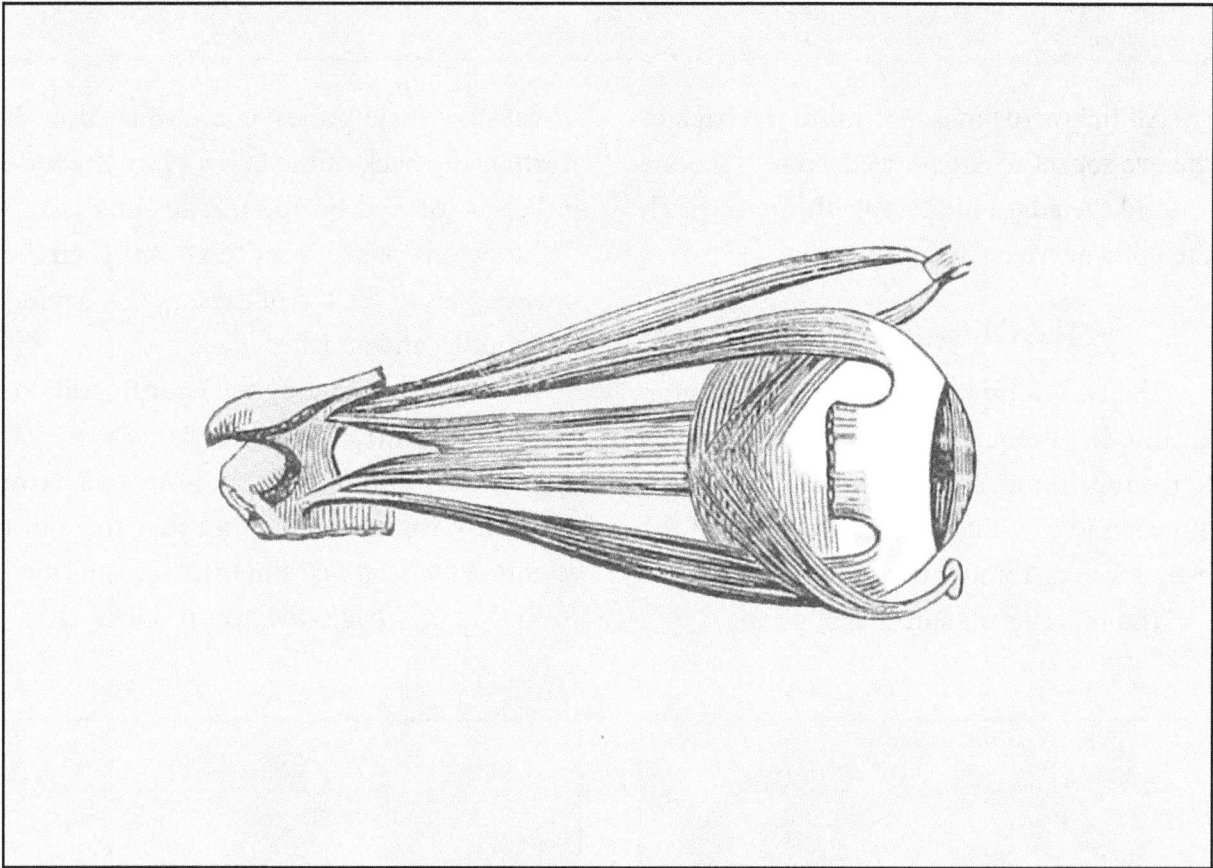

Figure 4.3: Lateral View of the Extraocular Muscles

This view is as if standing to the right of the person, looking at the outside of the right eye. The lateral rectus muscle is cut away to show the medial rectus muscle.

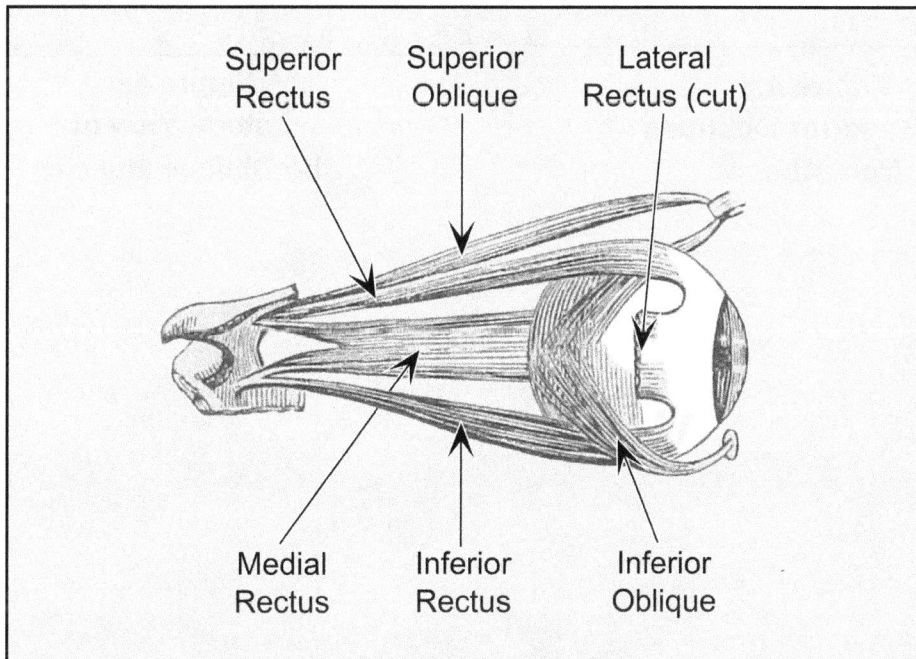

Figure 4.4: Extraocular Muscles, Lateral View, Labeled

All the rectus muscles run to the back of the eye socket where they attach to the bone around the edges of the hole through which the optic nerve passes.

The Oblique Muscles

The two oblique muscles basically wrap around the eyeball, top to bottom and back to the top, like a band. The inferior oblique is attached to the inner side of the bone of the eye socket, just under the front of the eye.

The superior oblique actually runs through a little pulley made of tendon. It starts at the back of the eye socket. The little pulley is located on the inside (medial) of the upper eye socket near the front. Then the muscle goes to the top of the eye, just behind the middle, and attaches there.

It is amazing that by the coordination of these twelve extraocular muscles, six in each eye, we can look about freely. Both eyes move smoothly together, keeping just the right alignment so that one single image is formed from the two images the eyes produce.

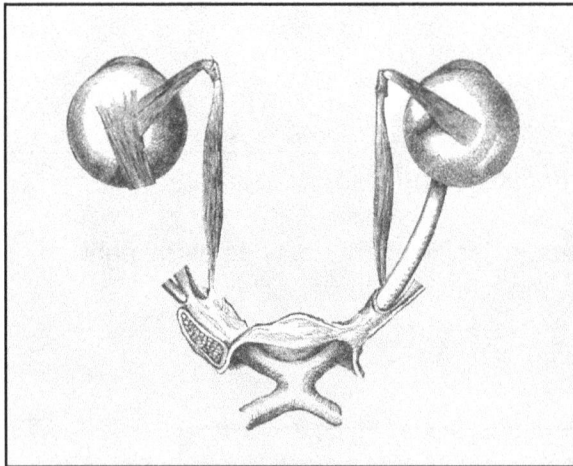

Figure 4.5
The Superior Obliques
from Above

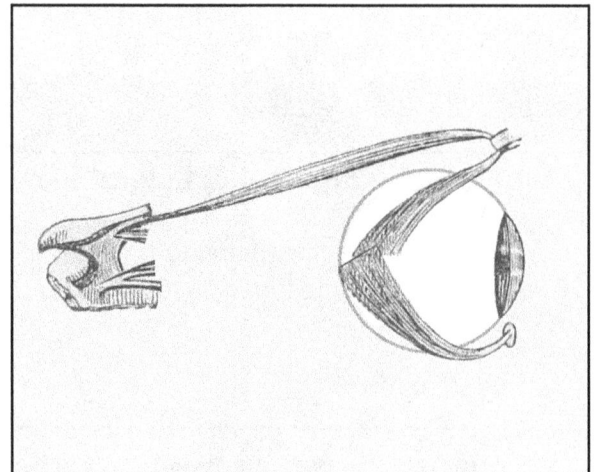

Figure 4.6
Lateral View of
the Oblique Muscles

The Heart of My Argument

And now we come to the heart of my argument. The eyeball is not a rigid thing. It is more like a little rubber ball. The shape of the eyeball can change. When the extraocular muscles pull on the eyeball, the shape of the eyeball must of necessity change. When the shape of the eyeball changes, the distance between the lens and the retina also changes. In a healthy eye, the extraocular muscles act to continuously change the shape of the eye to keep our world in focus.

While the subtleties of the actions of the extraocular muscles are complex, it is simple to see the basics of how these muscles focus the eye.

The Eyeball Elongates to Accommodate

The retina is the desired plane of focus. We want the clear image to fall on the retina. As an object approaches closer to a lens, the plane of focus of the image on the other side of that lens moves farther away from the lens. We need, then, to move the plane of focus, in this case the retina, back farther away from the lens. This is easily done by contraction of the two external oblique muscles; they squeeze the eye into a longer shape.

When the oblique muscles relax, the eyeball returns to its resting state, and the plane of focus moves up closer to the lens. In this state, the normal eye is focused more into the distance. If the rectus muscles contract, the eyeball shortens. The plane of focus in the eye moves closer to the lens and this focuses the eye further into the distance.

Vision Problems Are Due to Extraocular Muscle Dysfunction

Thus nearsightedness and farsightedness are errors of refraction that arise not from abnormally short or long eyeballs; they are instead the result of the habitual malfunction of the extraocular muscles. This malfunction can be corrected. The moment we relax the extraocular muscles and allow them to work freely and properly, the vision begins to improve.

[Dr. Bates is saying that many of us carry a mental habit of being tense. This habit makes us unconsciously use our eyes in a tense, staring way. This constant tension and staring interferes with our eyes' natural ability to focus using the extraocular muscles. **MA]**

If the oblique muscles are habitually in a pathological state of contraction, the eyeball is chronically lengthened, and the patient is nearsighted. If the rectus muscles are habitually in a pathological state of contraction, the eyeball is shortened, and the patient is farsighted.

In addition, this theory easily explains astigmatism. The cornea is firmly attached to the eyeball. If, for example, the superior rectus and inferior rectus are habitually in a pathological state of contraction, the eyeball will be flattened, and the cornea will flatten with it. This produces astigmatism in the horizontal plane. If the medial and lateral rectus muscles are habitually contracted, this produces astigmatism in the vertical plane. Indeed, astigmatism in any plane can be produced by various combinations of

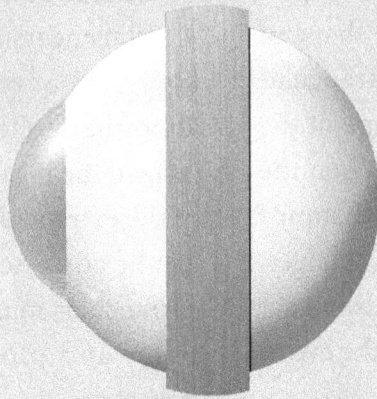

The oblique muscles are like
a band around the eyeball.

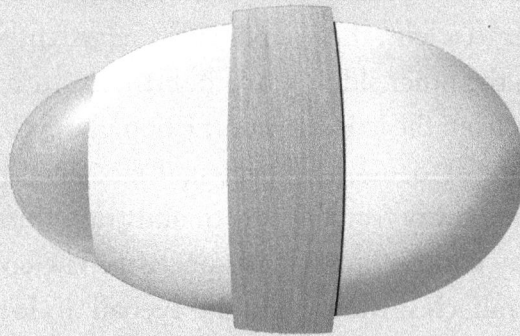

When both oblique muscles
contract together,
the eyeball gets longer.

Figure 4.7: The Oblique Muscles Can Make the Eyeball Longer

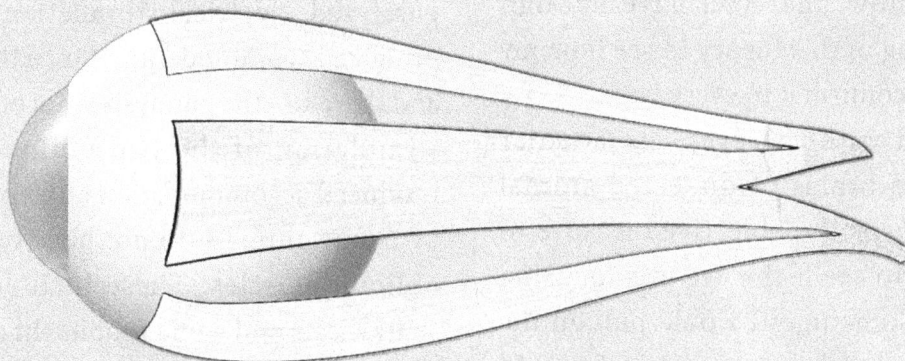

The four rectus muscles are like reins on a horse.

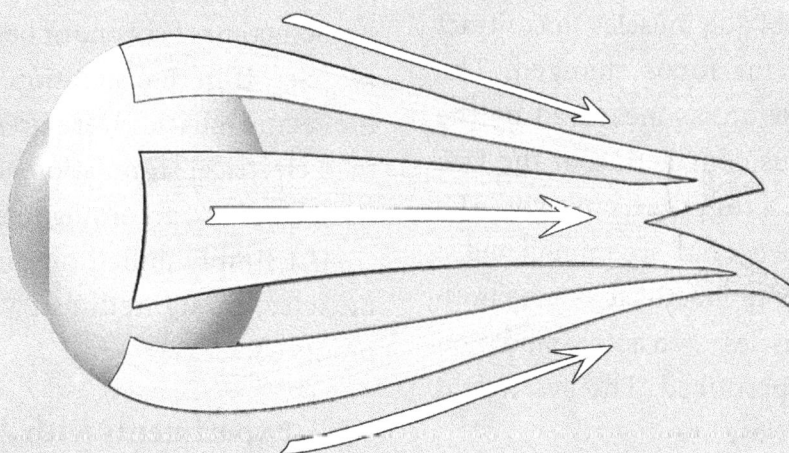

When they all contract together, the eyeball shortens.

Figure 4.8: The Rectus Muscles Can Make the Eyeball Shorter When They All Contract Together

inappropriate muscle contraction.

Many Experiments
Confirm This Theory

I hope, now, that you have enough understanding of this theory to see how my experiments confirm it in every way.

I worked with the eyes, extraocular muscles, and brains of dissected animal cadavers. I used the objective measure of retinoscopy to see if the eye was focusing near or far. Sometimes I would pull on the extraocular muscles. Sometimes I would shorten them by cutting out a bit of the muscle and sewing the loose ends together. Sometimes I would cause the muscles to contract by applying electrical stimulation to them. Sometimes I would cause them to contract by stimulating the part of the animal's brain which sends nerves to the muscle.

No matter how I approached it, when I caused the two oblique muscles to contract simultaneously, the focus changed: The eye focused close up, as measured by the retinoscope. Thus contraction of the two oblique muscles together changed the refraction as if the eye had accommodated.

If I took steps to inactivate one or both of the oblique muscles, then accommodation could never be produced. The eye would simply not focus close up.

Sometimes I inactivated one or both of the oblique muscles by cutting them. Then I would apply the same electrical current that produced accommodation before. There would be no change in focus. If I sewed the cut muscle or muscles back together and then applied the same electrical current, the eye

would accommodate as before.

Other times I used atropine to paralyze one or both of the oblique muscles. Once one or both of the oblique muscles were paralyzed, electrical stimulation could not produce accommodation. Once the atropine and therefore the paralysis wore off, electrical stimulation of the two oblique muscles produced accommodation as before.

Some animals do not have two distinct oblique muscles. These include dogfish, sharks, cats and some rabbits. In any animal lacking two distinct oblique muscles, near focus (accommodation) could not be produced by any electrical stimulation.

Sometimes if an animal had only one oblique muscle, I would supply the necessary counter-traction by sewing a thread from the eyeball to the lining of the eye socket. Once I did that, then accommodation could be produced by electrical stimulation.

Sometimes I cut one or both of the oblique muscles. If in that situation two or more of the rectus muscles were present and intact, then electrical stimulation always produced farsightedness, according to the retinoscope.

If I simply pulled on one of the rectus muscles, farsightedness was also always produced.

Experiments with Atropine

If I paralyzed the rectus muscles with atropine, or if I cut one or more of the rectus muscles, then electrical stimulation would no longer produce farsightedness. But after the effects of the atropine had passed away, or after the cut muscle or muscles had been sewed back together, farsightedness was produced as usual by electrical stimulation.

It should be emphasized that in order to paralyze either the rectus or the oblique muscles, it was found necessary to inject the atropine far back behind the eyeball with a hypodermic needle. Atropine is supposed to paralyze the ciliary muscles which surround the lens in the eye when dropped into the front of the eye as eye drops. But in all of my experiments, I found that atropine eye drops had very little effect on the power of the eye to change its focus.

Usually, when some manipulation of the muscles produced nearsightedness or farsightedness, some astigmatism would also occur. This makes sense because the forces I applied to the eyeball were crude and no doubt asymmetrical compared to what the living nervous system could produce.

Asymmetrical Extraocular Muscle Action Produces Errors of Refraction

That is to say, for a lens to focus an image properly, its surface must be a portion of a perfect sphere. Any other shape distorts the image or causes the image to be in focus in some areas and out of focus in other areas.

I've explained that in clinical situations, astigmatism can change, sometimes from moment to moment. This means that the shape of the cornea can change from moment to moment. Is it not likely, then, that as the extraocular muscles change the shape of the eyeball, the shape of the cornea changes along with it? As long as the extraocular muscles shorten or lengthen the eyeball symmetrically, a sharp image can still be focused on the

retina, and no astigmatism is produced.

When the action of the extraocular muscles is asymmetrical, it can cause the shape of the eyeball to become irregular. The shape of the cornea then becomes irregular and astigmatism is produced. The treatment is the same as for the other errors of refraction: Free up and relax the extraocular muscles.

Mixed astigmatism is a combination of nearsightedness in one axis and farsightedness in another. Mixed astigmatism always occurred when I applied traction on the insertion of the superior or inferior rectus in a direction parallel to the plane of the iris.

On the other hand, if either or both of the oblique muscles had been cut, the nearsighted part of this astigmatism disappeared. Similarly, when the superior or the inferior rectus was cut, the farsighted part of the astigmatism disappeared. Surgical shortening of the two oblique muscles combined with surgical shortening of the superior and inferior recti always produced mixed astigmatism.

Eyes from which the lens had been removed responded to electrical stimulation precisely as did normal eyes. But when the extraocular muscles were paralyzed by the injection of atropine deep into the eye socket, electrical stimulation had no effect on the refraction. The focus of the eye did not change at all.

In one experiment, I tested the refraction of the eyes of a live rabbit and found they could change focus normally. Then, using anesthesia, I performed the equivalent of cataract surgery on the right eye. In cataract surgery, the lens is simply removed. The wound was then allowed to heal.

Thereafter, for a period extending from one month to two years, electrical stimulation always produced accommodation in the lens-less eye precisely to the same extent as in the eye that had a lens. The same experiment with the same result was performed on a number of other rabbits, on dogs and on fish. The obvious conclusion is that the lens is not a factor in accommodation.

The Cranial Nerves

The cranial nerves are a set of twenty-four nerves, twelve on each side, that come out of the bottom of the brain. They go directly out of the skull to their destinations. (By contrast, all other nerves have to pass down the spinal cord.) The cranial nerves mostly serve functions in the face and head, especially sensory functions. For example, the second cranial nerve is the optic nerve. The optic nerve carries all the information about what we are seeing from the eye to the brain.

The cranial nerves numbered 3, 4 and 6 go to the extraocular muscles to move them about.

Most textbooks say that the third cranial nerve is responsible for focusing the eye because it goes to the ciliary muscle around the lens. But the third cranial nerve also goes to all the extraocular muscles except the superior oblique and lateral rectus.

Moreover, in my experiments, the fourth cranial nerve was just as responsible for changing focus in the eye as the third cranial nerve. Yet the fourth cranial nerve supplies only the superior oblique muscle.

Both third and fourth cranial nerves are easily found and stimulated at the point where they exit the underside of the brain. When either the third or the fourth nerve was stimulated with electricity, accommodation always resulted in the normal eye.

Then I tried paralyzing first one nerve then the other. I did this by putting a small wad of cotton soaked in atropine solution on the nerve at the point where it comes out of the bottom of the brain. Stimulation of the paralyzed nerve produced no accommodation, while stimulation of the unparalyzed nerve did produce accommodation. This was true both when the third nerve was paralyzed and the fourth nerve was not. It was also true when the fourth nerve was paralyzed and the third nerve was not.

When the origin (the point at which the nerve comes out of the brain) of both nerves was covered with cotton soaked in atropine, accommodation could not be produced by electrical stimulation of either or both nerves. When the cotton was removed and the nerves washed with normal salt solution, electrical stimulation of either or both nerves produced accommodation just as it did before the atropine had been applied. I did this over and over for more than an hour, alternately applying and removing the atropine. The results were always the same.

This experiment clearly demonstrates two new things. First, the fourth cranial nerve is involved in accommodation. Second, the superior oblique muscle is an important factor in accommodation.

I further found that when the action of the oblique muscles was prevented by cutting them, the stimulation of the third cranial nerve produced farsightedness instead of accommodation.

No Doubt That
The Crystalline Lens
Does Not Produce Accommodation

In all these experiments, I believe I eliminated every possible source of error. The experiments were all repeated many times and always with the same results. They seemed, therefore, to leave no room for doubt: neither the lens nor any muscle on the interior of the eyeball has anything to do with accommodation. These experiments show that the process whereby the eye adjusts itself for vision at different distances is entirely controlled by the action of the extraocular muscles on the outside of the eyeball.

CHAPTER 5

The Truth About Accommodation
as Demonstrated by
a Study of Images Reflected From the Eye

The conclusions I reached through the experiments described in Chapter 4 are diametrically opposed to those reached by Dr. Helmholtz. Recall that he studied the Purkinje images (Figure 3.1, p. 31), which are the reflections from the cornea and lens in the eye. I decided to repeat his experiments and find out, if possible, why his results were so different from my own.

I devoted four years to this work and was able to demonstrate that Dr. Helmholtz erred through defective technique. The images obtained by his method are so variable and uncertain that they lend themselves to the support of almost any theory.

I worked for a year or more using the techniques described by Dr. Helmholtz. I used a naked candle as the source of light. Clear and distinct images were obtained from the front of the cornea and the back of the lens. However, I was unable to obtain from the front of the lens an image which was sufficiently clear or distinct to be measured or photographed.

The image from the front of the lens was blurred, just as Dr. Helmholtz described. In addition, the size of the image from the front of the lens varied greatly in both size and intensity without any apparent cause. At times, no reflection at all could be obtained from the front of the lens. Changing the angle of the light or the position of the observer did not help.

I then used a photographer's diaphragm, as he had, which allowed me to control the size of the beam of light. With this, I got a clearer and more constant image, but it still was not sufficiently reliable to be measured.

Dr. Helmholtz wrote that the indistinct image of a naked flame seemed to show an appreciable change during accommodation. He wrote that the images obtained by the aid of the diaphragm showed it more clearly. I was unable, either with or without it, to obtain images which I considered sufficiently distinct to be reliable.

Men who had been teaching and demonstrating Dr. Helmholtz's theory repeated his experiments for my benefit. The images which they obtained on the front of the lens did not seem to me any better than my own.

No Reliable Findings
After a Year of Study

After studying these images almost daily for more than a year, I was unable to make any reliable observation regarding the effect of accommodation on them. In fact, it seemed that an infinite number of appearances might be obtained on the front of the lens when a candle was used as the source of illumination. At times, the image became smaller during accommodation and seemed to sustain the theory of Dr. Helmholtz. But just as frequently, the image became larger. At other times, it was impossible to tell what it did.

Increasing the brightness of the light was no help. A 30-watt lamp, then a 50-watt, then a 250-watt, and finally a 1000-watt lamp yielded no improvement in the quality of the images. The light of the sun reflected from the front of the lens produced an image just as cloudy and uncertain as the reflections from other sources of illumination and just as variable in shape, intensity and size.

To sum it all up, I was convinced that the front surface of the lens was a very poor reflector of light, and that no reliable images could be obtained from it by the means so far described.

Finally, a Clear Purkinje Image

After a year or more of failure, I began to work at an aquarium on the eyes of fish. It was a long story of failure. Finally I resorted to a very strong light: 1000 watts. I used a diaphragm and made the opening very small. Inspired by the use of condensers in microscopy, I added a condenser to focus the light to a small spot or point.

Under these circumstances, after some difficulty, I was able to obtain a clear and distinct image from the cornea of a fish. This image was sufficiently distinct to be measured, and after many months, a satisfactory photograph was obtained.

I then resumed the work on the eyes of human beings. The strong light, combined with the diaphragm and condenser, proved to be a decided improvement over Dr. Helmholtz's method. An image was at last obtained from the front of the lens that was sufficiently clear and distinct to be photographed. This was the first time, so far as published records show, that an image of any kind was ever photographed from the front of the lens.

I had asked professional photographers for help, and they had declined, assuring me that such an image could not be obtained. I had therefore been obliged to learn photography myself, from scratch.

I continued these experiments until, after almost four years of constant labor, I obtained satisfactory pictures. I obtained images before and after accommodation. I successfully photographed Purkinje images during the production of nearsightedness and farsightedness. I obtained not only images from the front of the lens but also images of reflections from the iris, the cornea, the front of the white of the eye and the side of the white of the eye.

I was also able to obtain images on any surface at will without any unwanted confounding reflections from the other parts. Before these results were obtained, however, many difficulties had still to be overcome.

Complicating Reflections

Complicating reflections were a perpetual source of trouble. Reflections from surrounding objects were easily eliminated, but reflections of light from the white of the eye were more difficult to deal with. Yet it was useless to try to obtain images from the front of the lens until, by a proper adjustment of the light, the images from the white of the eye had been greatly reduced or eliminated. The same apparent adjustment did not, however, always give similar results. Sometimes there would be no reflections for days. Then would come a day when, with the light apparently at the same angle, they would reappear.

With some adjustments of the light, multiple images were seen reflected from the front of the lens. Sometimes these images were arranged in a horizontal line, sometimes in a vertical one and sometimes at angles of different degrees. The distance of these reflections one from the other also varied. Usually there were three of them; sometimes there were more, and sometimes only two.

Occasionally the reflections were all of the same size, but usually they varied. There was apparently no limit to their possibilities of change in this and other respects.

Changes in the distance of the diaphragm from the light and from the condenser appeared to make no difference. Alterations in the size and shape of the diaphragm's opening also made no difference. Different adjustments of the condenser were equally without effect. Changes in the angle at which the light was adjusted sometimes lessened the number of images and sometimes increased them, until at last an angle was found at which but one image was seen. The images appear, in fact, to have been caused by reflections of the electric light off the eyeball.

Even after the light had been adjusted to

eliminate reflections, it was often difficult or impossible to get a clear and distinct image of the electric filament on the front of the lens. I rearranged the condenser and the diaphragm. I had the subject change the direction of the gaze. Yet despite all this, the image would still be clouded or obscured and its outline distorted.

The cause of the difficulty appeared to be that the light was not adjusted to the best angle. Yet it was not always possible to determine the exact axis at which a clear, distinct image would be produced. As in the case of the reflections from the sides of the eyeball, it seemed to vary without a known cause.

This was true, however: Some directions of gaze gave better images than others and what these directions were could not be determined with exactness.

I have labored with the light for two or three hours without finding the right angle. At other times, the ideal axis would remain unchanged for days, giving always a clear, distinct image.

Photographic Results Confirm the Cadaver Experiments

The results of these experiments confirmed the conclusions drawn from the experiments on the eye muscles of animal cadavers as discussed in Chapter 4. No change in the reflection of light from the front of the lens could be demonstrated during accommodation. Therefore, I conclude that the lens does not change shape during accommodation. And, therefore, the eye changes focus by changing the shape of the eyeball through the action of the extraocular muscles.

The images photographed from the front of the crystalline lens did not show any change in size or form during accommodation. This proves that the crystalline lens does not change shape during accommodation.

Images photographed from the iris before and during accommodation were also the same in size and form. This further confirms that the lens does not change shape during accommodation: If the lens changed during accommodation, the shape of the iris, which rests on the front of the lens, would change as well.

Four Well-Marked Changes

My theory is that the eyeball changes shape in order to change the focus of the eye. This was confirmed by images photographed from the cornea and from the front and side of the white of the eye (the sclera). These photographs showed a series of four well-marked changes, consistent with the changing shape of the eyeball:

1. In the normal eye during accommodation, the images from the cornea were smaller than when the eye was at rest. This shows that the eyeball elongated. As the eyeball elongates, the convexity of the cornea increases.

2. When the subject strained in an unsuccessful attempt to see the near point (the closest point at which one can focus), the image reflected from the front of the cornea became larger. This indicates that the cornea flattened and became less convex: The eyeball became shorter in the horizontal axis, which

is farsightedness.

3. When a strain was made to see at a distance, the image reflected from the front of the cornea became smaller than when the eye was at rest. This again indicates elongation of the eyeball and increased convexity of the cornea.

The images photographed from the front of the sclera showed the same series of changes as the corneal images.

Images Obtained from the Side of the White of the Eye

However images obtained from the side of the sclera were found to change in exactly the opposite manner than the images obtained from the front of it. This is exactly as expected, since if the front of the eyeball becomes more convex, the sides must of necessity flatten:

1. When the subject strained to see at a distance, the image reflected from the side of the sclera was larger than the image obtained when the eye was at rest. This shows that the side of the eyeball had flattened, which indicates that the eyeball had elongated.

2. When a normal eye focused up close, the image obtained from the side of the sclera was larger than when the eye was at rest. This shows that the side of the eyeball flattened, as it would when the eyeball got longer.

3. However, the image obtained in an unsuccessful effort to see near was much smaller than any of the other images. This indicates that the sclera had become more convex at the side. More convexity at the side means that the eyeball has shortened, as in farsightedness.

The most pronounced changes were

noted in the images reflected from the front of the sclera. Those from the side were less marked. It was difficult to photograph a white image on a white background, so these changes could not always be readily seen on the photographs. They were always plainly apparent, however, to the observer. They were even more apparent to the subject, who regarded them in a concave mirror.

The alterations in the size of the image reflected from the front of the cornea were so slight that they did not show at all in the photographs, except when the image was large. They were always apparent, however, to the subject and observer.

There is an instrument used to measure astigmatism called the ophthalmometer. Previously, physicians have noted that when the cornea is viewed through this instrument, no change in the reflection of light off the surface of the cornea is noted during accommodation. The explanation is that the ophthalmometer casts a very small light onto the cornea, too small for the changes to be noted.

The change in size of a large reflection from the front of the cornea was in fact one of the easiest of the series to produce. You can consult my original article for further details about technique.

CHAPTER 6

The Truth About Accommodation

as Demonstrated by Clinical Observations

As I explained in Chapter 4, I have shown by animal experiments that the lens is not a factor in accommodation. This fact is fully confirmed in clinical observations on every type of human eye—the eyes of adults, the eyes of children, the eyes of those with normal vision, the eyes of those with errors of refraction, and on the eyes of adults after the removal of the lens for cataract.

Atropine Does Not Act as Expected

I have pointed out that atropine eye drops are supposed to render the eye incapable of changing focus by paralyzing the ciliary muscle around the lens. Atropine is used to bring out the underlying condition of the eye's focus. They are supposed to eliminate any help with focusing that the ciliary muscle might be providing. These eye drops also widen the pupil by paralyzing the muscles that make the pupil smaller. This wider window into the eye allows a better examination of the retina at the back of the eye.

In about nine out of ten cases, atropine drops work as expected. But in the tenth case they do not. Every experienced ophthalmologist will have noted this. Many of these cases are reported in the literature, and many of them I have observed myself.

Latent Nearsightedness

According to the prevailing theory, there is a condition called latent nearsightedness. This occurs in people whose eyeballs are too short, which makes them farsighted. But they can apparently see normally at a distance because the ciliary muscles constantly contract to bring their vision into focus. In this theory, atropine ought to bring out latent farsightedness in some apparently normal eyes. That is, of course, provided that the patient is young enough for the lens to still be elastic.

The fact is, though, that the introduction of atropine into the front of the eye does not produce consistent results. Sometimes atropine drops produce farsightedness. Sometimes they produce nearsightedness. Sometimes they change farsightedness into nearsightedness.

The Action of Atropine on the Older Eye

In people over seventy, the lens is supposed to be as hard as a stone and unable to change the focus of the eye in any way. Yet in this age group, just as with others, atropine sometimes will produce nearsightedness and sometimes it will produce farsightedness.

When the elderly patient has the beginnings of a cataract, we call this incipient cataract. The crystalline lens is starting to harden. As the cataract develops more fully, the lens becomes rock hard. Yet atropine drops in this group can also sometimes produce nearsightedness and sometimes farsightedness.

Unpredictable Actions of Atropine

Some patients with apparently normal eyes will develop any one of the entire range of astigmatisms after the use of atropine eye drops. In other cases, atropine will not interfere with the eye's ability to focus or alter the refraction in any way.

Furthermore, there are cases where an adverse effect of atropine eye drops on near vision is easily overcome by briefly resting the eyes. *[This despite the fact that the action of atropine eye drops endures for a minimum of several hours.* **MA]** After a short rest, one patient could read very small type at six inches. Yet atropine is supposed to rest the eyes by paralyzing an overworked ciliary muscle.

In the treatment of double vision and lazy eye, I have often used atropine in the better eye for more than a year. This is to encourage the use of the weaker eye. At the end of this time, while still under the influence of atropine, such eyes have become able in a few hours or less, to read very small type at six inches (see Chapter 22).

Eye Still Accommodates When Ciliary Muscle is Paralyzed

To repeat, according to the current theory, atropine eye drops paralyze the ciliary muscle and thus, by preventing a change of curvature in the lens, prevent accommodation. Therefore, when accommodation occurs after the prolonged use of atropine, it is evident that it must be due to some factor or factors other than the lens and the ciliary muscle. All of these facts are in entire accord with the results of my experiments on the eye muscles of animals and my observations regarding the behavior of images reflected from various parts of the eyeball.

Clinical Results Confirm Experimental Results

The cases where atropine eye drops do not work as expected strikingly confirm the results of my experiments with atropine. The experiments with the cadavers of animals showed that accommodation could not be paralyzed completely unless the atropine was injected deep into the eye socket. *[Experiments of this kind are possible within a few hours of the death of the animal because all the nerves and muscles of the animal are still relatively intact.* **MA]** This deep injection paralyzed the real muscles of accommodation—the oblique extraocular muscles.

Similarly, farsightedness could not be prevented when the eyeball was stimulated with electricity without a similar injection of atropine deep into the eye socket so as to paralyze the rectus muscles.

As has also been noted, it is well known that after the removal of the lens for cataract, the eye often appears to accommodate just as well as it did before its removal. I have observed many such cases, where patients can read very small type with only their distance glasses on at ten inches or less. Indeed, one man was able to read very small type without any glasses at all. Many ophthalmologists have suggested that this accommodation occurs by some form of compensation. However, the retinoscope shows that in all these cases, the accommodation was real. There was indeed an accurate adjustment of the focus to the close distances.

As people age, they usually become farsighted. This is called presbyopia. The cure of presbyopia (see Chapter 20) must also be added to the clinical testimony against the accepted theory of accommodation. If the now so-called rock-hard lens were the mechanism of accommodation, such cures would be manifestly impossible. The fact that resting the eyes improves vision in presbyopia has been noted by others. It has been attributed to the supposed fact that the rested ciliary muscle is able for a brief period to influence the hardened lens. It is conceivable that this might happen briefly in the early stages of the condition. It is not conceivable that permanent relief from presbyopia should be obtained by this compensation. Neither is it conceivable that lenses that are as hard as a stone, as the saying goes, should be influenced, even momentarily, by any effort, however forceful, on the part of the ciliary muscle.

No Facts Challenge the Theory of Accommodation by Extraocular Muscle Action

The accepted theories of accommodation and of the cause of errors of refraction require a multitude of facts to be explained away. By contrast, during more than thirty years of clinical experience, I have not observed a single instance that challenges the theory that the lens and the ciliary muscle have nothing to do with accommodation. I also have seen nothing whatsoever to contradict the view that most errors of refraction are reversible.

I have seen how errors of refraction can be produced at will, and I have seen how errors of refraction may be cured. A temporary cure can often be obtained in a few minutes. A permanent cure may require continued treatment.

CHAPTER 7

The Variability of the Refraction of the Eye

The prevailing theory *[in 1923 MA]* is that errors of refraction, such as nearsightedness, farsightedness and astigmatism, are due to a permanent deformity of the eyeball. This leads naturally to two conclusions:

1. Errors of refraction are permanent states.

2. Normal refraction is also a continuous condition.

In this theory, the normal eye is generally regarded as a perfect machine, which is always in good working order. No matter whether the object regarded is strange or familiar, whether the light is good or imperfect, whether the surroundings are pleasant or disagreeable, the normal eye is expected to have normal refraction and normal sight all the time. Even when the person is under a strain or ill, vision is expected to be normal.

The facts do not harmonize with this view, but the facts are often explained away or simply ignored.

The Shape of the Eyeball Is Constantly Changing

In truth, the shape of the eyeball is controlled by the external ocular muscles and responds instantaneously to their action. No refractive state, whether normal or abnormal, is permanent or constant. This conclusion is confirmed by the retinoscope. I observed this truth long before I was able to explain it.

Everyone's Refraction Is Constantly Changing

During thirty years devoted to the study of refraction, I have found few people who could maintain perfect sight for more than a few minutes at a time, even under the most favorable conditions. Often I have seen the refraction change half a dozen times or more in a second. I have seen vision vary all the way from severe nearsightedness to normal in a fraction of a second.

Similarly, I have found no eyes with continuous or unchanging errors of refraction. All people with errors of refraction have, at frequent intervals during the day and night, moments of normal vision. In those moments, their nearsightedness, farsightedness or astigmatism, wholly disappears. The form of the error also changes. Nearsightedness can change into farsightedness. One form of astigmatism can change into another.

I examined 20,000 school children in one year. More than half had normal eyes, with sight that was perfect at times. But not one of them had perfect sight in each eye at all times of the day. Their sight might be good in the morning and imperfect in the afternoon, or imperfect in the morning and perfect in the afternoon. Many children could read one Snellen test chart with perfect sight while unable to see a different one as perfectly. Many could also read some letters of the alphabet perfectly but were unable to distinguish other letters of the same size under similar conditions.

The degree of this imperfect sight was quite variable in both severity and time. Under some conditions, it might continue for only a few minutes or less. Under other conditions, it might prevent the child from seeing the blackboard for days, weeks, or even longer. Frequently all the pupils in a classroom were similarly affected.

Among babies, I noted a similar situation. Most investigators have found babies farsighted. A few have found them nearsighted. My own observations indicate that the refraction of infants is continually changing. One child was examined under atropine on four successive days, beginning two hours after birth. The first examination showed a condition of mixed astigmatism. On the second day, there was compound farsighted astigmatism, and on the third day, compound nearsighted astigmatism. On the fourth day, one eye was normal and the other showed simple nearsightedness. Similar variations were noted in many other cases.

What is true of children and infants is equally true of adults of all ages. The vision of people over seventy years of age is entirely variable. For example, I found one eighty-year-old man with normal eyes and ordinarily normal sight. He did, however, have periods of imperfect sight lasting from a few minutes to half an hour or longer. Retinoscopy at such times always showed nearsightedness of 4 Diopters or more.

During sleep, the refractive condition of the eye is rarely, if ever, normal. People whose refraction is normal when they are awake will produce nearsightedness, farsightedness and astigmatism when they are asleep. People who have errors of refraction when they are awake will have increased errors of refraction during sleep. This is why some people wake in the morning with eyes more tired than at any other time. They may even wake up with severe headaches. When the subject is under anesthesia, or unconscious from any other cause, errors of refraction are also produced or increased.

Unfamiliar Objects Always Produce Errors of Refraction

When the eye regards an unfamiliar object, an error of refraction is always produced. Hence the proverbial fatigue caused by viewing pictures, or other objects, in a museum. Children with normal eyes who can read letters a quarter of an inch high at ten feet always have trouble reading strange writing on the blackboard, even though the letters may be eight times larger.

Maps have the same effect. I have never seen a child, or a teacher for that matter, who could look at a map from a distance without becoming nearsighted.

German type has been accused of being responsible for much of the poor sight once supposed to be a peculiarly German malady.

But if a German child attempts to read Roman print, the child will at once become temporarily farsighted. German print or Greek or Chinese characters will have the same effect on anyone accustomed to Roman letters.

A German ophthalmologist named Dr. Hermann Cohn repudiated the idea that German lettering was trying to the eyes. On the contrary, he always found it "pleasant, after a long reading of the monotonous Roman print, to return to our beloved German." Because the German characters were more familiar to him than any others, he found them restful to his eyes. "Use," he observed, "has much to do with the matter." Children learning to read, write, draw or sew always suffer from defective vision because of the unfamiliarity of the lines or objects with which they are working.

Any Challenging Stimulus Always Produces an Error of Refraction

A sudden exposure to strong light or rapid or sudden changes of light are also likely to produce imperfect sight in the normal eye, continuing in some cases for weeks and months (see Chapter 17).

Noise is also a frequent cause of defective vision in the normal eye. All people see imperfectly when they hear an unexpected loud noise. Familiar sounds do not lower the vision, but unfamiliar ones always do. Country children from quiet schools may suffer from defective vision for a long time after moving to a noisy city. They cannot do well in school because their sight is impaired.

It is, of course, a gross injustice for teachers and others to scold, punish or humiliate such children.

Under conditions of mental or physical discomfort, such as pain, cough, fever, discomfort from heat or cold, depression, anger, or anxiety, errors of refraction are always produced in the normal eye. If the eyes already have an error of refraction, adverse conditions make the error of refraction worse.

The variability of the refraction of the eye is responsible for many otherwise unaccountable accidents. When people are struck down in the street by automobiles or trolley cars, it is often due to the fact that they were suffering from a temporary loss of sight. Collisions on railroads or at sea, disasters in military operations, aviation accidents and so on, often occur because some responsible person suffered temporary loss of sight.

Statistics about errors of refraction are confusing because no one takes into account the conditions under which the vision is tested. It is possible to take the best eyes in the world and test them so that the subject will fail the Army standard. On the other hand, the test can be administered in a way to make eyes that are apparently much below normal at the beginning acquire normal vision during the course of the test.

CHAPTER 8

What Glasses Do to Us

The Romans must have known something of lenses, for Pliny tells us that Nero used to watch the games in the Colosseum through a concave gem that was set in a ring for that purpose.

While it is true that eyeglasses have brought improved vision and relief from pain and discomfort to some people, they have been simply an added torture to others. Eyeglasses always harm the vision to a greater or lesser degree. Even at their best, eyeglasses never improve the vision to normal.

Glasses Cannot Improve the Sight to Normal

That glasses cannot improve the sight to normal can be very simply demonstrated by looking at any color through a strong convex or concave glass. It will be noted that the color is always less intense than when seen with the naked eye. Since the perception of form depends on the perception of color *[or at least gradations of shading* **MA***]*, it follows that both color and form must be seen less distinctly with glasses than without them.

Even plane glass such as a clear window pane lowers the vision both for color and form, as everyone knows who has ever looked out of a window. Women who wear glasses for minor defects of vision often observe that they

are made more or less colorblind by them. In a shop, one may note that they remove their glasses when they want to match fabric samples. However, if the sight is seriously defective, the color may be seen better with glasses than without them.

Glasses Make the Refractive Error Chronic

The refraction of the eye varies continuously. That glasses must injure the eye becomes evident, then, because one cannot see through them unless one produces the degree of refractive error that they are designed to correct. But refractive errors, in the eye left to itself, are never constant. If one secures good vision by the aid of concave, convex, or astigmatic lenses, it therefore means that one is maintaining constantly a degree of refractive error that otherwise would not be maintained constantly. It is only to be expected that this should make the condition worse, and it is a matter of common experience that it does.

Generally, once people start wearing glasses, the strength has to be continually increased. Elders who put on glasses to read fine print soon find they need the same glasses to read print that was perfectly clear to them before.

A nearsighted woman who can see at

twenty feet what a normally sighted person can see at seventy feet (20/70 vision) may wear glasses that correct her vision to 20/20. But she may find in a week's time that her unaided vision has declined to where she can only see at 20 feet what a normally sighted person can see at 200 feet (20/200 vision).

When people break their glasses and go without them for a week or two, they frequently observe that their sight has improved. The sight always improves, to a greater or lesser degree, when glasses are discarded. However, this fact may not always be noted by the individual.

The Human Eye Resents Glasses

That the human eye resents glasses is a fact that no one would attempt to deny. Every ophthalmologist or optometrist knows that patients have to "get used" to their glasses. Sometimes they never succeed in doing so. Patients with high degrees of nearsightedness and farsightedness have great difficulty in accustoming themselves to full correction and often are never able to do so. The strong concave glasses required by those with severe nearsightedness make all objects seem much smaller than they really are. Convex lenses for farsightedness enlarge everything. These distortions are unpleasant.

Patients with high degrees of astigmatism suffer some very disagreeable sensations when they first put on glasses. They are even warned in an American Medical Association (AMA) pamphlet to "get used to your glasses at home before venturing where a misstep might cause a serious accident." Usually these difficulties are overcome, but often they are not. Indeed,

it sometimes happens that those who get on fairly well with their glasses in the daytime never succeed in getting used to them at night.

The Limitations and Inconveniences of Glasses

All glasses contract the field of vision to a greater or lesser degree. Even with very weak glasses, people are unable to see distinctly unless they look through the center of the lenses with the frames at right angles to the line of vision. Not only is their vision lowered if they fail to do this, but annoying nervous symptoms, such as dizziness and headache, are sometimes produced. Therefore, they are unable to turn their eyes freely in different directions. The extraocular muscles, then, do not move freely through their range of motion, and this lack of exercise makes them even more stiff and dysfunctional.

It is true that glasses are now ground in such a way that it is theoretically possible to look through them at any angle, but practically, they seldom accomplish the desired result.

The difficulty of keeping the lens clear is one of the minor discomforts of glasses, but nevertheless a most annoying one. On damp and rainy days, the atmosphere clouds them. On hot days, perspiration from the body may have a similar effect. On cold days, they are often clouded by the moisture of the breath. Every day, they are subject to contamination by dust and moisture and the touch of the fingers in unavoidable handling.

Reflections of strong light from eyeglasses are often very annoying. In the street these reflections may be very dangerous. Soldiers, sailors, athletes, workmen and children have great difficulty with glasses because of the activities of their lives. These activities may dislodge the lenses from their frames or cause them to break. If the glasses are not well settled on the face, it can throw the vision out of focus, particularly in the case of eyeglasses worn for astigmatism.

Cosmetic Considerations

The fact that glasses are considered to be very disfiguring by some people may seem a matter unworthy of consideration, but this mental discomfort does not improve either the person's general health or their vision. Some might consider glasses becoming. Huge round lenses in ugly tortoise shell frames are positively fashionable at the present time. However, there are still some minds to which the wearing of glasses is mental torture and the sight of them on others far from agreeable. As for putting glasses on a child, it is enough to make the angels weep.

Glasses Do Not Relieve Eye Strain

Up to a generation ago, glasses were used only as an aid to defective sight, but they are now prescribed for large numbers of people who can see as well or better without them. This is the group with "latent farsightedness." Remember the theory that some eyes see normally but are actually farsighted. Their normal sight is supposedly accomplished by constant effort of the ciliary muscle. In other words, even when they are looking far away, their eyes are accommodating as if they were looking up close.

Modern ophthalmology *[in 2017 as*

in 1920 **MA]** believes that this constant contraction of the ciliary muscle imposes a severe strain on the nervous system—a strain which is believed to be the cause of a host of functional nervous troubles. To relieve this strain, glasses are prescribed.

I have demonstrated, however, that the lens is not a factor either in the production of accommodation or in the correction of errors of refraction. Therefore, under no circumstances can there be a strain of the ciliary muscle to be relieved. I have also demonstrated that when the vision is normal, the extrinsic muscles of the eye are at rest while the eye is focused into the distance. Therefore, there can also be no strain of the extrinsic muscles to be relieved in these cases.

When a strain of the extrinsic muscles of the eye does exist, glasses only correct the effects of that strain on the refraction. Glasses do not relieve the strain itself. On the contrary, as has been shown, glasses only make the strain worse.

Placebo

Nevertheless, people with normal vision who wear glasses for the relief of a supposed muscular strain of the eyes are often benefited by them. This is because they expect these glasses to help them. It is a placebo effect. Plane glass (such as the glass in a clear window pane), if it could inspire the same faith, would produce the same result. In fact, many patients have told me that they had been relieved of various discomforts by glasses that I found to be simply plane glass. One of these patients was an optician who had fitted the glasses himself and was under no illusions whatever about them; yet he assured me that when he didn't wear them, he got headaches.

Some patients are so responsive to mental suggestion that you can relieve their discomfort or improve their sight with almost any glasses you like to put on them. I have seen people with farsightedness wearing concave lenses (which actually correct nearsightedness) with a great deal of comfort, and people with no astigmatism getting much satisfaction from glasses designed for the correction of astigmatism.

The Great Power of Imagination

Dr. Edmund Landolt mentions the case of a patient who had worn prisms for years. A prism is a form of lens used in glasses. The prism lens doesn't change the image, it just moves it over. In this case, the patient's medial rectus muscle was weak, which meant he had trouble turning the affected eye inward (medially). The prescription for a prism lens would move the image of that eye to the outside (laterally) so his two eyes could form one image. This patient found his glasses absolutely indispensable for work.

In fact, though, the optician had made a mistake, and the lens was backwards. Instead of moving the image to the side (laterally), the lens moved the image to the inside (medially). In theory, this would put more of a strain on the medial rectus muscle. Yet the patient was more than satisfied with their effect.

Dr. Landolt explained this case by "the slight effect of weak prisms and the great power of imagination." Doubtless the benefit derived from the glasses resulted from the patient's great faith in the specialist who prescribed them.

Some patients will even imagine that they see better with glasses that markedly lower the vision. A number of years ago, a patient for whom I had prescribed glasses consulted an ophthalmologist whose reputation was much greater than my own. This specialist gave him a different prescription and spoke slightingly of the ones that I had prescribed. The patient returned to me and told me how much better he could see with the second pair of glasses than he did with the first. I tested his vision with the new glasses, and found that while mine had given him a vision of 20/20, those of my colleague enabled him to see only 20/40.

The simple fact was that this patient had been hypnotized by a great reputation into thinking he could see better when he actually saw worse. It was hard to convince him that he was wrong, although he had to admit that when he looked at the test chart, he could see only half as much with the new glasses as with the old ones.

When glasses do not relieve headaches and other nervous symptoms, it is assumed to be because they were not properly fitted. Some practitioners and their patients exhibit an astounding degree of patience and perseverance in their joint attempts to arrive at the proper prescription.

A patient who suffered from severe pains at the base of his brain was fitted sixty times by one specialist alone. He had also visited many other eye and nerve specialists in this country and in Europe. He was relieved of his pain in five minutes by the methods presented in this book. As his pain was relieved, his vision became temporarily normal.

Many Refuse to Wear Glasses

Fortunately, many people refuse to wear their glasses. They thus escape not only much discomfort but also much injury to their eyes. Others, by wearing their glasses, submit to an amount of unnecessary torture that is scarcely conceivable.

One such woman wore glasses for twenty-five years, although they did not prevent her from suffering continual misery. In addition, her glasses lowered her vision to such an extent that she had to look over the tops when she wanted to see anything at a distance. Her oculist assured her that she might expect the most serious consequences if she did not wear the glasses. He was very severe about her practice of looking over instead of through them.

The Accurate Fitting of Glasses is Impossible

Even under the influence of atropine eye drops, refractive abnormalities are continually changing. One moment, the patient is nearsighted, the next farsighted, the next normally sighted. This makes the accurate fitting of glasses impossible. It completely invalidates the prevailing presumption that there is one correct prescription for any given eye.

In some cases, these fluctuations in visual acuity are so extreme that no relief whatever can be obtained from corrective lenses. The glasses just become an added discomfort.

Even at their best, glasses are nothing more than a very unsatisfactory substitute for normal vision.

CHAPTER 9

The Cause and Cure of Errors of Refraction

As I've previously explained, any strain or effort to see is accompanied by abnormal function of the external muscles of the eye. With relaxation of strain and effort, the extraocular muscles can function normally. At that point, all errors of refraction disappear. Thus we have the means by which all errors of refraction, so long held to be incurable, may actually be cured.

Even in the presence of other problems, the eye bends light normally if there is no straining to see. For example, there might be a problem with the retina such that the retina doesn't sense the light or transmit information about the image to the brain. There may be a cataract, which makes the image which falls on the retina cloudy. But so long as there is no struggle to see, the external ocular muscles act normally, and there is no error of refraction. That is to say, there is no error in the way in which the light that enters the eye is focused onto the plane of the retina. There is, therefore, no nearsightedness, no farsightedness, and no astigmatism. The objective test of retinoscopy confirms this.

There Is a Specific Type of Strain for Each Type of Error of Refraction

Furthermore, for each specific error of refraction, be it nearsightedness, farsightedness or astigmatism, there is a specific kind of strain. These facts can be verified in a few minutes by anyone who knows how to use a retinoscope (provided the instrument is not brought closer than six feet). The relationship of straining to see with specific errors of refraction is also confirmed by the study of images reflected from various parts of the eye, such as the reflection of a light off the white of the eye.

1. When a person strains to see into the distance, the eyeball always gets longer. The retina moves farther from the lens. Therefore,

– If the person has normal sight, they become nearsighted.

– If the person is nearsighted, they become more nearsighted.

– If the person is farsighted, they become less farsighted and may even pass over into nearsightedness.

2. When a person strains to see up close, the eyeball always becomes shorter. The retina moves closer to the lens. Therefore,

– If the person has normal sight, they become farsighted.

– If the person is farsighted, they become more farsighted.

– If the person is nearsighted, they become less nearsighted and may even pass over into farsightedness.

In other words, straining always produces the opposite of the effect for which a person is straining!

The Complex Case of Astigmatism

As just explained, when the eye strains, the shape of the eyeball changes in a reliably counterproductive manner. However, this change is not always uniform. If the eye shortens or elongates asymmetrically, the cornea will become asymmetric, and astigmatism will arise.

Remember that when the cornea becomes asymmetrical, the plane of focus of the image splits into two or more planes. A vertical slit of light may focus onto one plane; a horizontal slit of light may focus onto a different plane.

When straining does produce astigmatism, the astigmatism still always follows the two rules just stated:

1. If the person with normal vision strains to see up close, the eyeball may flatten asymmetrically, and farsighted astigmatism will be produced. *[Please see the glossary for a brief explanation of the different types of astigmatism.* **MA]**

2. If the person with normal vision strains to see faraway, the eyeball may elongate asymmetrically, and nearsighted astigmatism will be produced.

In clinical settings, there are some interesting associated findings:

In an eye that is already nearsighted, straining to see close objects lessens the nearsightedness. The eye may even refocus to see at a distance while it is straining to see up close. In some cases, while straining to see up close, the nearsighted eye may even pass over into farsightedness in one or all meridians.

However, all these changes are accompanied by signs of worsening strain, including eccentric fixation (see Chapter 11) and a subjective worsening of vision.

But strange to say, pain and fatigue are usually relieved to a marked degree.

In an eye which is already farsighted, straining to see far away objects lessens the farsightedness. Eccentric fixation is also improved, and there is a subjective improvement in vision. However, pain and fatigue may be produced or increased. This is the exact opposite of what happens when the nearsighted person strains to see up close.

In some cases, the farsightedness is completely relieved, and normal vision is produced, with a complete disappearance of all evidences of strain.

With continued straining to see far away, the eye may then pass over into nearsightedness, with an increase of strain as the nearsightedness increases.

Eyes That Have Had Cataract Surgery

What has been said of normal eyes applies equally to eyes from which the crystalline lens has been removed. After cataract surgery, the eye has no lens. Remember, the eye must bend light in order to focus. Most of that bending, called refraction, is done by the cornea. When the lens is removed, the eye still focuses light but not as powerfully. The plane of focus will move farther away from the cornea. In a person with normal sight and a crystalline lens, the plane of focus falls on the retina. If that person's lens is removed, the plane of focus will then fall behind the retina, and the person will be farsighted.

The eye with no lens still demonstrates the changes just described. To recap, when people strain to see up close, they become more farsighted. When they strain to look see far away, they become more nearsighted.

After cataract surgery, most people, having become more farsighted, strain to see up close. By this strain, they become even more farsighted. The power of accommodation appears to have been lost, and they require reading glasses. But later, the eyes become used to the absence of the lens. The eyes relax and again become able to focus up close. The eyeball elongates enough to compensate for the loss of the lens.

Animals show the same pattern. I have induced temporary nearsightedness in many dogs by getting them to strain to see a distant object. This change can be seen on the spot by the use of the retinoscope.

For example, I worked with one dog whose vision was normal. I could tell this by the retinoscopic exam, which requires no cooperation from the animal. However, the dog had a very nervous disposition.

When I allowed him to smell a piece of meat, he became very excited, pricked up his ears, arched his eyebrows and wagged his tail. The meat was then removed to a distance of twenty feet. The dog looked disappointed but didn't lose interest. While he was watching the meat, I dropped it into a box. A worried look came into his eyes. He strained to see what had become of it, and at that moment, the retinoscope showed that he had become nearsighted.

It should be added that this experiment would succeed only with an animal possessing two active oblique extraocular muscles. Animals in which one of these muscles is absent are unable to elongate the eyeball under any circumstances.

The Strain to See Is a Strain of the Mind

The strain to see is primarily a strain of the mind. When there is a strain of the mind, there is always loss of control. We freeze up. When we relax and see up close, the eye is focusing light to the same degree as when we tense up and strain to look far away. The shape of the eyeball is the same. The difference is that in one case, the eye is doing what the mind intends, and in the other it is not.

These facts appear sufficient to explain why visual acuity declines as civilization advances. Under the conditions of civilized life, our minds are under a continual strain *[in 1920!* **MA***]*. By comparison, preindustrial life was, if not necessarily more pleasant, at least more simple. In hunting and gathering cultures, physical performance was a necessity for survival. In modern society, physical ability is much less crucial.

When animals are subjected to civilized conditions, they respond to them in precisely the same way as humans. I have examined many domestic and zoo animals and in many cases have found them nearsighted, although they neither read nor write nor sew nor set type.

Some have argued that the constant demand for looking at things close up is responsible for the poor vision of our civilization. We lose our ability to see things far away. In fact, farsightedness is more common than nearsightedness in our society. Practically everyone who survives to the age of 45 suffers from it. Furthermore, nearsighted people, although they see better at the near point than they do at the distance, never see as well close up as does the normal healthy eye.

The Remedy Is to Get Rid of Strain

The remedy is not to avoid either near work or distant vision, but to get rid of the mental strain that underlies the imperfect functioning of the eye at both points. It has been demonstrated in thousands of cases that this can always be done. Fortunately, all people are able to relax at will under certain conditions.

All patients who are nearsighted or farsighted can temporarily improve their vision simply by looking at a blank wall without trying to see.

To secure permanent relaxation, though, sometimes requires considerable time and ingenuity. The same method cannot be used with everyone. The ways in which people strain to see are infinite, so the methods used to relieve the strain must be infinitely varied.

Whatever the method that brings relief, the desired end is always the same: relaxation. By constant repetition, frequent demonstration, and every other means possible, the fact must be impressed on the person that perfect sight can be obtained only by relaxation. Nothing else matters.

Most people ask, if relaxation will cure eye troubles, why does sleep not do so? The fact

is that the eyes are rarely, if ever, completely relaxed in sleep. The habitual strain we carry during the day continues into the sleeping state. This is actually true of many physical evidences of strain. Those with high blood pressure often have it higher in the night. Those with overly acid stomachs often have them more acidic in the night.

The idea that it rests the eyes not to use them is also erroneous. The eyes were made to see. If they do not see, it is because they are under such a great strain that they cannot see.

Near vision, although accomplished by a muscular act, is no more a strain on the eyes than distant vision. The use of the muscles does not necessarily produce fatigue. Some men can run for hours without becoming tired. Many birds support themselves on one foot during sleep, the toes tightly clasping the swaying bough, and the muscles remaining unfatigued by the apparent strain. In truth, when the mind is at rest, nothing can tire the eyes. When the mind is under a strain, nothing can rest them. Anything that rests the mind will benefit the eyes.

We See Better When We Are Interested

Almost everyone has observed that the eyes last longer when reading an interesting book than when perusing something tiresome or difficult to comprehend. A schoolboy can sit up all night reading a novel without even thinking of his eyes. If that same schoolboy tries to sit up half the night studying his lessons, he soon finds his eyes completely exhausted.

I worked with a child whose vision was

ordinarily so acute that she could see the moons of Jupiter with the naked eye. She was very much interested in astronomy. She detested arithmetic. The retinoscope showed that when asked to do a mathematical sum in her mind, she immediately became nearsighted.

Sometimes the conditions that produce mental relaxation are very curious. For instance, one woman was able to correct her error of refraction when she looked at the test chart with her body bent over at an angle of about forty-five degrees. The improvement continued after she sat back up. Although the position was an unfavorable one, she had somehow got the idea that it improved her sight, and therefore it did so.

Time to Cure

The time required to effect a permanent cure varies greatly. In some cases, five, ten, or fifteen minutes is sufficient. I believe the time is coming when it will be possible to cure everyone quickly. It is only a question of accumulating more facts and presenting these facts in such a way that the person can grasp them quickly. At present, however, it is often necessary to continue the treatment for weeks and months. The time needed for cure is not proportional to the severity of the problem or its duration.

In most cases, after cure, the treatment must be continued for a few minutes every day to prevent relapse. The eye relaxes when viewing familiar objects that have good associations. The daily reading of the Snellen test chart is usually sufficient for this purpose.

It is also useful, particularly for farsightedness, to read fine print every day,

as close to the eyes as it can be done.

Complete Cure Is Permanent

When a cure is complete, it is always permanent. Complete cures, however, are rare. They involve attaining more than what is ordinarily called normal sight. Complete cures go on to show the true potential of the human: some measure of telescopic and microscopic vision.

Even in these rare cases, the treatment can be continued with benefit, for it is impossible to place limits to the visual powers of the human. No matter how good the sight, it is always possible to improve it.

Even in those with perfect sight, the vision can decline under strain. Daily practice of the art of vision is necessary to prevent this. No system of training will provide an absolute safeguard against such lapses in all circumstances. Nevertheless, the daily reading of small distant, familiar letters will do much to lessen the tendency to strain when disturbing circumstances do arise. All people who need good eyesight to work safely should be required to do this.

Generally, people who have never worn glasses are more easily cured than those who have. Glasses should be discarded at the beginning of the treatment, if possible. When this cannot be done safely, their use always delays the cure.

Children usually, though not invariably, respond much more quickly. Children younger than sixteen who have never worn glasses are usually cured in a few days, weeks, or months. All such children are cured within a year. They have simply to read the Snellen test chart every day.

CHAPTER 10

Strain

The foundation of straining to see lies in wrong habits of thought. We believe that to do anything well requires effort. This idea is drilled into us from the cradle. The whole educational system is based on it. Montessori has obtained wonderful results in education by the total elimination of every species of compulsion. Still, educators who call themselves modern cling to the bludgeon of forcing the child to learn through effort.

It is as natural for the eye to see as it is for the mind to acquire knowledge. Any effort in either case is not only useless but self-defeating. You may force a few facts into a child's mind by various kinds of compulsion, but you cannot make the child learn anything. The facts remain, if they remain at all, as dead lumber in the brain. They contribute nothing to the vitality of thought and understanding. This type of "learning" destroys the natural impulse of the mind toward the acquisition of knowledge. By the time the child leaves school or college, he or she not only knows nothing but is no longer capable of learning anything.

In the same way, you may temporarily improve your sight by effort, but you cannot improve it to normal. If the effort is allowed to become continuous, sight will steadily deteriorate and may eventually be destroyed. Very seldom is the impairment or destruction

of vision due to any fault in the construction of the eye. Of two equally good pairs of eyes, one will retain perfect sight to the end of life and the other will lose it in kindergarten. This is simply because one pair looks at things without effort and the other does not.

The Act of Seeing Is Passive

Eyes with normal sight never try to see. If for any reason, such as dim light or distance, they cannot see a particular point, they simply shift to another. Healthy eyes never try to bring out a point by staring at it. Eyes with imperfect sight are constantly doing just that

Whenever eyes try to see, they at once cease to have normal vision. A person may look at the stars with normal vision. Strain to count the stars, and the vision becomes nearsighted.

A male patient was able to look at the letter K on the Snellen test chart with normal vision, but when asked to count its twenty-seven corners, he lost his normal vision completely.

It obviously requires a strain to fail to see into the distance, because the eyes at rest are adjusted for distant vision. If one does anything to see into the distance, it is the wrong thing. The shape of the eyeballs cannot be altered during distant vision without strain.

There must equally be strain if one fails

to see up close. When the muscles respond to the mind's desire, they do it without strain. Only by an effort can one prevent eyes from elongating to see close up.

Eyes possess perfect vision only when absolutely at rest. When there is any movement, either in the eyes or the object of vision, the eyes must realign and refocus. Therefore, any movement produces, at least momentarily, an error of refraction. When the movement is slow, these dynamic errors of refraction are mild and go unnoticed in daily life. Nevertheless, they can still be observed with the retinoscope.

When movement is rapid, vision becomes a blur. It is impossible to see a moving object perfectly.

The moving pictures *[of 1920* **MA***]* illustrate this well. They are actually a series of still pictures that flash on the screen for 1/24 of a second, one after another. The image is blocked from being projected during the time it is moving into place, for during this time, the viewer would only see a blur. Once in place, the film halts for a fraction of a second while the image is projected onto the screen. So moving pictures (movies) are never actually seen in motion!

The act of seeing is passive. Things are seen just as they are felt, heard, or tasted, without any effort or volition on the part of the subject. When sight is perfect, the letters on the test chart are waiting, perfectly black and perfectly distinct, to be recognized. They do not have to be sought; they are there. In imperfect sight, the letters are sought and chased. Eyes go after them. An effort is made to see them.

The muscles of the body are supposed never to be at rest. The blood vessels, with their muscular coats, are never at rest. Even in sleep, thought does not cease. But the normal condition of the nerves of the senses— hearing, sight, taste, smell and touch—is one of rest. They cannot act. They can only be acted upon. The optic nerve, the retina, and the visual centers of the brain are as passive as the finger nail. They have nothing whatever in their structure that makes it possible for them to do anything. When they are the subject of effort from outside sources, their efficiency is always impaired.

Any Strain Impairs the Vision

For eyes, this fact can easily be demonstrated. If patients can read all the small letters on the 20/20 line of the test chart, their visual acuity is normal. But if, while reading the 20/20 line, they either deliberately or carelessly say any of them incorrectly, the retinoscope will show an error of refraction. This is because in the moment they realize that they have made a mistake, they tighten up.

As an experiment, I have asked many people to state their ages incorrectly or to try to imagine that they were a year older or a year younger than they actually were. In every case, when they do so, the retinoscope indicates an error of refraction.

A patient twenty-five years old had no error of refraction when he looked at a blank wall without trying to see. But when he said he was twenty-six years old, or someone else said it in his hearing, or even when he tried to imagine it, he immediately became nearsighted. The same thing happened when he stated or tried to imagine that he was twenty-four. When he stated or remembered the truth, his vision was normal, but when he stated or imagined an error, he had an error of refraction.

One day, two little girls who were my patients arrived one after the other. The first accused the second of having stopped at Huyler's for an ice-cream soda. She had been told that she was not allowed to do this, since she was somewhat too much addicted to sweets. The accused denied the charge. The first little girl knew that the retinoscope could detect changes when people lied. She said, "Do take the retinoscope and find out."

I followed her suggestion. Having thrown the light into the second child's eyes, I asked, "Did you go to Huyler's?"

"Yes," was the response. The retinoscope showed no error of refraction.

"Did you have an ice-cream soda?"

"No," said the child; but the telltale shadow cast in the eye by the retinoscope moved in a direction opposite to normal, showing that she had become nearsighted and was not telling the truth.

The child blushed when I told her this. She acknowledged that the retinoscope was right, for she had heard of the ways of the uncanny instrument before.

If a normally sighted man pronounces the initials of his name correctly while looking at a blank surface without trying to see, there will be no error of refraction. If he miscalls one initial, even without any consciousness of effort and with full knowledge that he is deceiving no one, nearsightedness will be

immediately produced.

A Different Kind of Strain for Each Error of Refraction

Mental strain may produce many different kinds of eye strain. According to the statement of most authorities, there is only one kind of eye strain. In fact, I have described how there is not a different strain for nearsightedness as opposed to farsightedness. To go further, there is in fact a different strain for most other abnormal conditions of the eye. The strain that produces an error of refraction is not the same as the strain that produces amblyopia (crossed eyes), or cataract, or glaucoma, or inflammation of the white of the eye or inflammation of the margins of the eyelids, or disease of the optic nerve, or disease of the retina. All these other conditions may exist with only a slight error of refraction.

The relief of one strain usually means the relief of many others that may coexist with it. However, it sometimes happens that the strain associated with such conditions as cataract and glaucoma can be relieved without the complete relief of the strain that causes the error of refraction. Even the pain that so often accompanies errors of refraction is never caused by the same strain that causes the actual nearsightedness or farsightedness.

Some nearsighted people cannot read without pain or discomfort, but most of them suffer no inconvenience. Farsightedness behaves quite differently. When a farsighted person looks at a distant object, the farsightedness is lessened, but pain and discomfort may be increased.

While there are many kinds of strain, there

is only one cure for all of them: relaxation. The health of the eye depends on the blood, and blood circulation is very largely influenced by thought. When thought is without excitement or strain, the circulation in the brain is normal, the blood supply to the optic nerve and visual brain centers is normal, and the vision is perfect. When thought is abnormal, tense, and neurotic, then the circulation is disturbed, the supply of blood to the optic nerve and visual centers in the brain is impaired, and vision is lowered.

The Cure Is as Quick as the Thought That Relaxes

We can consciously think thoughts that disturb the circulation and lower the visual power. We can also consciously think thoughts that restore normal circulation and cure all errors of refraction as well as many other abnormal conditions of the eyes.

We cannot by any amount of effort make ourselves see better but by learning to control our thoughts. We can, however, accomplish that end indirectly.

You can teach people how to produce any error of refraction: how to see two images of an object, one above another, side by side, or at any desired angle from one another. You can do all this simply by teaching them how to think disturbing thoughts in a particular way. When the disturbing thought is replaced by one that relaxes, all the disturbances in vision disappear. This is as true of abnormalities of long standing as of those produced voluntarily. No matter what the degree or duration, the cure is accomplished just as soon as the patient is able to secure mental control. Be it any particular error of refraction or any other functional disturbance of the eye, the cause is simply a thought, a wrong thought. Therefore, the cure is as quick as the thought that relaxes [my underlining **MA**]. In a fraction of a second, the highest degrees of refractive error may be corrected, strabismus may disappear, or the blindness of a lazy eye may be relieved. If the relaxation is only momentary, the correction is momentary. When the relaxation becomes permanent, the correction is permanent.

This relaxation cannot, however, be obtained by any sort of effort. It is fundamental for people to understand this. So long as they think, consciously or unconsciously, that relief from strain may be obtained by another strain, their cure will be delayed.

CHAPTER 11

Central Fixation

The eye is in many ways like a tiny camera. There is one very important difference, though. Camera film is the same throughout. By contrast, the retina has one small point at which it is most sensitive to detail. Every other part of the retina is less able to perceive detail. In fact, the farther from that one incredibly sensitive spot one goes, the less sensitive the retina becomes. This point of maximum sensitivity to detail is called the **fovea**. The fovea is tiny—about 1.5 mm in diameter. *[For comparison, the diameter of a grain of sand is about 0.5 mm. The thickness of a dime is about 1.0 mm. The thickness of a credit card is about 0.75 mm. A sheet of paper is on average a little less than .10 mm. MA]*

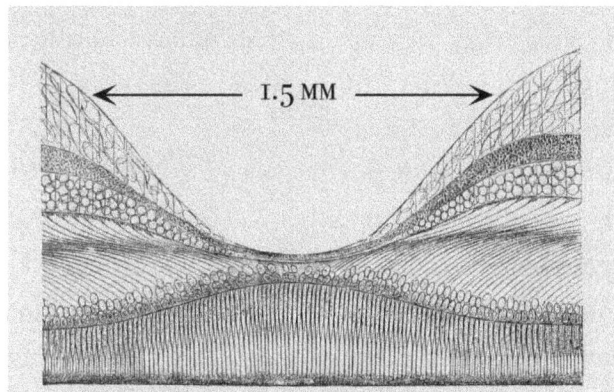

**Figure 11.1: Fovea in Cross Section
(19th Century Drawing)**

membrane are nine layers. Only one of these layers actually perceives light. This layer is composed of microscopic cells, some shaped like rods, some like cones. In the center of the retina is a small circular elevation. This spot is called the macula, which is just Latin for "spot." The fovea, which perceives such vivid detail and color, is in the center of this spot. The fovea is a little pit in the center of the macula.

The structure of the fovea is very specialized and different from the rest of the retina. The cone cells are packed in tight, and there are no rods. That is because cones perceive color while rods see only black and white. In addition, the other eight layers of the retina become extremely thin or even absent in the fovea.

The center of the fovea is the seat of the most accurate and detailed vision. As an image falls farther away from the fovea on the retina, the fine detail of the visual perceptions of that image rapidly decreases. Eyes with

The Fovea

The retina is an extremely delicate membrane that coats the inside of the eyeball. It is only from 1/80 of an inch to 1/40 of an inch thick. That's about 1/3 to 2/3 of a millimeter. Within that extremely thin normal vision, therefore, see only one small area with exquisite detail. Everything else in the field of vision is not as clear. The farther away from the fovea the image of a detail falls, the less clearly that detail is seen. *[The eyes naturally look about, from spot to spot, and it is the mind that assembles a clear image based on the many clear spots the fovea sees.* **MA]**

Central Fixation

To repeat, the center of vision is the fovea, which lies at the center of the macula. When we direct our attention to something, say a bird in the sky, we automatically move our eyes in such a way that the image falls exactly on the fovea. This activity of naturally moving the eyes so that the image of the object of interest falls on the fovea is called central fixation. *[Eccentric fixation means that the image of the object of interest falls not on the fovea but on some more peripheral area of the retina. Eccentric in this context does not imply "odd" or "peculiar;" it simply means "not at the center."* **MA]**

Central Fixation Lost

It is an invariable symptom of all abnormal conditions of the eyes that central fixation is lost. This is true whether there is some physical problem in the eye or whether the eye is simply not functioning correctly.

Why is central fixation lost? When the sight is normal, the sensitivity of the fovea is normal. When the sight is imperfect, regardless of the cause, the sensitivity of the fovea is lowered. When the fovea does not see as well, then other parts of the retina see just as well or even better.

The Tiny Area of Maximum Vision

Contrary to what is generally believed, the area that the fovea sees is extremely small. Textbooks say that at a distance of twenty feet, the area the fovea sees is about half an inch in diameter—slightly smaller than a dime.

In my experience, the area of maximum vision is even smaller. The smallest letters of the Snellen test chart are only 1/4 of an inch high. Yet at twenty feet, anyone who tries to see every part of one of these letters equally well at one time will immediately become nearsighted. The fact is that the nearer the point of maximum vision approaches a mathematical point, a tiny point that has no area or diameter, the better the sight.

Strain Blinds the Fovea

The cause of loss of central fixation is mental strain. As all abnormal conditions of the eyes are accompanied by mental strain, all such conditions must necessarily be accompanied by loss of central fixation. When the mind is under a strain, eyes usually go more or less blind. The center of sight goes blind first, partially or completely, according to the degree of the strain. If the strain is great enough, then the major part or even the whole of the retina may suffer this loss of vision.

When vision at the center of sight has been suppressed, either partially or completely, people no longer see best what they are looking at directly. Instead, they see objects not regarded directly just as well, or even better. The sensitivity of the fovea to detail has been lost. The sensitivity of the retina has now become approximately equal in every part. Indeed, the sensitivity of the retina might even be better in the outer areas than in the fovea. Therefore, in all cases of defective vision, people are unable to see best where they are looking.

This condition is sometimes so extreme that a person may look as far away from an object as possible to see it and yet see it just as well as when looking directly at it.

In one case, a patient could see only with the edge of the retina on the nasal side. She could not see her fingers at all if she held them up in front of her face. She could only see them if she held them up at the outer side of her eye (which is the area the nasal side of the retina can see). This lady had only a slight error of refraction, which confirms that different kinds of strain produce different visual problems. Every error of refraction is accompanied by eccentric fixation, but the strain that causes an error of refraction is different from that which produces eccentric fixation.

This woman had been examined by specialists in this country and Europe. They attributed her blindness to disease of the optic nerve or brain. In my clinic, her vision was restored simply by relaxation, which demonstrates that her condition was due simply to mental strain.

Eccentric fixation, even in its lesser degrees, is completely unnatural. When acute, eccentric fixation produces great discomfort or even pain. But when eccentric fixation is chronic, discomfort and pain may be absent. In this situation, it is actually a good sign if discomfort returns temporarily as the vision heals.

You can confirm for yourself that eccentric fixation quickly causes pain by trying to see all parts of even a very small area equally well at the same time. As the pain arises, the retinoscope would demonstrate that an error of refraction has also been produced.

When the strain of eccentric fixation is habitual, it leads to all sorts of abnormal conditions. In fact, it is at the bottom of most eye troubles, both functional and organic.

Eyes with Central Fixation Are Tireless

When the eye possesses central fixation, it not only possesses perfect sight, but it is perfectly at rest. In this state, the eyes can be used indefinitely without fatigue. They are open and quiet. No nervous eye movements are observable. When they regard a point in the distance, the visual axes are parallel. In other words, there are no muscular insufficiencies.

The textbooks state that muscular insufficiencies do occur in eyes having normal sight, but I have never seen such a case. If the eye is relaxed and central fixation is present, I find that the muscles of the face and of the whole body are also at rest. When this healthy condition is habitual, there are no wrinkles or dark circles around the eyes.

Eyes with Eccentric Fixation Tire Quickly

By contrast, when there is eccentric fixation, the eyes quickly tire. The eyes and the face are expressive of effort or strain. Seeing an eye close up with an ophthalmoscope, it becomes apparent that the eyeball moves at irregular intervals, be it from side to side, vertically, or in other directions. These movements are often so extensive as to be easily seen by an observer's naked eye. Sometimes the movements are so intense that they resemble a neurological condition called nystagmus.

When eccentric fixation is present, nervous movements of the eyelids may also be noted. Also, they eyes never point exactly in the same direction. This deviation from the normal may become so marked as to constitute strabismus (cross-eyed). Other signs of eccentric fixation include redness of the white of the eyes, redness of the lid margins, and tearing.

Eccentric fixation is a symptom of strain, and it is relieved by any method that relieves strain. In some cases, though, patients are cured the moment they realize that they do not see best where they are trying to focus. Ask them to pick a point and note that they do not see it as clearly when they look away from that point. This leads them to a direct experience that their peripheral vision is not as clear as their central vision.

Once people have this experience, they can reduce little by little the distance that they have to look away in order to see a point less clearly. Finally, they can look directly at the top of a small letter and see the bottom less well, or look at the bottom and see the top less well. The smaller the letter regarded in this way, the greater the visual relaxation and the better the sight.

When it becomes possible to look at the bottom of a letter and see the top less well or to look at the top and see the bottom less well, it is then possible to see the letter as it

is—perfectly black and distinct. At first such vision may come only in flashes. The letter will come out distinctly for a moment and then disappear. But gradually, if the practice is continued, central fixation will become habitual.

Most patients can readily look at the bottom of the largest C on the Snellen chart and realize that they then see the top less well. In a few rare cases, they just cannot appreciate any difference. These extreme cases sometimes require considerable ingenuity in demonstrating to them that the area to which they are directing their gaze is not the area that their eye sees most clearly.

The use of a strong light as one of the points of fixation or of two lights five or ten feet apart has been found helpful. It is easier to see that a point of light is less bright as one looks away from it than to see that a black letter is less sharp.

The highest degrees of eccentric fixation occur in the severely nearsighted. In these cases, the patients do best by practicing close up. Distance can then be gradually extended until it becomes possible to practice achieving central fixation at twenty feet.

CASE: One woman was very nearsighted. She said that the farther she looked away from an electric point of light, the better she saw it. This is severe eccentric fixation. I had her work close up with a pinpoint of light. By alternately looking at, then away from the light, she became able, in a short time, to appreciate that it looked brighter when she looked directly at it than when she looked away from it. Later she became able to do the same thing at twenty feet. At that point, she experienced a wonderful feeling of relief. No words, she said, could adequately describe it. Every nerve seemed to be relaxed and a feeling of comfort and rest permeated her whole body. Afterward, her progress was rapid. She soon became able to look at one part of the smallest letters on the chart and see the rest of the letter less well. Soon she could read the letters on the 20/20 line at twenty feet.

Some patients are benefited by consciously making their sight worse. When they learn by actual demonstration just how their visual defects are produced, they can then avoid the unconscious strain that causes them. I have taught patients how to deliberately worsen their eccentric fixation. When they do this and experience the discomfort and pain that results, they become better able to correct the unconscious habit of eccentric fixation.

In general, people find it more relaxing to focus on how the point not being looked at is less clear. When they focus on how clear the point being looked at is, they tend to intensify the strain under which the eye is already laboring.

Benefits of Central Fixation

One part of an object is seen most clearly only when the mind is content to see the greater part of it indistinctly. As the degree of relaxation increases, the area of the part seen less well increases. In the end, the part seen best becomes merely a point.

The limits of vision depend on the degree of central fixation. A man may be able to read a sign half a mile away when he sees the letters all alike, but when taught to see one letter best, he will be able to read smaller letters that he didn't even know were there. The vision of some indigenous peoples is remarkable. They can see with the naked eye objects for which most of the rest of us require a telescope. This is just a matter of central fixation.

Some people can see the moons of Jupiter with the naked eye. It is not because of any superiority in the structure of their eyes but because they have attained a higher degree of central fixation than most people.

Not only do all errors of refraction and all functional disturbances of the eye disappear when it sees by central fixation, but many physical conditions are relieved or cured. I am unable to set any limits to its possibilities. I would not have ventured to predict that glaucoma, incipient cataract and syphilitic iritis could be cured by central fixation. The fact is, though, that I have seen these conditions disappear when central fixation was attained. Often, relief is obtained in a few minutes. In rare cases, this immediate relief was permanent. Usually, however, a permanent cure has required more prolonged treatment.

Inflammatory conditions of all kinds, including inflammation of the cornea, iris, conjunctiva, and even the optic nerve itself, have benefited by practicing central fixation after other methods have failed. Infections as well as diseases caused by metabolic imbalances, or the poisons of typhoid fever, influenza, syphilis and gonorrhea, have also benefited by it. Even with a foreign body in the eye, there is no redness and no pain so long as central fixation is retained.

Central fixation is impossible without mental control. Therefore, central fixation of the eye means central fixation of the mind. It means, therefore, health in all parts of the body. Why? Because all the operations of the physical mechanism depend on the mind. Not only the sight but all the other senses—touch, taste, hearing and smell—are benefited by good central fixation. All the vital processes—digestion, assimilation, elimination, etc.—are improved by it. The efficiency of the mind is enormously increased. The benefits of well-developed central fixation already observed are, in short, so great that the subject merits further investigation.

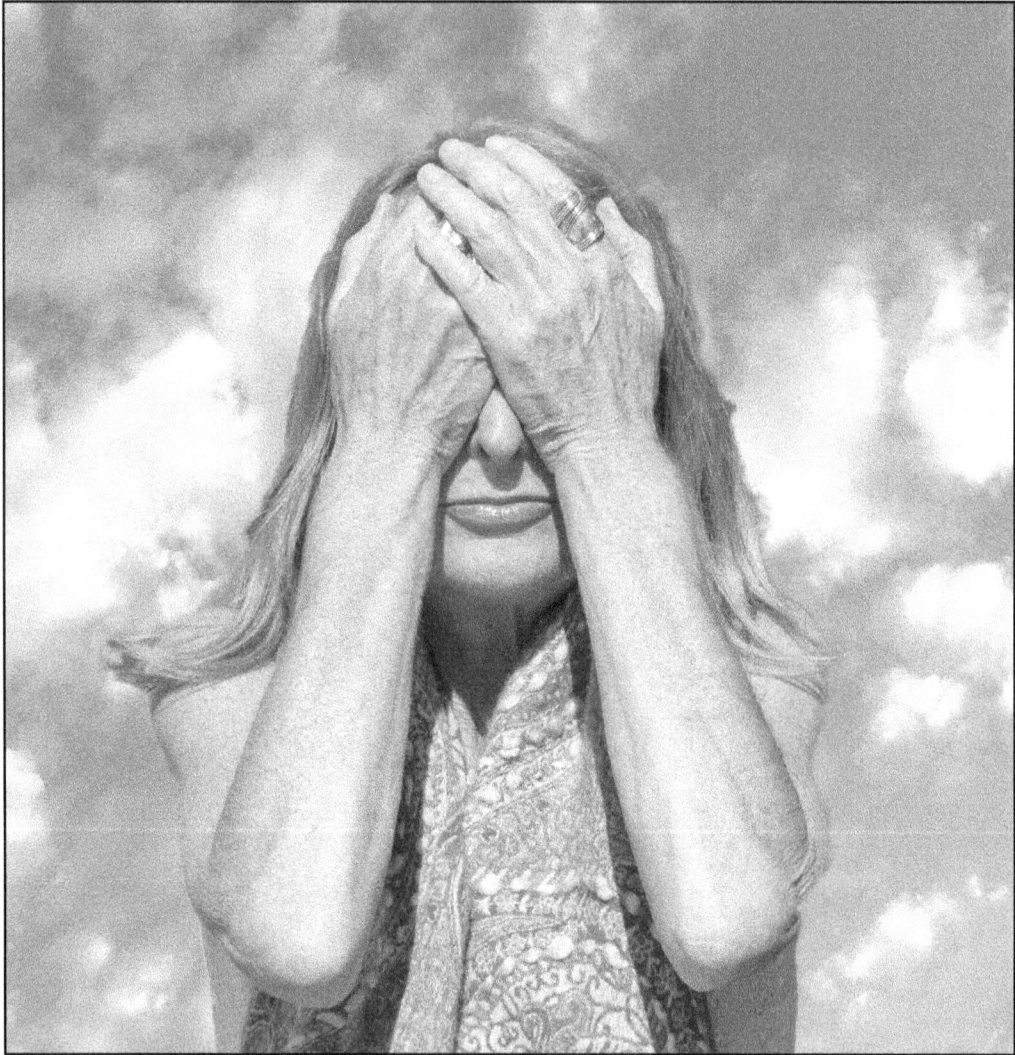

CHAPTER 12

Palming

All methods used in the cure of errors of refraction are simply different ways of obtaining relaxation. Most (but not all) people find it easiest to relax with their eyes shut.

Most people benefit simply by closing the eyes. Flashes of improved vision usually can be obtained as follows: Alternately rest the vision with the eyes closed, then open them briefly to look at a test chart in this relaxed state, then return to resting with the eyes closed. Repeat over and over.

Some temporarily obtain almost normal vision by this means. In rare cases, a complete cure has been effected, sometimes in less than an hour.

But since some light comes through closed eyelids, a still greater degree of relaxation can be obtained by excluding that light. This can be done by covering the closed eyes with the palms of the hands (the fingers being crossed on the forehead) in such a way as to avoid pressure on the eyeballs. I call this palming.

The Practice of Palming

The practice of palming is so effective in relieving strain that we all instinctively resort to it at times. While palming, one ought to see a field so black that it is impossible to remember, imagine, or see anything blacker.

But even with the eyes closed and covered, the visual centers of the brain may still be disturbed, and the eyes may still strain to see. Then, instead of black, the a person is likely to see illusions of lights and colors, ranging all the way from an imperfect black to kaleidoscopic appearances so vivid that they seem to be actually seen with the eyes. As a rule, the worse the condition of the eyesight, the more numerous, vivid and persistent these appearances are.

Any disturbance of mind or body, such as fatigue, hunger, anger, worry or depression, also makes it difficult for people to see black when they palm. People who can see black perfectly under ordinary conditions are often unable to do so without assistance when they are ill or in pain.

It is impossible to see a perfect black unless the eyesight is perfect. This is because only when the eyesight is perfect is the mind at rest. But some people can approximate a perfect black nearly enough to improve their eyesight without difficulty. As the eyesight improves, the deepness of the black increases. Some people with very imperfect sight are, surprisingly, able to palm almost perfectly from the beginning. They are very quickly cured.

People who fail to see even an approximate

black when they palm state that, instead of black, they see streaks or floating clouds of gray, flashes of light, patches of red, blue, green, yellow, and so on. Sometimes, instead of an immovable black, clouds of black will be seen moving across the field of vision. In other cases, the black will be seen for a few seconds and then some other color will take its place. The different ways in which people can fail to see black when their eyes are closed and covered are, in fact, very numerous and often very peculiar.

Some people have been so impressed with the vividness of the colors they saw while palming that no amount of argument could, or did, convince them that these colors were not actually there. They asserted this reality even while acknowledging that if others saw bright lights or colors while palming, these things must be illusions.

In more difficult cases they may have to practice all of the methods described in this book before they can palm successfully.

Remembering a Black Object

The majority of people who have difficulty gaining improvement are greatly helped by remembering a black object. The reasons for this will be given in the next chapter.

The person is directed to look at a black object from the distance at which they see best. They then close their eyes and are asked to remember the color. This activity is repeated until the memory of black is as clear as the actual sight of black.

Then they are instructed, while still holding the memory of black, to palm. If the memory of black is perfect, the whole

background will be black. If it is not, it may become so in the course of a few seconds. If the memory of black does not become perfect, the eyes are opened and the black object is regarded again. Repeat as needed.

By this method, many people become able to see black almost perfectly for a short time. Most, even those whose eyes are not very bad, have great difficulty in seeing black continuously. Being unable to remember black for more than three to five seconds, they cannot see black for longer than this.

Central Fixation and Shifting While Palming

Such people are helped by central fixation. Black is seen most perfectly at the very center of the visual field where details are also seen most perfectly. When people have become able to see one part of a black object as darker than the whole, then they are able to remember the black of that smaller area for a longer time than they could the larger one. They thus become able to see black for a longer period when they palm.

People who have trouble palming and remembering perfect black can also be helped by doing mental shifting from one black object to another. (This exercise is described in Chapter 15.)

As I've explained, the fovea, at the center of the macula, is the very center of visual clarity. It is impossible to see, remember, or imagine anything, even for so much as a second, without the fovea shifting. It may shift from one part of the object to another or to some other object and back again. If there is an attempt to see or visualize something without moving the gaze, the attempt will always produce strain. Those who think they are remembering a black object continuously are unconsciously comparing it with something not so black. It only seems pure black by comparison. Or in their perception, the color and position of the object are constantly changing, but they do not notice this.

In healthy eyes, shifting occurs constantly and unconsciously. It is therefore impossible to remember even such a simple thing as a perfectly black and stationary period for more than a fraction of a second. Those with visual problems stare instead of shifting. When shifting is not done unconsciously, then people must be encouraged to do it consciously. They may be directed, for instance, to remember successively a black hat, a black shoe, a black velvet dress, a black plush curtain, or a fold in a black dress or a black curtain. They are to hold the image of each one for not more than a fraction of a second. Many people have benefited by remembering all the letters of the alphabet in rapid sequence perfectly black. Others prefer to shift from one small black object, such as a period or a small letter, to another. Still others benefit when they "swing" such an object (the exercise of swinging will be described in Chapter 15).

Exercise: This exercise in some cases has proved successful: When you see what you think is a perfect black, remember a piece of white starch on this background. *[Starch was probably the whitest thing imaginable in Dr. Bate's era. MA]* Visualize the letter F on the starch as black as the background. Then let go of the starch

and remember only the blackest part of the F, on the black background. In a short time, the whole visual field may become as black as the blackest part of the F. The process can be repeated many times with a constant increase of blackness in the visual field.

CASE: In one case, a woman saw gray so vividly when she palmed that she was positive she was really seeing it with her eyes. She could not believe that the gray was not actually there. She was able to obliterate nearly all the gray by first imagining a black C on the grey field, then two black C's, and finally a multitude of overlapping black C's.

Palming in the Nearsighted

As a rule, nearsighted people more readily become able to see black while palming than those with farsightedness or astigmatism. This holds true no matter how severe their nearsightedness or how much the interior of the eye may be diseased. If they can read tiny print close up, they more readily come to the experience of seeing pure black while palming.

Why is this so? Because it is impossible to remember black perfectly when it is not seen perfectly. If one sees black imperfectly, the best one can do is to remember it imperfectly. People who are nearsighted cannot see anything perfectly, even close up. Nearsighted people, however, see better close up than people with farsightedness or astigmatism see at any distance. Therefore, the nearsighted have an advantage over those with farsightedness or astigmatism in the practice of remembering black.

On the other hand, the severely nearsighted often find palming very difficult because of the effort they are making to see. They often cannot remember black for more than one or two seconds.

Any other condition of the eyes that prevents people from seeing black perfectly also makes palming difficult. In some cases, black is never seen as black. Instead, black may appear as gray, yellow, brown, or even bright red. In such cases it is usually best for them to improve their sight by other methods before trying to palm.

People who have lost their sight and become blind usually have more trouble in seeing black than those who can see. These people may be helped by the memory of a black object familiar to them from before they lost their sight. I worked with a blind painter who saw grey continually when he first tried to palm. He had no perception of light whatever and was in terrible pain. He finally became able to see black by the aid of the memory of black paint. The pain then vanished, and when he opened his eyes he saw light.

Even the imperfect memory of black is useful as a stepping stone to both seeing and remembering a still blacker black.

EXERCISE: Regard a black letter on a Snellen test chart from the distance at which you see best. Then close your eyes, palm, and remember it. If the palming has produced relaxation, it will then be possible to imagine a deeper shade of black than was previously seen. Holding the memory of this black, open your eyes and again regard the letter. You will able to see it as blacker than before. Return to palming—a still deeper black can then be imagined. This deeper black can, in turn, be transferred to the letter on the test chart.

By continuing this process, a perfect perception of black, and hence perfect sight, are sometimes very quickly obtained. The deeper the shade of black obtained with the eyes closed, the more easily it can be remembered when regarding the letters on the test chart.

Once Strain Creeps in, Stop Palming

For some people, the longer they palm the more they relax. The more they relax, the darker the shade of black they can both remember and see. Others are able to palm successfully for short periods but begin to strain if they keep it up too long. Once strain creeps in, it is useless to continue to palm.

It is impossible to succeed by effort or by attempting to "concentrate" on the black. As popularly understood, concentration means to do or think one thing only. This is impossible, and any attempt to do the impossible is a strain, which defeats its own end. The human mind is not capable of thinking of one thing only. True, the mind can think of one thing best. In fact, the mind is only at rest when it does so. But the mind cannot think of one thing only.

CASE: I had a woman who tried to see black only. She struggled to ignore the kaleidoscopic colors that intruded themselves on her field of vision. Her symptoms became worse and worse. She actually went into convulsions from the strain of trying to ignore these kaleidoscopic colors and only see black. She had to be attended every day for a month by her family physician before she was able to resume treatment with me.

I advised her to stop palming. Instead, with her eyes open, she was to recall as many colors as possible. I asked her to remember each color as perfectly and vividly as possible. By thus taking the bull by the horns and consciously making the mind wander from black more than it did unconsciously, she became able to palm for short periods.

Visualize Black Optimums

For many, some black objects are more easily remembered than others. Any object that improves our vision when we look at it is called an optimum (more of this in Chapter 18).

Optimums vary by individual, but for many, black plush of a high grade is an optimum. These people see black plush better than they see the black of velvet, silk, broadcloth, ink or the letters on the Snellen test chart. In fact, black plush is no blacker than these other blacks. It is just that for these

individuals, the eyes relax when they regard black plush.

A familiar black object can often be remembered more easily than one that is unfamiliar. I treated a dressmaker, for instance, who was able to remember a thread of black silk when she could not remember any other black object.

When a black letter is regarded before palming, the patient will usually remember not only the blackness of the letter but the whiteness of the background as well. If the memory of the black is held for a few seconds, however, the white background usually fades away, and the whole field of vision becomes black.

People often say that they remember black perfectly when they do not. If there is no improvement after palming, then they are usually not remembering black perfectly. They can be helped to realize this by bringing the black object closer.

EXERCISE: Black is the easiest color to remember, as a rule. If the memory of black fails to improve the vision, try this: Remember a variety of colors: bright red, yellow, green, blue, purple, and especially white. Remember each of them in the most intense shade possible. Do not attempt to hold any color for more than a second. Keep this up for five or ten minutes. Then remember a piece of white starch *[or some other perfectly white thing - MA]* about half an inch in diameter. Remember the most vivid white possible. Then note the color of the background. Usually the background will be a shade of black. If it is, note whether it is possible to remember anything blacker, or to see anything blacker with the eyes open. In all cases, if the white starch is remembered perfectly, the background will be so black that it will be impossible to remember anything blacker with the eyes closed or to see anything blacker with them open.

Palming is One of the Best Methods

When palming is successful, it is one of the best methods I know of for securing relaxation of all the sensory nerves, including those of sight. We know when perfect relaxation is gained in this way because the person can then see a perfect black. Once this relaxation is retained completely when the eyes are opened, the person is permanently cured. At the same time, pain in the eyes and head, and even in other parts of the body, is permanently relieved.

Such cases of dramatic and global cure are very rare, but they do occur. With a lesser degree of relaxation, much of the relaxation is lost when the eyes are opened. The relaxation that is retained is usually not held permanently. In other words, the greater the degree of the relaxation produced by palming, the more of it is retained when the eyes are opened and the longer it lasts. If you palm perfectly, you retain all of the relaxation that you gained when you open your eyes, and you do not lose it again. If you palm imperfectly, you retain only part of what you gained and retain it only temporarily. You may even retain the relaxation for only for a few moments. However, even the smallest degree of relaxation is useful. By means of slight

relaxation, a still greater degree of relaxation may be obtained.

People who succeed with palming from the beginning are to be congratulated, for they are always cured very quickly.

CASE: A very remarkable case of this kind was that of a man nearly seventy years of age. He had astigmatism and presbyopia. A cataract was in the process of forming in his lens. For more than forty years he had worn glasses to improve his distant vision. For twenty years he had worn glasses for reading and desk work. Because of the cloudiness of the lenses of his eyes, he had now become unable to see well enough to do his work, even with glasses. The other physicians whom he had consulted had given him no hope of relief except by operation when the cataract was ripe.

When he found that palming helped him, he asked:

"Can I do that too much?"

"No," he was told. "Palming is simply a means of resting your eyes, and you cannot rest them too much."

A few days later he returned and said, "Doctor, it was tedious, very tedious, but I did it."

"What was tedious?" I asked.

"Palming," he replied. "I did it continuously for twenty hours."

"But you couldn't have kept it up for twenty hours continuously," I said incredulously. "You must have stopped to eat."

And then he related that from four

o'clock in the morning until twelve at night he had eaten nothing, only drinking large quantities of water. He had devoted practically all of this time to palming. It must have been tedious, as he said, but it was also worthwhile. When he looked at the test chart he read the 20/20 line at twenty feet without using glasses. He also read fine print at six inches and at twenty inches. The cloudiness of the lens had become much less. In the center of the lens the cloudiness had entirely disappeared. I followed up with him two years later, and there had been no relapse.

If You Feel Stuck, Try Some Other Exercise

Most people are helped by palming, but some are simply unable to see black. These people only increase their strain by trying to get relaxation in this way. If much difficulty is experienced, it is usually better and more expeditious to drop the method until the sight has been improved by other means. The patient may then become able to see black when palming. Even then, some never succeed in seeing black until they are cured.

CHAPTER 13

Memory as an Aid to Vision

When the mind is able to remember perfectly any sense experience, it is always perfectly relaxed. In these circumstances, sight is normal. When the mind is perfectly relaxed and the eyes are closed and covered, one sees a perfectly black field. That is, one sees nothing at all.

If you can remember the ticking of a watch, or an odor or a taste perfectly, then your mind is perfectly at rest. In that state you will see a perfect black when your eyes are closed and covered. If your memory of a sensation of touch could be equal to the reality, you would see nothing but black when the light was excluded from your eyes. If you were to remember a bar of music perfectly, then when your eyes were closed and covered, you would see nothing but black.

But in the case of any of these sensory experiences, it is not easy to test the correctness of the memory. The same is true of the memory of any color other than black. All other colors, including white, are altered by the amount of light to which they are exposed. All other colors are seldom seen as perfectly as it is possible for the normal eye to see them. But when sight is normal, black is just as black in a dim light as in a bright one. It is also just as black at the distance as at the near point. A small area of black is just as black as a large

one, and in fact, appears blacker. Moreover, black is more readily available than any other color. There is nothing blacker than printer's ink, and that is practically ubiquitous.

Perfect Black
Means Perfectly Relaxed

By means of the memory of black, therefore, it is possible to measure accurately one's own relaxation. If the color is remembered perfectly, one is perfectly relaxed. If it is remembered almost perfectly, one's relaxation is almost perfect. If it cannot be remembered at all, then one has very little or no relaxation.

These facts can be readily demonstrated by means of simultaneous retinoscopy. An absolutely perfect memory is very rare, but a practically perfect memory is normal and attainable by everyone under certain conditions. With such a memory of black, the retinoscope shows that all errors of refraction are corrected. If the memory is less than normal, the retinoscope will show that the vision is less than normal. If the memory of black fluctuates, the shadow of the retinoscope will fluctuate. The testimony of the retinoscope is, in fact, more reliable than the statements of the person.

People often believe and state that they

remember black perfectly, or normally, when the retinoscope indicates an error of refraction. In such cases it can usually be demonstrated that the memory is not equal to the sight by bringing a test chart to the point at which the black letters can be seen best.

You can easily demonstrate for yourself that the color black cannot be remembered perfectly when the eyes and mind are under a strain. Simply try to remember a perfect black while making a conscious effort to see. Stare, or partly close the eyes and squint, or frown, or just make an effort to see all the letters of a line of print equally well at one time. You will find that black either cannot be remembered at all under these conditions or that it is only remembered very imperfectly.

If one eye is better than the other, the memory is better when the good eye is open and worse when the weaker eye is open in exact proportion to the difference in the vision between the two eyes. This is perfectly reflected by how long the person can remember a black period. Say a woman has normal vision in the right eye and half-normal vision in the left. Now say that she, while looking at the Snellen test chart, can remember a black period perfectly for 20 seconds if both eyes are open. If she covers the good eye, she will only be able to remember a black period perfectly for 10 seconds.

One person with half-normal vision in the right eye and one-quarter normal in the left could remember a period twelve seconds with both eyes open and only six seconds with the better eye closed. A third patient, with normal sight in the right eye and vision of one-tenth in the left, could remember a period twenty seconds with both eyes open and only two seconds when the better eye was closed.

This relationship between relaxation and memory is of great practical importance in the treatment of eye troubles. The sensations and discomforts of the eye and mind supply very little information as to the degree of strain to which both are being subjected. Those who strain most often suffer the least discomfort. But by means of their ability to remember black, they can always know whether they are straining or not. They will therefore be able to avoid the conditions that produce strain.

Whatever method of improving sight people are using, they are advised to constantly carry with them the memory of a small area of black, such as a period. In this way they may recognize and avoid the conditions that produce strain. As I've mentioned, in some cases people have obtained a complete cure in a very short time by this means alone. One advantage of this method is that it does not require a test chart. At any hour of the day or night, whatever people may be doing, they can always place themselves in the conditions favorable to the perfect memory of a period.

Effort is Useless

The state of mind in which a black period can be remembered cannot be attained by any sort of effort. The memory is not the cause of the relaxation but must be preceded by it. The memory is obtained only during moments of relaxation and retained only as long as the causes of strain are avoided. How this is accomplished cannot be fully explained, just as many other psychological phenomena cannot be explained. We only know that under certain conditions that might be called favorable, a degree of relaxation sufficient for the memory of a black period is possible. We also know that by persistently seeking these conditions, people become able to increase the degree of relaxation and prolong its duration. Finally, they become able to retain the relaxation under unfavorable conditions.

Prolonging the Relaxation

For most people, palming provides the most favorable condition for the memory of black. When the strain to see is lessened by the exclusion of light, people usually become able to remember a black object for a few seconds or longer. This period of relaxation can be prolonged in one of two ways. First, they can open the eyes and look at a black object from whatever distance they see best, using central fixation. The distance from which they see best is the distance at which their eyes are the most relaxed. Alternatively, they can shift mentally from one black object to another or from one part of a black object to another. By these means, and perhaps also through other influences that are not clearly understood, most people become able, sooner or later, to remember black for an indefinite length of time with their eyes closed and covered.

Looking at a blank surface is another approach that can help the vision. If a person looks at a blank surface without trying to see, then the unconscious strain to see is lessened. The person then becomes able to remember a black period. In this state, the retinoscope shows that all errors of refraction vanish. If the mind drifts and the memory of a black period is lost, or if the person begins to think

about things seen imperfectly, then the errors of refraction return.

It also happens that, with the improved vision, details on the blank surface begin to come out. If a person strains to see them, the memory of the black period will immediately be lost and the error of refraction will return.

When looking at a surface on which there is nothing to see, distance makes no difference to the memory. Near or far, a person can always look at such a surface without straining to see it. However, when looking at letters or other details, memory is best at the distance at which the patient's sight is best. At that distance, the eyes and mind are most relaxed. By practicing central fixation at the most favorable distance, therefore, the memory of the period may be improved, in some cases, very rapidly.

If the relaxation gained under these favorable conditions is perfect, a person will be able to retain it when the mind is conscious of objects at unfavorable distances. Such cases are very rare, however. Usually the degree of relaxation gained is markedly imperfect. The relaxation is, therefore, lost to a greater or lesser degree when conditions become unfavorable. Conditions are unfavorable when the nearsighted regard objects far away or the farsighted regard objects close up.

Seeing More Disturbs Us

Also, when we see that which we previously could not see, we become disturbed. Just as soon as details begin to come out at distances at which they have not previously been seen, people usually lose their relaxation and with it the memory of the perfectly black period.

In fact, the strain to see may even return before they have had time to become conscious of the clear image, as the following case strikingly illustrates:

CASE: A woman of fifty-five had nearsightedness of 15 Diopters. Six Diopters is already considered severe. She also had other conditions that, in sum, made it impossible for her to see the largest letter on the Snellen chart at more than one foot. She was unable to go about without an attendant, either in her house or on the street.

By looking at a blank green wall without trying to see it, she became able to remember a perfectly black period. Soon she could see a small area of the wallpaper at a distance as well as she could at the near point.

At a point when she was close to a wall, I asked her to put her hand on the doorknob, which she did without hesitation. "But I don't see the knob," she hastened to explain. As a matter of fact, she had seen it long enough to put her hand on it. But as soon as the idea of seeing it was suggested to her, she lost the memory of the period and with it her improved vision. When she again tried to find the knob she could not do so.

If a black period is remembered perfectly while a letter on the Snellen test chart is being regarded, the clarity of the letter improves. This occurs whether or not the patient is conscious of it. Why? Because it is impossible to strain and relax at the same time. If one

relaxes sufficiently to remember the period, consciously or unconsciously, one must also relax sufficiently to see the letter. The clarity of letters on either side of the one regarded or on the lines above and below it also improves. At first, when people become conscious of seeing the letters, it is very distracting. It usually causes them to immediately forget the period. As described earlier, for some, the strain to see returns even before the letters are consciously recognized.

The Horns of a Dilemma

Thus people find themselves on the horns of a dilemma. The things they see with their improved vision cause them to lose their relaxation and memory. The moment they lose their relaxation and memory, their vision becomes as bad as it ever was. It is very remarkable to me that this difficulty is ever overcome. Nevertheless, some people are able to overcome it in five minutes or half an hour. With others, the process is long and tedious.

To review, the more people's vision improves, the more they see. The more they see, the more they tense up. The more they tense up, the more their vision returns to its original state of imperfection.

There are various ways of helping people deal with this situation. One is to remember the period while looking a little to one side of the test chart, say a foot or more. Then look a little nearer to the test chart. Finally, look between the lines of letters. In this way you may become able to see the letters in the peripheral vision without losing the memory of the period. Once you can do this, you may become able to go a step further and look directly at a letter without losing control of the memory of the black period.

Variations on the Period

You can also try looking at only one part of a letter—usually the bottom.

Some people benefit by imagining the period as part of the letter while noting that the rest of the letter is less black and less distinct than the part directly regarded. *[This is basically an exercise in central fixation.* **MA]** When they can do this, they become able to remember the period better than when the letter is seen as having the same degree of blackness all over. In that instance the perfect memory of the period is always lost.

The next step is to note whether the bottom of the letter is straight, curved, or open, without losing the visualization of the period superimposed onto the bottom of the letter. Once you can do this, then do the same with the sides and top of the letter, still visualizing the period on the bottom. Usually when the parts can be observed separately in this way, the whole letter can be seen without losing the memory of the period.

It does occasionally happen that this approach is unsuccessful. Then further practice is needed before a person can become conscious of all sides of the letter at once without losing the period. This may require moments, hours, days or months.

CASE: In one case, the following method succeeded: A man had 15 Diopters of nearsightedness, which is quite severe. He was very much disturbed by what he saw when his vision improved by the memory of a black period. I directed him to look away from the object he was regarding when he found the details coming out more clearly. For about a week, he went around persistently dodging his improved sight. As his memory improved, it became more and more difficult for him to do this. By the end of the week it was impossible. When he looked at the 20/20 line of the Snellen test chart at a distance of twenty feet, he remembered the period perfectly, and when asked if he could see the letters, he replied, "I cannot help but see them."

Some people retard their recovery by decorating the scenery with periods as they go about during the day instead of simply remembering a period in their minds. This does them no good. On the contrary, it is a cause of strain. The period cannot be imagined perfectly on any surface that is not black. The attempt to imagine it on such surfaces defeats the end in view. The reason that it is beneficial to imagine the black period as forming part of a black letter on the test chart is because this merely means imagining that one sees one part of the black letter best.

The ability to remember a smaller area of black indicates a greater degree of relaxation. In the beginning, some people find it easier to remember a somewhat larger area. For example, they could start with the largest letter on the Snellen test chart and imagine one part of that letter blacker than the rest. With practice they can then proceed to the smaller letters and finally to a period. Once they achieve the memory of a period, I have found that they remember this small area more easily than the larger ones and that its black is more intense.

Instead of a period, some people find it easier to remember a colon, with one period blacker than the other. Some do better remembering a collection of periods, with one blacker than all the others. Others do well remembering the dot over an i or j. Others prefer a comma to a period.

In the beginning, most people find it helpful to shift consciously from one of these black areas to another or from one part of such an area to another. While they do this, it helps to realize the swing, or pulsation, produced by such shifting (see Chapter 15). When the memory finally becomes perfect, one object may be held continuously, without conscious shifting, while the swing is realized only when attention is directed to the matter.

Whatever is Easy is Best

Whatever the patient finds easiest to remember is the best to remember, because the memory can never be perfect unless it is easy. Although black is the best color to remember, as a rule, some people are bored or depressed by it and prefer to remember white or some other color. A familiar object or one with pleasant associations is often easier to remember than one that has no particular interest. One person was cured by the memory of a yellow buttercup. Another woman was able to remember the opal of her ring when she could not remember a period.

When the memory of the period becomes habitual, it is no burden. In fact, it becomes a great help to other mental processes. The mind, when it remembers one thing better than all other things, possesses central fixation. The mind's efficiency is thereby increased, just as the efficiency of the eye is increased by central fixation.

In other words, the mind attains its greatest efficiency when it is at rest. The mind is never at rest unless one thing is remembered better than all others. When the mind is such that a period is remembered perfectly, the memory for other things is improved.

A high school girl reports that when she was unable to remember the answer to a question in an examination, she remembered the period, and the answer came to her. When I cannot remember the name of a patient, I remember a period and, behold, I have it! A musician who had perfect sight and could remember a period perfectly, had a perfect memory for music. Another musician with imperfect sight could not remember a period. He could play nothing without his notes. Once his sight and visual memory became normal, he gained the ability to play without looking at the sheet music.

Some people have told me that they strained so hard to see the letters on the Snellen test chart that they couldn't even remember their own names, much less a black period.

Tests of the Accuracy of the Memory of Black

People may measure the accuracy of their memory of the period not only by comparing it with the sight of one but also by the following tests:

1. When the memory of the period is

perfect, it is instantaneous. If a few seconds or longer are necessary to obtain the memory, it is never perfect.

2. A perfect memory is both instantaneous and continuous.

3. When the period is remembered perfectly, perfect sight comes instantaneously. If good vision is obtained only after a second or two, it can always be demonstrated that both the memory of the period and the sight are imperfect.

The memory of a period is a test of relaxation. It is the evidence by which people can know that their eyes and mind are at rest. It may be compared to the steam gauge of an engine. A steam gauge has no effect on the machinery. It simply gives information of great importance about the machinery. When the period is black, one knows that the engine of the eye is in good working order. When the period fades or is lost, one knows that the eye is out of order. Once a cure is effected, one does not need a period or any other aid to vision.

One man who had gained telescopic and microscopic vision said that he had done nothing to prevent a relapse. Indeed, he said he had even forgotten how he was cured. When people are cured, they do not need to do anything consciously to stay cured. However, the treatment can always be continued with benefit, since even supernormal vision can be improved.

CHAPTER 14

Imagination as an Aid to Vision

Perfect imagination not only corrects all errors of refraction, it also corrects any false interpretations of the retinal image we receive.

We see very largely with the mind and only partly with the eyes. The phenomena of vision depend on the mind's interpretation of light's impression on the retina. We do not see the image on the retina. We see our interpretation of that image. Our impressions of size, color, form and location can be shown to depend on the interpretation by the mind of the retinal picture. The figure of a man on a high building or on the topmast of a vessel looks small to the land lover. To sailors, the figure appears to be of ordinary size, because they are accustomed to seeing the human figure in such positions.

One might think that when there is an error of refraction it accounts for all the defects in the image of what is seen. This is not true. When sight is imperfect, it is not just the eye that is at fault. Memory and imagination are also impaired, so that the mind adds imperfections to the already imperfect retinal image.

People with normal vision use their memory and imagination as an aid to sight. No two people with normal sight will get the same visual impressions from the same object.

Each one's interpretation of the retinal picture will differ as much as their individualities differ.

When the sight is imperfect, the interpretation is even more variable. It reflects the loss of mental control responsible for the error of refraction. When the eye is out of focus, the mind is also out of focus.

The Eye is Not Just a Camera

There is a great difference between an image from an out-of-focus camera and the image in the mind when the eye is out of focus. When the camera is out of focus, it turns black into gray and the lines in the image are blurred. However, the camera produces these results uniformly and constantly. On the screen of the camera, an imperfect picture of a black letter would be equally imperfect in all its parts. The same error of focus would always produce the same blurred picture.

But when the eye is out of focus, the imperfect picture in the person's mind is always changing, whether the focus changes or not. There will be more gray on one part than on another. Both the shade and the position of the gray may vary within wide limits in a very short space of time. One part of a letter may appear gray and the rest black. Certain outlines may be seen more clearly than others.

Vertical lines may appear black and diagonal lines gray, or vice versa. Black may be changed into brown, yellow, green or even red. There may be spots of color or black on the gray, or on the white openings in a letter. There may also be spots of white or color on the black. All these transmutations are possible to the impaired human vision but impossible to the camera.

When the camera is out of focus, the picture it produces of any object is always slightly larger than the image produced when the focus is correct. When the eyes are out of focus, the picture the mind sees may be either larger or smaller than it normally would be. I had one patient for whom the largest letter on the Snellen test chart at ten feet appeared smaller than at either twenty feet or four inches. To some people, the largest letter on the Snellen test chart appears larger than it actually is at twenty feet, and to others it seems smaller.

When the human eye is out of focus, the forms frequently appear to be distorted, and their location may appear to change as well. The image may be doubled, tripled, or still further multiplied. One object, or part of an object, may appear multiplied while other objects or parts of objects may remain single. The location of these multiple images is sometimes constant and at other times subject to continual change. Nothing like this could ever happen with a camera out of focus.

If two cameras are out of focus to the same degree, they will take two imperfect pictures exactly alike. If two eyes are out of focus to the same degree, similar impressions will be made on the retina of each eye. However, the impressions made on the mind may be totally different. This is true even when the two different eyes belong to the same person. If the normal eye looks at an object through glasses that change its refraction, the grayness and blurring produced are uniform and constant. With the eye that has an error of refraction equivalent to that produced by these same glasses, the grayness and blurring are variable and not at all uniform.

Understanding is Fundamental

It is fundamental that the person should understand that these aberrations of vision are illusions produced by the mind. They are not at all produced by a fault in the eye. When we know that a thing is an illusion, we are less likely to see it again. When we become convinced that what we see is imaginary, it helps to bring the imagination under control. Perfect imagination is impossible without perfect relaxation. Perfect imagination not only corrects the error of refraction, it also corrects the false interpretation of the retinal image.

Imagination is closely allied to memory, although distinct from it. Imagination depends on memory, because a thing can be imagined only as well as it can be remembered. You cannot imagine a sunset unless you have seen one. If you attempt to imagine a blue sun, which you have never seen, you will immediately become nearsighted. This can be detected by simultaneous retinoscopy. Neither imagination nor memory can be perfect unless the mind is perfectly relaxed. Therefore, when the imagination and memory are perfect, the sight is perfect. Imagination, memory and sight are, in fact, synchronized. When one is perfect, all are perfect. When one is imperfect, all are imperfect. If you imagine a letter perfectly, you will see the letter perfectly. In addition, other letters in its neighborhood will come out more distinctly. Why? Because it is impossible for you to relax and imagine you see a perfect letter and at the same time strain and actually see an imperfect one. If you imagine a perfect period on the bottom of a letter, you will see the letter perfectly because you cannot take the mental picture of a perfect period and put it on an imperfect letter.

It is possible, however, for a person not to be conscious that they are seeing perfectly. In some cases, people may imagine a period perfectly, as demonstrated by the retinoscope, without being conscious of seeing the letter. For these people, it is often some time before they are able to be conscious of the letter without losing the period.

Remarkable Results Through Imagination

Very remarkable results are sometimes obtained by the aid of the imagination. People must be willing to believe that the letters can be imagined. They must be content to imagine without trying to see. Comparing what they see with what they imagine always brings back the strain. Some people at once become able to read all the letters on the 20/20 line of a test chart after they become able to imagine that they see one letter perfectly black and distinct. The majority, however, are so distracted by what they see when their vision improves by imagination that they lose the improvement.

It is one thing to be able to imagine perfect sight of a letter. It is quite another to be able to see the letter and other letters without losing control of the imagination.

EXERCISE: In nearsightedness the following method is often successful:

First look at a letter from the distance at which it is best seen. For nearsighted people, this is usually the closest point at which they can still focus. Then close the eyes and remember the letter. Repeat until the memory is almost as good as the real experience. Then, with the test chart at a distance of twenty feet, look at a blank surface a foot or more to one side of the letter, and again remember the letter. Do the same at six inches to one side and again at three inches to one side. When you look three inches to one side, note the appearance of the letters on the chart. You are seeing them in your peripheral vision. If the memory is still perfect, they will appear to be a dim black, not gray. Those nearest the point at which you are looking directly will appear more deeply black than those more distant. Gradually reduce the distance between where you look and the letter until you are able to look straight at the letter and imagine that it is seen as well as it is remembered.

Occasionally it is helpful during the practice to close and cover the eyes and remember the letter, or a period, perfectly black. The rest and mental control gained in this way help in gaining control when one looks at the test chart.

People who succeed with this method are not conscious of seeing an imperfect letter while imagining a perfect one. They are thus not distracted when their vision is improved by their imagination.

Many people can remember a letter perfectly with their eyes closed or when they are looking at a place where they cannot see the letter. But just as soon as they actually look at the letter, they begin to strain and lose control of their memory. Therefore, as the imagination depends on the memory, they cannot imagine that they see the letter while actually looking at it. In such cases, it has been my custom to proceed somewhat in the manner described in Chapter 13. I begin by saying to the person,

"Can you imagine a black period on the bottom of this letter? Now at the same time, while imagining the period perfectly, are you able to imagine that you see the letter?"

Sometimes they are able to do this, but usually they are not. In that case, they are asked to imagine part of the letter, usually the bottom. When they have become able to imagine this part, they become able to imagine the sides and top, while still holding the period on the bottom.

Even after they have done this, they may still not be able to imagine the whole letter without losing the period. Sometimes I have had to coax them along by bringing the chart up a little closer, then moving it farther away. The eyes are most relaxed at the distance from which they see best. The imagination therefore improves in proportion as one approaches the point where the sight is best, assuming there is something to see. When there is nothing in particular to see, the distance makes no difference because no effort is being made to see.

To encourage people to imagine they see the letter, it seems helpful to keep saying to them over and over again,

"Of course you do not see the letter. I am not asking you to see it. I am just asking you to imagine that you see it perfectly black and perfectly distinct."

When people become able to see a known letter by the aid of their imagination, they become able to apply the same method to an unknown letter. Just as soon as any part of a letter, such as an area equal to a period, can be imagined to be perfectly black, the whole letter is seen to be black. At first this visual perception may not last long enough for the person to become conscious of it.

In trying to distinguish unknown letters, the person discovers that it is impossible to imagine perfectly unless one imagines the truth. If a letter, or any part of a letter, is imagined to be other than it is, the mental picture is foggy and inconstant, just like a letter which is seen imperfectly.

Things That Interfere with Imagination

The ways in which the imagination can be interfered with are very numerous. There is one way of imagining perfectly and an infinite number of ways of imagining imperfectly. The right way is easy. The mental picture of the thing imagined comes as quick as thought and can be held more or less continuously. The wrong way is difficult. The picture comes slowly, and is both variable and discontinuous.

This can be demonstrated by asking a person to first imagine or remember a black letter as perfectly as possible with the eyes closed, and then to imagine the same letter imperfectly. This is usually easily done. On the other hand, they can find it very difficult to imagine a sharp black letter to be gray, with fuzzy edges and clouded openings. It will be impossible for them to form a mental picture of it that remains constant for any appreciable length of time. The letter will vary in color, shape and location in the visual field, precisely as a letter does when it is seen imperfectly. Also, just as the strain of imperfect sight produces discomfort and pain, the effort to imagine imperfectly will sometimes produce pain. The more nearly perfect the mental picture of the letter, the more easily and quickly it comes and the more constant it is.

CASE: Some very dramatic cures have been effected by means of the imagination. One patient, a physician, had worn glasses for forty years. At twenty feet, he could not see the largest letter on the Snellen test chart without his glasses. This gentleman was cured in fifteen minutes simply by imagining that he saw the letters black.

When first asked to describe the largest letter on the Snellen test chart with unaided vision, he said it looked gray to him. In his vision, the opening of the letter was obscured by a gray cloud to such an extent that he had to guess that it had an opening. He was told that the letter was black, perfectly black, and that the opening was perfectly white, with no gray cloud. The chart was brought close

to him so that he could see that this was so. When he again regarded the letter at a distance, he remembered its blackness vividly. He was able to imagine that he saw the letter just as black as he had seen it at the near point, with the opening perfectly white. He therefore saw the letter on the chart perfectly black and distinct.

Using this same approach, he became able to read the seventy line (for 20/70 vision). He continued to go down the chart and, in about five minutes, he became able to read at twenty feet the line that the normal eye is supposed to read at ten feet (20/10 vision).

Next, very small type was given to him to read. The letters appeared gray to him, and he could not read them. His attention was called to the fact that the letters were really black, and immediately he imagined that he saw them black and became able to read them at ten inches.

The explanation of this remarkable occurrence is simply relaxation. All the nerves of the patient's body were relaxed when he imagined that he saw the letters black. When he became conscious of seeing the letters on the chart, he still retained control of his imagination. Therefore, he did not begin to strain again and actually saw the letters as black as he imagined them.

The patient not only had no relapse, but continued to improve. About a year later, I visited him in his office and asked him how he was getting on. He replied that his sight was perfect, both for distance and the near point. He could see the motor cars on the other side of the Hudson River and the people in them. He could read the names of boats on the river, which other people could make out only with a telescope. At the same time, he had no difficulty in reading the newspapers. To prove the point, he picked up a newspaper and read a few sentences aloud. I was astonished, and asked him how he did it.

"I did what you told me to do," he said.

"What did I tell you to do?" I asked.

"You told me to read the Snellen test chart every day, which I have done, and to read fine print every day in a dim light, which I have also done."

CASE: Another patient had a high degree of nearsightedness complicated by optic nerve atrophy. He had been discouraged by many physicians. The practice of imagination benefited him so wonderfully and rapidly that one day while in the office, he lost control of himself completely. Raising a test chart which he held in his hand, he threw it across the room.

"It is too good to be true," he exclaimed. "I cannot believe it. The possibility of being cured and the fear of disappointment are more than I can stand."

He was calmed down with some difficulty and encouraged to continue. Later he became able to read the small letters on the test chart with normal vision. He was then given fine print to read. When he looked at the very small type, he at once said that it was impossible for him to read it. However, he was told to follow the same procedure that had benefited his distance sight. That is, he was to imagine a period on one part of the small letters while holding the type at six inches. After testing his memory of the period a number of times, he became able to imagine he saw a period perfectly black on one of the small letters.

Then he lost control of his nerves again, and on being asked, "What is the trouble?" he said: "I am beginning to read the fine print, and I am so overwhelmed that I lose my self-control."

CASE: In another case, a woman with severe nearsightedness also had an incipient cataract. Her vision improved in a few days from 3/200 to 20/50. This is to say that at first she could only see at three feet what a normal person could see from 200 feet away. Then she could see at 20 feet what a normal person could see at 50 feet.

From there, instead of improving gradually, she jumped from the 20/50 to 20/10. In that session, the chart was brought up close to her, and she was asked to look at the letter O at three inches— the distance at which she saw it best. She was then asked to imagine that she saw a period on the bottom of it and that the bottom was the blackest part. When she was able to do this at the near point, the distance was gradually increased until she became able to see the "O" at three feet.

Then I placed the chart at ten feet, and she exclaimed: "Oh, doctor, it is impossible! The letter is too small. It is too great a thing for me to do. Let me try a larger letter first." Nevertheless, in fifteen minutes she became able to read the small "O" on the ten line at twenty feet.

CHAPTER 15

Shifting and Swinging

When a letter is regarded by the eye with normal vision, that letter may appear to pulsate or to move in various directions. When the normal eye looks about, moving from one thing to another, the whole scene may appear to shift. This apparent movement is due to shifting of the direction in which the eye is looking. This apparent shifting is always in a direction contrary to the movement of the eye.

If one looks at the top of a letter, the letter appears to move downward. If one looks at the bottom, the letter appears to move upward. If one looks to the left of the letter it appears to move to the right. If one looks to the right, it appears to move to the left.

People with normal vision are rarely conscious of this illusion. They may even have difficulty in consciously perceiving it. Nevertheless, in all the cases that have come under my observation, everyone is eventually able to see this movement. By contrast, when the sight is imperfect, the letters may appear to remain stationary or even to move in the same direction that the eye moves.

It is impossible for the eye to fix a point for longer than a fraction of a second. If it tries to do so, it begins to strain and the visual acuity is lowered. This can readily be demonstrated by trying to hold the gaze on one part of a letter for any appreciable length of time. No matter how good the sight, the image will begin to blur very quickly. The letter may even disappear. Sometimes the effort to hold the gaze absolutely steady will produce pain.

In the case of a few exceptional people, a point may appear to be held for a considerable length of time. The subjects themselves may think that they are holding it. In fact, the eye is shifting subtly and unconsciously. These tiny movements are so rapid that the object may seem steady.

The shifting of the eye with normal vision is usually not conspicuous. However, the retinoscope always reveals it. The eyes move together. If one eye is examined with the retinoscope while the other looks straight ahead, the eye under examination is seen to move in various directions. If the vision is normal, these movements are extremely rapid and unaccompanied by any appearance of effort. The shifting of the eye with imperfect sight, on the other hand, is slower. The excursions are wider, and the movements are jerky and made with apparent effort.

The Eye Shifts with Incredible Rapidity

We can also infer that the eye is capable of shifting with a rapidity that the ophthalmoscope cannot measure. From ten or fifteen feet away in dim light, the normal eye can read the 20/20 line of the Snellen test chart so rapidly that the letters seem to be seen all at once. But the area seen most clearly by the fovea is very small, a little less than a dime at the distance of twenty feet. If you do the math for this example, it turns out that the eye must shift about four times per letter. One must also shift from one letter to another. So while it may seem that the letters are seen all at once, in fact the eye has shifted about 70 times in a fraction of a second.

A line of small letters on the Snellen test chart may be less than a foot long by a quarter of an inch in height. If it requires seventy shifts in a fraction of a second to see this apparently all at once, it must require many thousands of shifts to see an area the size of a movie screen. Think of all the details—people, animals, houses, or trees. Then to see sixteen such areas a second, as is done in viewing moving pictures, must require a rapidity of shifting that can scarcely be imagined. Yet it is admitted that the present rate of taking and projecting moving pictures is too slow. The results would be more satisfactory, authorities say, if the rate were raised to twenty, twenty-two, or twenty-four frames a second. *[In 2017, the usual frame rate is around 24 per second.* **MA***]*

The human eye and mind are quite capable of this rapidity of action without any effort or strain. Indeed, it is only when the eye is able to shift so rapidly that the eye and mind are at rest and the efficiency of both is at a maximum. It is true that every motion of the eye produces an error of refraction, because the eye then has to refocus. But when the

movement is short, the error is very slight. Usually the shifts are so rapid that the error does not last long enough to be detected by the retinoscope. When the eye movements are reduced to less than four or five per second, it becomes possible to detect the errors in refraction produced by shifts in gaze with the retinoscope.

Perfect Sight Requires Continuous Shifting

Basically, each time the eye looks somewhere different, it takes a fraction of a second to refocus. The period during which the eye is at rest is much longer than the period during which the eye is refocusing. Hence, when the eye shifts normally, no error of refraction is manifest. The more rapid the unconscious shifting of the eye, the better the vision. But if one tries to consciously shift too rapidly, a strain will be produced.

Perfect sight is impossible without continual shifting, and such shifting is a striking illustration of the mental control necessary for normal vision. It requires perfect mental control to think of thousands of things in a fraction of a second. Each point of fixation has to be thought of separately, because it is impossible to think of two things perfectly at the same time. The eye with imperfect sight tries to accomplish the impossible by looking fixedly at one point for an appreciable length of time; that is, by staring. When it looks at a strange letter and does not see it, it keeps on looking at it in an effort to see it better. Such efforts always fail, and are an important factor in the production of imperfect sight.

Shifting Among the Best of Methods to Improve the Sight

Shifting is one of the best methods of improving the sight. When we shift, we consciously imitate the unconscious shifting of normal vision. We consciously appreciate the apparent motion produced when the eyes move about. Whether one has imperfect or normal sight, conscious shifting and swinging are a great help and advantage to the eye. Both imperfect and normal sight can be improved by shifting. When the sight is imperfect, shifting, if done properly, rests the eye as much as palming. Proper shifting always lessens or corrects the error of refraction.

An eye with normal sight never attempts to hold a point more than a fraction of a second. The gaze is directed so that the point of interest falls on the fovea, which is where the most detail is seen. When the eye shifts, the previous point always then falls on some other part of the retina. Therefore, the previous point of fixation is always seen less clearly. When vision is impaired, the eye ceases to shift rapidly. The point in the peripheral vision is no longer perceived as less clear as when it was at the center of the visual field. The person no longer experiences the fact that when we shift our eyes in one direction the world seems to swing in the opposite direction. These facts are the keynote of the treatment by shifting.

To reiterate, the previous point of fixation is not seen as clearly as the current point of fixation. This is because the image from the point of fixation in a healthy eye falls on the fovea. When the eye moves, that point then falls on a peripheral area of the retina. To appreciate that the previous point of fixation is seen less clearly, the eye with imperfect sight has to look farther away from it than does the eye with normal sight. If the eye shifts the gaze only a quarter of an inch, for instance, the eye with imperfect sight may see the previous point of fixation as well as or better than before. Instead of being rested by such a shift, the eye strain will be increased. There will be no perception of swing, and the vision will be lowered.

When the shift is a couple of inches, the eye may be able to let go of the first point. If neither point is held more than a fraction of a second, the eye will be rested by such a shift, and the illusion of swinging may be produced. The shorter the shift, the greater the benefit; but even a very long shift —as much as three feet or more—is a help to those who cannot accomplish a shorter one. When patient person is capable of a short shift, on the other hand, the long shift lowers the vision. The perception of swing is evidence that the shifting is being done properly, and when it occurs, the vision is always improved.

Swinging

It is possible to shift without improvement. It is not possible to produce the illusion of a swing without improvement. When this can be done with a long shift, the movement gradually can be shortened until the person can shift from the top to the bottom of the smallest letter on the Snellen test chart or elsewhere and maintain the perception of swing. Later, the person may become able to be conscious of the swinging of the letters without conscious shifting.

No matter how imperfect the sight, it is always possible to shift and produce a swing, so long as the previous point of fixation is seen poorly. Even double vision and multiple images seen by the eye do not prevent swinging producing some improvement of vision. Usually, the eye with imperfect vision is able to shift from one side of the test chart to the other and observe that the chart appears to move from side to side. Similarly, the eye with perfect vision is usually able to shift from a point above the test chart to a point below it and observe that it appears to move up and down.

Shift at the Near Point

Shift at the nearest point at which the eyes can focus. Sight is best at the near point, not only for the nearsighted but often for the farsighted as well. People who cannot see that the periphery is less sharp at distance can usually do it readily at the near point. Once the swing can be produced at the near point, the distance can be gradually increased until the same thing can be done at twenty feet.

If the degree of eccentric fixation is severe, it may be necessary to use some of the methods described in Chapter 11, "Central Fixation."

Shifting and swinging are often more successful after resting the eyes by closing them or palming. By alternately resting the eyes and then shifting, people with very imperfect sight have sometimes obtained a temporary or even permanent cure in a few weeks.

Shifting may be done slowly or rapidly. At the beginning, shifting too rapidly is likely to cause strain. In that case, the point shifted away from will not be seen less well, and there will be no perception of the swing. As improvement is made, the speed of shifting can be increased. It is usually impossible, however, to perceive the swing if the shifting is more rapid than two or three times a second.

A mental picture of a letter can, as a rule, be made to swing as precisely as can an actual letter on the test chart. Indeed, for most people, the mental swing is easier at first than the visual swing. When they become able to swing in the imagination, it becomes easier for them to swing the letters on the test chart.

Rapid progress is sometimes made by alternating the mental exercise with the visual one. As relaxation becomes more perfect, the mental swing can be shortened until it becomes possible to conceive and swing a letter the size of a period in a newspaper. This is easier, once it is accomplished, than swinging a larger letter. Many people have derived great benefit from this approach.

Transient Improvement

Without exception, everyone who shifts and swings successfully decreases their error of refraction. The retinoscope shows this. The improvement may be momentary or partial, but it is always there.

A moment of improvement may be so transitory that the person is not conscious of it. But once it is possible to imagine the shift and swing, it then becomes easier to maintain relaxation long enough to be conscious of improved sight.

For instance, a woman, after looking away from the chart, may look back to the largest

C. For a fraction of a second, the error of refraction may be lessened or corrected, as demonstrated by the retinoscope, yet she may not be conscious of the improved vision. By imagining that the C is seen better, however, the moment of relaxation may be prolonged enough for her to become conscious of it.

Universal Swinging

When mental or visual swinging is successful, a person may become conscious of a feeling of relaxation manifested as a sensation of universal swinging. Everything seems to be swinging. The motion may be imagined in any part of the body to which the attention is directed. It may be felt in the chair in which the person is sitting or seen in any object in the room. It may also be appreciated in any object that arises in the memory. The building, the city, the whole world, in fact, may appear to be swinging.

When a person becomes conscious of this universal swinging, the memory of the object with which it started is lost. So long as the person is able to maintain the vision or memory of movement in a direction contrary to the original movement of the eyes, relaxation is maintained.

It is easy to imagine the universal swing with the eyes closed, and some people soon become able to do it with the eyes open. Later, the feeling of relaxation that accompanies the swing may be realized without consciousness of the swing, but the swing can always be perceived when the person thinks of it.

There is but one cause of failure to produce a swing, and that is strain. Some people try to make the letters swing by effort. Such efforts

always fail. The eyes and mind do not swing the letters. The letters swing of themselves. The eye can shift voluntarily. This is a muscular act resulting from a motor impulse. But the swing comes of its own accord when the shifting is normal. The swing itself does not produce relaxation. The swing is an evidence of relaxation. The swing in and of itself has no value. It is only valuable as an indication that relaxation is being maintained.

EXERCISES:

The following methods of shifting have been found useful in various cases:

Exercise 1:

A. Regard a letter.

B. Shift to a letter on the same line far enough away so that the first is seen worse.

C. Look back at No. 1 and see No. 2 less clearly.

D. Look at the letters alternately for a few seconds, seeing the one not regarded less well.

When successful, both letters improve and appear to move from side to side in a direction opposite to the movement of the eye.

Exercise 2:

A. Look at a large letter on a test chart.

B. Look at a smaller one a long distance away from the large letter. The large one is then seen less well.

C. Look back and see the large letter better.

D. Repeat half a dozen times.

When successful, both letters improve, and the chart appears to move up and down (because the small letters are on the lower lines).

Shifting by these methods usually allows flashes of improved vision.

Exercise 3:

In order to see the letter well continuously, it is necessary to become able to shift from the top of the letter to the bottom, or from the bottom of the letter to the top. The person must see the part not directly regarded less well and must produce the illusion of a vertical swing.

A. Look at a point far enough above the top of the letter to see the bottom, or the whole letter, less well.

B. Look at a point far enough below the bottom of the letter to see the top, or the whole letter, worse.

C. Repeat half a dozen times.

If successful, the letter will appear to move up and down, and the vision will improve. The shift can then be shortened until it becomes possible to shift between the top and the bottom of the letter and maintain the swing. The letter is now seen continuously. If the method fails, rest the eyes, palm, and try again.

One may also practice by shifting from one side of a letter to a point beyond the other side, or from one corner of a letter to a point beyond the other corner.

Exercise 4:

A. Regard a letter at the distance at which it is seen best. In nearsightedness this will be at the near point, which is the closest point at which you can still focus.

Shift from the top to the bottom of the letter until you are able to see each point worse alternately. Then the letter will appear blacker than before, and an illusion of swinging will be produced.

B. Now close the eyes, and shift from the top to the bottom of the letter mentally.

C. Regard a blank wall with the eyes open and do the same. Compare the ability to shift and swing mentally with the ability to do the same visually at the near point.

D. Then regard the letter at a distance, and shift from the top to the bottom. If successful, the letter will improve and an illusion of swinging will be produced.

Exercise 5:

Some people, particularly children, are able to see better when the letters are pointed to. In other cases, this is a distraction. When pointing is helpful, one can proceed as follows:

A. Place the tip of a finger three or four inches below the letter. Regard the letter, and shift the sight to the tip of the finger, seeing the letter less well.

B. Reduce the distance between the finger and the letter, first to two or three inches, then to one or two, and finally to half an inch, proceeding each time as in Step A.

If successful, you will become able to look from the top to the bottom of the letter, seeing each peripheral spot less well and producing the illusion of swinging. It will then be possible to see the letter continuously.

Exercise 6:

When vision is imperfect, it often happens that the larger letters on an eye chart look more deeply black, even when vision is focused on the smaller letters. This makes it impossible to see the smaller letters perfectly. The cause of this appearance is eccentric fixation. In this situation, look at the letter seen best, then shift to the smaller letter. After a few repetitions, the smaller letter regarded directly will appear blacker than the larger one in the periphery. If you are not successful after a few trials, rest the eyes by closing and palming, and try again.

One may also shift from the large letter to a point some distance below the smaller letter, gradually approaching the small letter as vision improves.

Exercise 7:

Shifting focus alternately from a chart three to five feet away to a chart ten to twenty feet away often proves helpful. The unconscious memory of the letter seen at the near point helps to bring out the one in the distance.

It is a mistake to continue the practice of any method that does not yield prompt results. Different people will find the various methods of shifting more or less useful. If any method does not succeed, abandon it after one or two trials. Try something else. The cause of the failure is strain, and it does no good to continue the strain.

When it is not possible to practice with a Snellen test chart, other objects may be used.

One can shift from one window of a distant building to another or from one part of a window to another part of the same window. One can shift from one auto to another or from one part of an auto to another part. When talking to people, one can shift from one person to another or from one part of the face to another part. When reading a book or newspaper, one can shift consciously from one word or letter to another or from one part of a letter to another. In each case, it is possible to produce the illusion that objects are moving in a direction contrary to the movement of the eye.

Shifting and swinging give a person something definite to do. For this reason, they are often more successful than other methods of obtaining relaxation. In some cases, remarkable results have been obtained simply by demonstrating that staring lowers the vision and shifting improves it.

CASE: One patient, a girl of sixteen with progressive nearsightedness, obtained very prompt relief by shifting. She came to the office wearing a pair of glasses tinted a pale yellow and with shaded side panels.

In spite of this protection, she was so annoyed by the light that her eyes were almost closed, and she had great difficulty in finding her way about the room. Her vision without glasses was 3/200: She could see at three feet what a normally sighted person could see from 200 feet away. All reading had been forbidden. Looking at the notes on sheet music while playing the piano was not allowed. She had been obliged to give up the idea of going to college. Her hypersensitivity to light was relieved in a few minutes by

> *I STRONGLY RECOMMEND AGAINST SUN GAZING. IT MAY DAMAGE THE EYE. MA*

focusing the light of the sun on the upper part of the eyeball when she looked far down (see Chapter 17).

The patient was then seated before a Snellen test chart and directed to look away from it, rest her eyes, and then look at the largest C. For a fraction of a second, her vision improved. By frequent demonstrations, she came to realize that any effort to see the letters always lowered the vision. By alternately looking away and then looking back at the letters for a fraction of a second, her vision improved so rapidly that in the course of half an hour, it was almost normal for distance.

Then very small type was given her to read. Her attempt to read it at once brought on severe pain. She was directed to proceed as she had in reading the Snellen test chart. In a few minutes, by alternately looking away from and then at the first letter of each word in turn, she became able to read without fatigue, discomfort, or pain. She left the office without her glasses and was able to see her way without difficulty. Other people have benefited as promptly by this simple method.

CHAPTER 16

The Illusions of Imperfect Sight and of Normal Sight

People with imperfect sight always have illusions of vision; so do people with normal sight. But while the illusions of normal sight are evidence of relaxation, the illusions of imperfect sight are evidence of strain. Some people with errors of refraction have few illusions. Others have many. This is because the strain that causes the error of refraction is not the same as the strain that is responsible for the illusions.

The illusions of imperfect sight may relate to the color, size, location and form of the objects regarded. They may include appearances of things that have no existence at all, as well as various other curious and interesting manifestations.

Illusions of Color

When people regard a black letter and believe it to be gray, yellow, brown, blue or green, they are suffering from an illusion of color. This phenomenon differs from colorblindness. Colorblind people are unable to differentiate between different colors, usually blue and green, and the limitation is constant. People suffering from illusions of color do not see the false colors constantly or uniformly. When they look at a Snellen test chart, the black letters may appear to be gray. At another moment, they may appear to be a shade of yellow, blue, or brown. Some people

always see the black letters as red. To others, the black letters appear red only occasionally. Although the letters on the test chart are all of the same deep black, some may see the large letters black and the smaller ones yellow or blue. Usually the large letters are seen as darker than the small ones, whatever color they might appear to be.

Often different colors appear in the same letter. Part of the letter seems to be black, and the rest might appear gray or some other color. Spots of black, or of color, may appear on the white background. Spots of white, or of color, may appear on the black letters.

Illusions of Size

Large letters may appear small or small letters large. One letter may appear to be of normal size, while another of the same size and at the same distance may appear larger or smaller than the first.

A letter may appear to be of normal size at the near point and at the far distance. In the middle distance, though, it may appear only half of its actual size.

When people can judge the size of a letter correctly at all distances up to twenty feet, their vision is normal. If the size appears different at different distances, they are suffering from an illusion of size.

At great distances, the judgment of size

is always imperfect because sight at such distances is imperfect. This is true even for those with perfect sight at ordinary distances. The stars appear to be dots because eyes do not possess perfect vision for objects at such distances. A candle seen half a mile away appears smaller than at the near point, but seen through a telescope (which gives perfect vision at that distance), it will seem to be the same size as at the near point.

With improved vision, the ability to judge size improves. Errors of refraction have very little to do with incorrect perceptions of size. The correction of an error of refraction by glasses seldom enables people to judge size as correctly as the normal eye does. Different people with the same error of refraction and the same strength of lenses may differ greatly in their ability to perceive size. Take a person with 10 Diopters of nearsightedness. This is fairly severe. One such person with corrective lenses may be able to judge the sizes of objects correctly, although this is rare. Another person with the same degree of nearsightedness and the same strength glasses may see objects as only one-half or one-third their actual size.

Illusions of Form

When there are illusions of form, round letters may appear square or triangular. Straight letters may appear curved. Letters of regular form may appear very irregular. A round letter may appear to have a checkerboard or a cross in the center. In short, an infinite variety of changing forms may be seen.

Illumination, distance and environment are all factors in illusions of form. Many people can see the form of a letter correctly on the chart when the other letters are covered. When the other letters are uncovered, they suddenly cannot see the form of the letter in question.

The indication of the position of a letter by a pointer helps some people to see it. Others are so disturbed by the pointer that they cannot see the letter as well as when the pointer is absent.

Illusions of Number

Multiple images of a single object are frequently seen by people with imperfect sight. Multiple images may be seen with both eyes together, with each eye separately, or with only one eye.

The manner in which these multiple images make their appearance is sometimes very curious. For instance, a man with presbyopia read the word HAS normally with both eyes. The word PHONES he read correctly with the left eye alone. When he tried to read the word PHONES with the right eye alone, he saw the letter P as double. The imaginary image was a little distance to the left of the real one.

In this same gentleman, the left eye, while it had normal vision for the word PHONES, multiplied images when looking at a pin. When the shaft of the pin was in a vertical position, he saw multiple images of the shaft but only a single image of the head. When the shaft of the pin was in a horizontal position, he saw only a single shaft, but the image of the head of the pin was multiplied. When the point of the pin was placed below a very small letter, the point was sometimes doubled but the image of the letter remained single.

No physical error of refraction can

account for these phenomena. They are tricks of the mind only.

The ways in which multiple images can be arranged are endless. They are sometimes placed vertically, sometimes horizontally, sometimes obliquely. Sometimes the multiple images form circles, triangles or other geometrical forms. The number of false images seen may also vary from two or three to four or more. They may be stationary, or they may change their position with more or less rapidity. They also show an infinite variety of color, including a white even whiter than that of a white background.

Illusions of Location

A period following a letter on the same line may appear to change its position in a great variety of curious ways. The distance of the period from the letter may appear to vary. The period may even appear to be on the other side of the letter. It may also appear to be above or below the line.

Some people can see all the letters of a word, but they appear to be arranged in the wrong order. In the case of the word "AND," for instance, the word may appear as "ADN" or as "DNA."

The letters on a Snellen chart sometimes appear to be farther away than they really are. At a distance of twenty feet, the small letters may appear to be a mile away. People troubled by illusions of distance sometimes ask if the position of the chart has been changed.

All these things are mental illusions.

Illusions of Non-Existent Objects

When the eye has imperfect sight, the mind often imagines that it sees things that do not exist. One common illusion is that of "floaters." These are specks in the visual field. These specks are known scientifically as muscae volitantes, or "flying flies." They are of no real importance, being symptoms of nothing except mental strain. However, they have attracted so much attention and caused so much alarm that they will be discussed at length in Chapter 23.

Illusions of Complementary Colors

Many people with imperfect sight see afterimages in a complementary color. If they look at a white circle and then close their eyes, they then see a black circle. If they look at a green square and then close their eyes, they see a red square and so forth. Afterimages usually last only a short time.

These afterimages may also be seen with the eyes open, on any background at which the subject happens to look. They are often so vivid that they appear to be real.

Illusions of the Color of the Sun

People with normal sight see the sun as white, the whitest white there is. When the sight is imperfect, it may appear to be any color in the spectrum: red, blue, green, purple, yellow, etc. In fact, it has even been described by some people with imperfect vision as totally black.

The setting sun commonly appears to be red because of atmospheric conditions. But even when these conditions are absent and the setting sun is actually white, it may still appear red to people with imperfect vision. When the redness of a red sun is an illusion not due to atmospheric conditions, its image on the ground glass of a camera lens will be white, not red. The rays of the sun focused with a magnifying glass will also be white. The same is true of a red moon.

**I STRONGLY RECOMMEND
AGAINST SUN GAZING.
IT MAY DAMAGE THE EYE.
MA**

Blind Spots After Looking at the Sun

**CAUTION: ALL MODERN
PHYSICIANS WARN AGAINST
LOOKING DIRECTLY AT THE SUN.
I COUNSEL AGAINST DR. BATES'S
ADVICE HERE. MA**

After looking at the sun, most people see black or colored spots that may last from a few minutes to a year or longer but are never permanent. These spots are also illusions. They are not due, as is commonly supposed, to any organic change in the eye. Even the total blindness that sometimes results temporarily from looking at the sun is only an illusion.

The Cause of Illusions in Those with Imperfect Sight

All the illusions of imperfect sight are the result of strain in the mind. When the mind is disturbed for any reason, illusions of all kinds are very likely to occur. The strain that produces illusions is different from the strain that produces errors of refraction.

There is a different kind of strain for each and every one of the visual illusions. For example, if we strain to see color, there will be illusions of color. If we strain to see forms, there will be illusions of forms.

With a little practice, anyone can learn to produce illusions of form and color by straining consciously in the same way that one strains unconsciously. Whenever illusions are produced deliberately, it will be found that eccentric fixation and an error of refraction have also been produced.

The strain that produces multiple images is different again from the strain that produces illusions of color, size and form. After a few attempts most people easily learn to produce multiple images at will. Staring or squinting will usually make one see double if the strain is great enough. One can produce the illusion of several lights arranged vertically by looking above a light and straining to see it as well as when looking at it directly. If the strain is great enough, there may be as many as a dozen false images. By straining to see while looking to the side of a light or looking away obliquely at any angle, the false images can be made to arrange themselves horizontally or obliquely at any angle. The same is true of straining to look at a letter.

To see objects in the wrong location, as when the first letter of a word occupies the place of the last, is more difficult. This requires an ingenuity of eccentric fixation and an unusual education of the imagination.

The black or colored spots seen after looking at the sun, and the strange colors that the sun sometimes seems to assume, are also the result of mental strain. When one becomes able to look at the sun without strain, these phenomena immediately disappear.

> *AGAIN, I RECOMMEND AGAINST SUN GAZING. IT IS THE CONSENSUS OF THE MODERN MEDICAL COMMUNITY THAT GAZING AT THE SUN WILL CAUSE BLINDNESS. MA*

Afterimages have been attributed to fatigue of the retina, which is supposed to have been overstimulated by a color. The retina therefore seeks relief in the hue that is complementary to the original color. If the retina gets tired looking at the black C on a Snellen test chart, for instance, it is supposed to seek relief by seeing the C as white.

This explanation of the phenomenon is very ingenious but scarcely plausible. The eyes cannot see when they are closed. If they appear to see while closed, it is obvious that the subject is suffering from a mental illusion and that the retina has nothing to do with the matter.

Neither can the retina see what does not exist. If a white C appears on a green wall where there is no such object, it is obvious again that the subject is suffering from a mental illusion.

The afterimage simply indicates a loss of mental control. It occurs when there is an error of refraction, because errors of refraction are also due to a loss of mental control. Anyone can produce an afterimage at will by straining to see all parts of the largest C on the chart equally well simultaneously. If

one is relaxed and gazes with central fixation, one can look at the letter indefinitely without any such result.

Illusions of Twinkling Stars

The idea that the stars twinkle has been embodied in song and story and is generally accepted as part of the natural order of things. It can be demonstrated that this appearance is simply an illusion of the mind. While people with imperfect sight usually see the stars twinkle, the stars do not necessarily do so. Therefore it is evident that the strain that causes the twinkling is different from that which causes the error of refraction. If one can look at a star without trying to see it, then it does not twinkle. When the illusion of twinkling has been produced, one can usually stop it by "swinging" the star. On the other hand, one can start the planets or even the moon to twinkling if one strains sufficiently to see them.

Illusions of Normal Sight

The illusions of normal sight include all the healthy phenomena of central fixation. The letters on a test chart are perfectly black and distinct, but normal eyes see the point at the center of the vision most clearly. Everything else in the field of vision appears less distinct.

Healthy eyes may form the impression that one letter is blacker than the others or that one part of a letter is blacker than the rest. This is an illusion.

On the other hand, normal eyes may shift so rapidly that they seem to see a whole line of small letters all alike simultaneously. There is, in fact, no such picture on the retina. Each letter has been seen separately. If the letters are seen at a distance of fifteen or twenty feet, they could not be recognized unless about four shifts were made on each letter. To produce the impression of a simultaneous picture of fourteen letters, some sixty or seventy pictures, each with one point more distinct than the rest, must have been produced on the retina in sequence. The mind then assembles all those pictures into one clear picture. The idea that the letters are seen all alike simultaneously is, therefore, an illusion.

In illusions of normal sight, we have two different kinds of illusions. In the case of unhealthy vision, the impression made on the brain is in accordance with the picture on the retina but not in accordance with the fact. In healthy eyes, the mental impression is in accordance with the fact but not with the pictures on the retina. To be more specific, in unhealthy eyes, the retina receives a blurred image and the mind sees that image as blurred, which does not reflect the fact of the object seen. In healthy eyes, the mental image of what is seen is sharp, but the eyes have really seen many images in which only the center is sharp. It is the mind that assembles all these images into the illusion of one sharp image consistent with the fact.

Normal eyes usually see the background of a letter as whiter than it really is. In looking at the letters on a Snellen test chart, normal eyes see white streaks at the margins of the letters and between the lines. If the lines of fine type are covered, the illusion of white streaks between the lines disappears. In reading fine print, healthy eyes see a white more intense than the reality in the area between the lines

and the letters and in the openings of the letters. People who cannot read fine print may see this illusion, but they see it less clearly. The more clearly it is seen, the better the vision.

In healthy vision, the illusion of increased whiteness in the gaps is imagined unconsciously. In those with errors of refraction, imagining this illusion consciously can improve the vision.

One can of course use a magnifying glass to see small letters. When a person with normal sight does this, the illusion of increased whiteness in the gaps is not destroyed. However, the intensity of the increased white and black is lessened. With imperfect sight, the intensity of the white and black may be increased to some extent by a magnifying glass. However, it will remain less intense than the white and black seen by the normal eye. These facts demonstrate that perfect sight cannot be obtained with glasses.

The illusion of movement produced by shifting the eye (as described in detail in Chapter 15: "Shifting and Swinging") must also be numbered among the illusions of normal sight.

The appearance of objects as upright is also an illusion, since their image on the retina is actually inverted. This is the most curious illusion of all. No matter what the position of the head and regardless of the fact that the image on the retina is inverted, the mind always sees things as right side up.

CHAPTER 17

Vision Under Adverse Conditions Benefits the Eyes

According to accepted ideas of vision health, it is important to protect the eyes from a great variety of influences. These influences are often very difficult to avoid. Most people resign themselves to the visual demands of life, but with the uneasy sense that they are thereby "ruining their eyesight."

Bright lights, artificial lights, dim lights, sudden fluctuations of light, fine print, reading in moving vehicles, reading lying down and more have long been considered "bad for the eyes." Libraries of literature have been produced about the supposedly direful effects on the vision of such activities.

The truth is quite different. When the eyes are properly used, vision under adverse conditions does not injure them. In fact, vision under adverse conditions actually benefits the eyes because a greater degree of relaxation is required to see under such conditions. It is true that the conditions in question may at first cause discomfort, even to people with normal vision. But a careful study of the facts has demonstrated that only people with imperfect sight suffer seriously from using their vision under adverse conditions. If those with imperfect vision practice central fixation, they can quickly become accustomed to seeing under adverse conditions and derive great benefit from doing so.

Although the eyes were made to react to light, both the laity and the medical profession have a very general fear of the effect of light on the eyes. Extraordinary precautions are taken in our homes, offices and schools to temper the light, whether natural or artificial, and to ensure that it shall not shine directly into the eyes. Smoked and amber glasses, eye shades, as well as broad-brimmed hats and parasols are commonly used to protect the eyes from what is considered an excess of light. When actual disease is present, it is no uncommon thing for people to be kept for weeks, months and even years in dark rooms. Some even wear bandages over their eyes for long periods.

Little Evidence That Light Harms

There is only the slightest evidence on which to base this universal fear of light. Within the voluminous literature on the subject, one finds a tremendous lack of information. In 1910, Dr. J. Herbert Parsons of the Royal Ophthalmic Hospital of London addressed a meeting of the Ophthalmological Section of the American Medical Association. He said that ophthalmologists, if they were honest with themselves, "must confess to a lamentable ignorance of the conditions which render bright light deleterious to the eyes."

Since then, Drs. Verhoeff and Bell have

reported an exhaustive series of experiments carried on at the Pathological Laboratory of the Massachusetts Charitable Eye and Ear Infirmary. These experiments indicate that the danger of injury to the eye from light has been "very greatly exaggerated."

That brilliant sources of light sometimes temporarily produce unpleasant symptoms cannot, of course, be denied. But Drs. Verhoeff and Bell were unable to find, either clinically or experimentally, any evidence of injury to the eyes from exposure to light alone.

As for danger from the heat that may accompany bright light, they consider this to be "ruled out of consideration by the immediate discomfort produced by excessive heat." Drs. Verhoeff and Bell conclude, in short, that "the eye in the process of evolution has acquired the ability to take care of itself under extreme conditions of illumination to a degree hitherto deemed highly improbable."

In their experiments, humans as well as rabbits and monkeys were flooded for an hour or more with light of extreme intensity. They found no sign of permanent injury. The resulting blind spots in the field of vision disappeared within a few hours.

Commercial light sources were found to be entirely free of danger under any ordinary conditions of use. It was even found impossible to damage the retina with any artificial light source, except by exposures and intensities enormously greater than any likely to occur outside the laboratory.

Exaggerated importance has been attached by many recent writers to the ultraviolet part of the spectrum. Nevertheless, the situation was found to be much the same for ultraviolet

as for the rest of the spectrum: "under all practicable conditions found in actual use of artificial sources of light for illumination the ultraviolet part of the spectrum may be left out as a possible source of injury."

My Own Experience

The results of these experiments are in complete accord with my own observations as to the effect of strong light on the eyes. In my experience, such light has never been

> *AGAIN, I RECOMMEND AGAINST THIS. THIS MAY IN FACT INJURE THE EYES. ALSO, PLEASE REMEMBER THAT THE OZONE LAYER IS NOW THINNER THAN A CENTURY AGO AND UV RADIATION IS MORE INTENSE. MA*

permanently injurious. People with normal sight have been able to look at the sun for an indefinite length of time, even an hour or longer, without any discomfort or loss of vision.

Immediately afterward, these people were able to read a Snellen test chart with improved vision, their sight having actually become better than what is ordinarily considered normal. Some people with normal sight do suffer discomfort and loss of vision when they look at the sun. In such cases, the retinoscope always indicates an error of refraction, showing that this condition is due not to the light but to strain.

In exceptional cases, people with defective sight have been able to look at the sun, or have thought that they have looked at it, without discomfort and without loss of vision. However, as a rule, the strain in such eyes is enormously increased and the vision decidedly lowered by sun gazing. This is confirmed by the fact that afterward they are unable to read the Snellen test chart. In addition, blind areas and apparent spots (scotomata) may develop in various parts of the visual field. The sun may appear to be slate-colored, yellow, red, blue or even totally black instead of appearing perfectly white. After looking away from the sun, they may see patches of color of various kinds and sizes. These patches of color may continue for a variable length of time, from a few seconds to a few minutes, hours, or even months. In fact, one person was troubled in this way for a year or more after looking at the sun for only a few seconds. Even total blindness lasting a few hours has been produced.

Visible physical changes may also be produced by looking at the sun. I have seen sun gazing produce inflammation and redness of the white of the eye, cloudiness of the lens, cloudiness of the gel that fills the eyeball, congestion of the retina, swelling of the optic nerve and swelling of the blood circulation layer just behind the retina. These effects, however, are always temporary. The blind spots, the strange colors, even the total blindness that may occur are in fact only mental illusions. No matter how much the sight may have been impaired by sun gazing, or how long the impairment may have lasted, a return to normal has always occurred.

In addition, as soon as eye strain is relieved, there is prompt relief from all the symptoms mentioned. This shows that the adverse effects of sun gazing are the result not of the light but of strain.

Some people who believed their eyes to be permanently injured by the sun have been promptly cured by central fixation. This demonstrates that their blindness was simply

AGAIN, I RECOMMEND AGAINST SUN GAZING. THIS MAY IN FACT INJURE THE EYES. ALSO, PLEASE REMEMBER THAT THE OZONE LAYER IS NOW THINNER THAN A CENTURY AGO AND UV RADIATION IS MORE INTENSE. MA

functional *[i.e., that there was no physical injury.* **MA***]*

By persistence in looking at the sun, a person with normal sight soon becomes able to do so without any loss of vision. People with imperfect sight usually find it impossible to accustom themselves to such a strong light until their vision has been improved by other means. One has to be very careful in recommending sun gazing to people with imperfect sight. Although no permanent harm can result from it, great temporary discomfort may be produced with no permanent benefit. In some rare cases, however, complete cures have been effected by means of sun gazing alone.

CASE: One woman was extremely sensitive to normal daylight. An eminent specialist felt justified in putting a black bandage over one eye and covering the other with a smoked glass so dark as to be nearly opaque. She was kept in this condition of almost total blindness for two years without any improvement. Other treatments also failed to produce satisfactory results.

I advised her to look directly at the sun. The immediate result was total blindness, which lasted several hours. However, the next day the vision was improved. The sun gazing was repeated, and each time the blindness lasted for a shorter period. At the end of a week, she was able to look directly at the sun without discomfort. Before treatment, her vision had been 20/200 without glasses and 20/70 with them. After treatment, her vision improved to 20/10—twice the accepted standard for normal vision.

People of this class have also been greatly benefited by focusing the rays of the sun

> *AGAIN, I RECOMMEND AGAINST SUN GAZING. THIS MAY IN FACT INJURE THE EYES. ALSO, PLEASE REMEMBER THAT THE OZONE LAYER IS NOW THINNER THAN A CENTURY AGO AND UV RADIATION IS MORE INTENSE.*
> *MA*

directly on their eyes, marked relief being often obtained in a few minutes.

Like the sun, a strong electric light may also lower the vision temporarily, but it never does any permanent harm. In those exceptional cases in which the person can become accustomed to the light, it is beneficial. After looking at a strong electric light, some people have been able to read the Snellen test chart better.

Darkness Is Dangerous to the Eyes

It is not light but darkness that is dangerous to the eye. Prolonged exclusion from light always lowers the vision and may produce serious inflammatory conditions.

Among young children living in tenements, light deprivation is a somewhat frequent cause of ulcers on the cornea. These ulcers can ultimately cause blindness. The children, finding their eyes sensitive to light, bury them in their pillows and thus shut out the light entirely.

The universal fear of reading or doing fine work in a dim light is, however, unfounded. So long as the light is sufficient so that one can see without discomfort, this practice is not only harmless, but it may be beneficial.

Sudden Fluctuations of Light Are Not Harmful to the Eyes

Sudden contrasts of light are supposed to be particularly harmful. The theory on which this idea is based is summed up as follows by Fletcher B. Dresslar, a specialist in school hygiene and sanitation for the United States Bureau of Education:

"The muscles of the iris are automatic in their movements, but rather slow. Sudden contrasts of strong light and dim light are painful and harmful to the retina. For example, if the eye, adjusted to a dim light, is suddenly turned toward a brilliantly lit object, the retina will receive too much light and will be shocked before the muscles controlling the iris can react to shut out the superabundance of light. If contrasting changes in light are not strong, but are frequently made, the muscles controlling the iris become fatigued. They then respond more slowly and less perfectly. As a result, the retina is over-stimulated. This is one cause of headaches and tired eyes."

There is no evidence whatever to support these statements. Sudden fluctuations of light undoubtedly cause discomfort to many people. However, such fluctuations are not injurious. Indeed, I have found them to actually be beneficial in all cases observed.

The pupil of a normal eye, when it has normal sight, does not change appreciably under the influence of changes in the intensity of light. People with normal vision are not inconvenienced by such changes in brightness. I have seen a woman look directly at the sun after coming from a poorly lit room. Then, returning to the room, she was immediately able to pick up a newspaper and read it.

When eyes have imperfect sight, the pupils usually contract in the light and expand in the dark. However, I have also seen pupils contract to the size of a pinhole in the dark. Whether the contraction takes place under the influence of light or of darkness, the cause is the same: strain. People with imperfect sight may suffer great inconvenience and lowered vision from changes in the intensity of the light. But the lowered vision is always temporary, and when the eye is persistently exposed to these changes, the sight is benefited.

Such practices as reading alternately in a bright and a dim light, or going from a dark room to a well-lit one and vice versa, are to be recommended. During a movie, bright light rapidly alternates with the total darkness that occurs between frames. Even such rapid and violent fluctuations of light are, in the long run, beneficial to all eyes.

Other Activities That Are Also Not Harmful

I always advise people under treatment for the cure of defective vision to go to the movies frequently and practice central fixation there. They soon become accustomed to the flickering light. After the movies, other lights and reflections cause less annoyance.

Reading is supposed to be one of the necessary evils of civilization. It is believed that the deleterious influence of reading can be minimized by avoiding fine print and taking care to read only under certain favorable conditions. Extensive investigations as to the effect of various styles of print on the eyesight of school children have been made. Detailed rules have been laid down as to the size of the print, its shading, the distance of the letters from each other, the spaces between the lines, the length of the lines, and so forth. Various sizes and fonts are considered more or less damaging than others, especially for children.

All this is directly contrary to my own experience. Children might be bored by books in excessively small print, but I have never seen any reason to suppose that their eyes would be harmed by such type. On the contrary, the reading of fine print, when it can be done without discomfort, has invariably proven to be beneficial to the sight. The more dim the light and the closer to the eyes the fine print is held, the greater the benefit. Provided, of course, that the reader does not feel strain. By means of small type in dim light, I have seen severe pain in the eyes relieved in a few minutes or even instantly. The reason is that fine print cannot be read in dim light and close to the eyes unless the eyes are relaxed. By contrast, the eyes can strain when reading large print in good light at an ordinary reading distance.

When fine print can be read under adverse conditions, the reading of ordinary print under ordinary conditions is vastly improved.

Nearsightedness is always lessened when there is strain to see near objects. Nearsightedness is always made worse when there is a strain to see distant objects. Therefore, the nearsighted may actually benefit by straining to see fine print up close. This activity may counteract the tendency to strain in looking at distant objects. Even straining to see print so fine that it cannot be read is a benefit to some nearsighted people.

People who wish to preserve their eyesight are frequently warned not to read in moving vehicles. Many find no other time to read, so one cannot expect that they will ever discontinue the practice. Fortunately, reading in moving vehicles does not injure the vision. The vibration of the vehicle makes the book move about rapidly. At first, strain and lowered vision are always produced. But this is always temporary. Ultimately the vision is improved by reading in moving vehicles.

There is probably no visual habit against which we have been more persistently warned than that of reading while lying down. So

delightful is the practice that few, probably, have ever been deterred from it by fear of the consequences. It is gratifying to be able to state, therefore, that I have found these consequences to be beneficial rather than injurious. As with other difficult conditions, it is good to read lying down. The ability to read lying down improves with practice. In an upright position with good light coming over the left shoulder, one can read with the eyes under a considerable degree of strain. By contrast, lying down in dim light with the angle of the page to the eye unfavorable, one cannot read unless one relaxes. Anyone who can read lying down without discomfort is not likely to have any difficulty in reading under ordinary conditions.

Vision Under Difficult Conditions May Be Good Mental Training

The fact is that vision under difficult conditions is good mental training. The mind may be disturbed at first by the unfavorable environment. But after the mind has become accustomed to such environments, mental control and therefore eyesight is improved. To advise against using the eyes under unfavorable conditions is like telling a person who has been in bed for a few weeks to refrain from exercise. Of course, discretion must be used initially in both cases. The convalescent must not at once try to run a marathon. Neither must the person with defective vision attempt, without preparation, to out-stare the sun at noonday. But just as invalids may gradually increase their strength until the marathon has no terrors for them, so may eyes with defective sight be educated until all

the inconvenient rules of "eye hygiene" may
be disregarded.

CHAPTER 18

Optimums and Pessimums

Nearly all those with errors of refraction can see certain objects with normal vision. Such objects I have called optimums. Optimums are unique to each individual.

Everyone with normal sight has certain objects that they always see imperfectly. Such objects I have called pessimums. These objects are unique to each individual. The very sight of them produces an error of refraction that can be seen by the retinoscope.

An object is an optimum or pessimum according to the effect it produces on the individual's mind. In some cases this effect is easily accounted for. For many children their mother's face is an optimum, and the face of a stranger is a pessimum.

I knew a dressmaker who was always able to thread a No. 10 needle with a fine thread of silk without glasses. Then, when she had to sew on buttons, she could not see the buttonholes without glasses. Her color vision was so good that she could match samples without holding them up side by side. Yet even though she could see a black thread to thread a needle, she could not see a black line in a book. The line was no thinner than the thread. So needle and thread were optimums for her.

An employee in a barrel-making factory had been engaged for years in picking out defective barrels as they went rapidly past him on an inclined plane. He was able to continue this work after his sight for most other objects had declined greatly. By contrast, people with much better visual acuity when tested were unable to detect the same defective barrels.

In these cases, the familiarity of the objects made it possible for the subjects to look at them without strain – that is, without trying to see them. Therefore the barrels were to the barrel maker optimums. The needle's eye and the colors of fabrics were optimums to the dressmaker.

Unfamiliar objects, on the other hand, are always pessimums. The eye always goes out of focus when it tries to see something unfamiliar.

Optimums and Pessimums Are Unpredictable

In other cases there is no accounting for the idiosyncrasies of the mind that make one object a pessimum and another an optimum. Indeed, an object may be an optimum for one eye and not for the other. An object may be an optimum at one time and not another. An object may be an optimum at one distance and not at others.

Among these unaccountable optimums one often finds a particular letter on the

Snellen test chart. One patient, for instance, was able to see the letter K on the forty, fifteen and ten lines, but could see none of the other letters on these lines. This is unusual because many other letters have a more simple outline and most people see them more clearly than the "K".

Pessimums may be as curious and unpredictable as optimums. The letter V is simple in its outlines. Many people can see the V when they cannot see other letters on the same line. Yet some people are unable to distinguish "V" at any distance, although they are able to read other letters in the same word or on the same line of the Snellen test chart. Some other people will not only be unable to recognize the letter V in a word, but they are even unable to read any word that contains it. In this instance the pessimum lowers their sight not only for the pessimum itself but for other surrounding objects as well.

Some letters or objects become pessimums only in particular situations. A letter, for instance, may be a pessimum when located at the end or at the beginning of a line or sentence, and not in other places. When the attention of the patient is called to the fact that a letter seen in one location ought logically to be seen equally well in others, the letter often ceases to be a pessimum in any situation.

A pessimum, like an optimum, may be lost and later return. It may vary according to the light and distance. An object that is a pessimum in moderate light may not be so when the light is increased or diminished. A pessimum at twenty feet may not be one at two feet or thirty feet. An object that is a pessimum when directly regarded may be

seen with normal vision in the peripheral vision.

For Most, the Snellen Chart Is a Pessimum

For most people, the Snellen test chart is a pessimum. *[This means that most people are walking around with glasses that are too strong for them.* **MA***]* If you can see the Snellen test chart with normal vision, you can see almost anything else in the world.

Patients who cannot see the letters on the Snellen test chart can often see with normal sight other objects of the same size and at the same distance. When there are letters that are hard to see in the field of vision, the retinoscope shows that the error of refraction is always increased. The patient may regard a blank white poster without any error of refraction. The lower part of a Snellen test chart may appear to him just as blank because his vision is so poor and the letters are so small. But when he looks at the apparently blank test chart an error of refraction can always be demonstrated with the retinoscope. Even when the larger visible letters of the Snellen test chart are covered, an error of refraction is produced just because the patient knows that the letters are there behind the covering.

The pessimum may, in short, be letters or objects that the patient is not conscious of seeing. This phenomenon is very common. The clarity of the point in the center of the visual field may decline the moment the Snellen test chart is seen subliminally in the periphery of the vision.

For instance, a patient may regard an area

of green wallpaper at a distance. She may see the green color as well as she does at the near point. If I then place a Snellen test chart in the neighborhood of the green wallpaper, the retinoscope may suddenly show an error of refraction.

When the vision improves, the number of letters on the Snellen test chart that are pessimums diminishes and the number of letters that are optimums increases. Eventually, the whole chart becomes an optimum.

A pessimum, like an optimum, is a manifestation of the mind. It is something associated with a strain to see. An optimum is something that has no such association. A pessimum is not caused by an error of refraction. The pessimum produces an error of refraction. When the visual strain has been relieved, the object ceases to be a pessimum and becomes an optimum.

CHAPTER 19

The Relief of Pain and Other Symptoms

by the Aid of Memory

People who cure their vision are also often relieved of pain. They are often relieved of pain not only in the eyes and head, but in other parts of the body as well. Even pain caused by some physical disease or physical injury is often relieved.

In many patients, this relief was so striking that I investigated some thousands of cases. I found it to be a fact that people with perfect sight, or the memory of perfect sight, do not suffer pain in any part of the body. By contrast I have been able to produce pain in various parts of the body by a strain or effort to see.

For the relief of pain, we do not need perfect visual perception of form. We need only see a color perfectly, and the easiest color to see perfectly is black.

Perfect sight is never continuous. Careful scientific tests have shown that perfect sight is seldom maintained for more than even a few minutes. For practical purposes in the relief of pain, therefore, the memory is more useful than sight.

When black is remembered perfectly, a temporary, if not a permanent, relief of pain always results. The skin may then be pricked by a sharp instrument without causing discomfort. The lobe of the ear may be pinched between the nails of the thumb and first finger and no pain will be felt. At the

same time, the sense of touch becomes more acute. The senses of taste, smell and hearing are also improved, while the efficiency of the mind is increased. The ability to distinguish different temperatures is increased, but one does not suffer from heat or cold. Physical conditions may not be changed, but all of the functional consequences, such as fever, weakness, and shock, are relieved.

Patients who have learned to remember black under all circumstances no longer dread the dentist. When they remember a perfectly black period, the drill causes them no pain. They are not annoyed even by the extraction of teeth. It is possible to perform surgical operations without anesthetics when the patient is able to remember black perfectly

The following are only a few of many striking cases that demonstrate relief or prevention of pain by this means:

CASE: A woman suffered from ulcerations of the eyeball. These occurred intermittently and finally resulted in the formation of holes through which the fluids inside the eyeball were escaping. These openings had to be closed by surgery. At first these operations were performed under the influence of cocaine,

141

which is a local anesthetic. Eventually the progression of the disease caused so much congestion of the circulation that local anesthetics no longer worked. General anesthetics such as ether and chloroform had to be used.

As so many surgeries were needed, it became desirable to get along, if possible, without anesthetics. The patient's success in relieving her everyday pain by the memory of black suggested that she might also be able to prevent the pain of surgery in the same way. Her ability to do this was tested by touching her eyeball lightly with a blunt instrument. At first she forgot the black as soon as the instrument touched her eye. Later she became able to remember it. The operation was then successfully performed. The patient felt no pain, and her self-control was better than when cocaine had been used.

Later, fourteen more operations were performed under the same conditions. The patient suffered no pain. More remarkably, she had no pain or soreness afterward.

The patient stated that knowing the surgeon and having confidence in him was very helpful. She felt that if she had been operated on by a stranger, she would have been too nervous to maintain the memory of the black period. However, later she was treated by a strange dentist. He made two extractions and did some other work, all without causing her any discomfort. She had been able to remember the period perfectly even under these circumstances.

CASE: A man who had been extremely nervous in the dentist's chair had undergone four extractions made under anesthetic gas. When he learned how to relieve pain by the memory of a black period, he surprised his dentist. He was able to have an extraction without any anesthesia. The dentist complimented him on his nerve and looked incredulous when the patient said he had felt no pain at all.

CASE: In another case, that of a woman, the dentist removed the nerve from three teeth without causing the patient any pain.

CASE: A boy of fourteen came to the Emergency Room with a foreign body deeply embedded in his cornea. He was in great pain. Using local anesthetics, a number of physicians tried to remove the foreign body. They were unable to do so because the child could not hold still.

The boy was told to look at a black object, then to close and cover his eyes. He was told to think of the black object until he saw black. He was soon able to do this, and the pain in his eye was relieved. He was next taught to remember the black with his eyes open. The foreign body was then removed from the cornea. The operation was one of much difficulty and required considerable time, but the boy felt no pain. While the operation was in progress he was asked if he was still remembering black. "You bet I am," he replied.

CASE: In the same hospital, a surgeon from the accident ward visited the eye clinic with a friend suffering from pain in his eyes and head. The patient was benefited very quickly by these relaxation methods. The surgeon said this was unusual, and spoke slightingly of my methods. I challenged him to bring me a patient with pain that I could not relieve in five minutes.

"All right," he said. "I want you to understand that I am from Missouri."

He returned soon with a woman who had a brain tumor. She had suffered severe pain in her head for several years. She had been operated on a number of times and had been hospitalized for many months.

I doubted the existence of a brain tumor, but I said: "Brain tumor or no brain tumor, my assistant will stop the pain in five minutes."

The surgeon took out his watch, opened it, looked at the time, and told my assistant to go ahead. The patient was directed to look at a large black letter, note its blackness, then to cover her closed eyes with the palms of her hands, shutting out all the light. She was then told to remember the blackness of the letter until she saw nothing but black.

In less than three minutes she said, "I now see everything perfectly black. I feel no pain in my head. I am completely relieved, and I thank you very much."

The surgeon looked bewildered and left the room without a word.

To prevent a relapse, the patient was advised to palm every day six times or more. The pain did not return, and she came to the clinic some weeks later to express her gratitude.

Sometimes the memory of perfect sight not only relieves pain but actually causes the cure of an illness. Coughs, colds, hay fever, rheumatism and glaucoma are among the conditions that I have seen relieved in this way.

CASE: A woman under treatment for imperfect sight from a high degree of mixed astigmatism one day came to the office with a severe cold. She coughed continually, and there was a profuse discharge from both eyes and nose. There was severe pain in the eyes and head as well as some fever. She was unable to breathe through her nose because of the inflammatory swelling.

Palming was successful in half an hour. The pain and discharge ceased, the nose opened, and the breathing and body temperature became normal. The benefit was permanent—a very unusual thing after one treatment.

CASE: A boy of four years had whooping cough. The cough was always relieved by covering his eyes and remembering black. The relapses became less frequent, and in a few weeks he had completely recovered.

CASE: A man suffered every summer from attacks of hay fever. They began in June and lasted throughout the season. All his symptoms were completely relieved by palming for half an hour. After three years, there were no relapses.

CASE: A man of sixty-five was treated for rheumatism for six months with no improvement. He obtained temporary relief by palming. By the time his vision had become normal, the relief of the rheumatism was complete.

In many cases of glaucoma, both the pain and the increased pressure inside the eye have been completely relieved by palming. In some cases, permanent relief of the increased pressure inside the eye has followed one treatment. In other cases, many treatments have been required.

The mechanism of action of many medicines has not yet been explained. In the same way, I cannot as yet explain why the memory of black should have the effect of relieving pain. It is evident that the body must be less susceptible to disturbances of all kinds when the mind is under control. Only when the mind is under control can black be remembered perfectly.

That pain can be produced in any part of the body by the action of the mind is not a new observation. If the mind can produce pain, it is not surprising that it should also be able to relieve pain and the conditions that produce it. This, doubtless, is the explanation of some of the remarkable cures reported by Faith Curists and Christian Scientists. Whatever the explanation, however, the facts have been attested to by numerous proofs and are of the greatest practical value.

With a little training, anyone with good sight can be taught to remember black perfectly with the eyes closed and covered. With a little more training, anyone can learn to remember black perfectly with the eyes open.

When one is suffering extreme pain, however, the control of the memory may be difficult. The assistance of someone who understands the method may be necessary. With such assistance, improvement in pain is almost always possible.

CHAPTER 20

Presbyopia: Its Cause and Cure

To change the focus of the eyes from far away to close up is to accommodate. Among people living under civilized conditions, the accommodative power of the eye gradually declines with age. In most cases, by the age of sixty or seventy, it appears to have been entirely lost. The individual becomes absolutely dependent on glasses for vision at the near point. This onset of farsightedness with age is called presbyopia.

As to whether the same thing happens among indigenous people or people living under indigenous conditions, very little information is available. One authority says that the power of accommodation diminishes at the same rate regardless of how we use our eyes. People who use their eyes a lot at the near point get presbyopia at the same age as farmers, sailors and others who use their eyes mainly for distant vision. Other authorities say the contrary.

The eye always goes out of focus when it looks at something unfamiliar. This is a fact: Individuals who cannot read will manifest a failure of near vision when asked to look at printed characters. This occurs regardless of age and even when the subject's vision is otherwise perfect at the near point. If you test the vision of elderly indigenous people who cannot read, the fact that they cannot make out letters at the near point does not show they have presbyopia. It only shows that they are looking at something unfamiliar. A young illiterate would do no better.

Even among young students, the attempt to read unfamiliar type always results in imperfect sight, at least for a moment. Young students may be able to read Roman characters at the near point easily. These same students will always and immediately develop symptoms of imperfect sight the first time they attempt to read old English, Greek, or Chinese characters.

The Onset of Presbyopia

When the accommodative power has declined to the point at which reading and writing become difficult, the patient is said to have presbyopia. This condition is generally accepted, both by popular and scientific minds, as one of the unavoidable inconveniences of old age.

"Presbyopia is the normal quality of the normal eye in advanced age," says one expert. An endless number of similar statements can be easily found.

The decline of the ability to focus up close is commonly attributed to a number of factors. Most important is the idea that the lens hardens with age, so it cannot become more round to change focus. Also, it is thought that the resting shape of the lens naturally flattens with age. This focuses the eye more into the distance. To this is added the idea that, with advancing age, the physical composition of the crystalline lens changes in such a way that it does not bend light as much as it used to. Finally, it is theorized that the muscle responsible for causing the lens to change shape (the ciliary muscle) weakens and shrivels up with age.

The Progression of Presbyopia Is Not Always Predictable

So regular is the decline of the eye's ability to focus up close that tables have been compiled showing the near point that can be expected at various ages. From these tables, one might almost fit glasses for presbyopia without testing the vision of the subject. Conversely, one might judge people's age within a year or two from their glasses.

According to the depressing numbers in these tables, one must expect at thirty to have lost no less than half of one's original ability to accommodate. At forty, two-thirds of it would be gone. At sixty, the eye's ability to accommodate would be practically nonexistent.

There are many people, however, who do not fit this schedule. Many people at forty can read fine print at four inches distance. According to the tables, they should have lost that power shortly after twenty. Worse still, there are people who refuse to become presbyopic at all. Oliver Wendell Holmes mentions one of these cases in "The Autocrat of the Breakfast Table."

"There is now living in New York State," he says, "An old gentleman who, perceiving his sight to fail, immediately took to exercising it on the finest print. In this way he fairly bullied Nature out of her foolish habit of taking liberties at the age of five-and-forty, or thereabout. And now this old gentleman performs the most extraordinary feats with his pen, showing that his eyes must be a pair of microscopes. I should be afraid to say how much he writes in the compass of a half-dime—whether the Psalms or the Gospels, or the Psalms and the Gospels, I won't be positive."

There are also people who regain their near vision after having lost it for ten, fifteen, or more years. There are people who, in accordance with their optimums and pessimums, are presbyopic for some objects but have perfect sight for others. Many dressmakers, for instance, can thread a needle with the naked eye. With the retinoscope, it can be demonstrated that, in the moment they are threading the needle, their eyes are accurately focused up close. Yet these same people cannot read or write without reading glasses.

Every ophthalmologist of any experience has seen cases where the eyes do not become presbyopic. One hears of them at the meetings of ophthalmological societies. They are even reported in the medical journals. But such is the force of authority that when it comes to writing books, these cases are either ignored or explained away. Every new treatise that comes out repeats the old superstition that presbyopia is a normal result of growing old.

German Science

We have beaten Germany *[in World War I* **MA***]*, but the dead hand of German science still oppresses our intellects and prevents us from believing the plainest evidence of our senses.

Some of us are so filled with repugnance for Germans that we can no longer endure the music of Bach or the language of Goethe and Schiller. Nevertheless, German ophthalmology is still sacred, and no facts are allowed to cast discredit upon it.

Fortunately, for those who feel called on to defend the old theories, nearsightedness postpones the advent of presbyopia. Also, a decrease in the size of the pupil, which is said to often take place in old age, has some effect in facilitating vision at the near point. This is because as light passes by an edge, it is bent outward. In this case, the edge is the edge of the pupil. Reported cases of people reading without glasses when over fifty or fifty-five years of age, therefore, can be easily disposed of by assuming that the subjects must be nearsighted or that their pupils are unusually small.

If such cases come under actual observation, the matter may not be so simple. It may be found that actually these people are not nearsighted at all. They may in fact have normal vision or even be farsighted. The pupil may be of normal size. For the orthodox in ophthalmology, there is nothing to do with these cases but to ignore them.

Abnormal changes in the form of the lens have also been held responsible for the retention of near vision beyond the prescribed age. Some cases, for example, are explained by incipient cataract. When a cataract is developing, the lens swells. A thicker, swollen lens will have a closer focal point.

There are also cases of premature presbyopia. The theory then is that there is accelerated hardening of the lens and premature weakness of the ciliary muscle.

The final fact on the explanation of presbyopia is one of human behavior. No matter what the observation or how poorly it fits the prevailing theory, some explanation consistent with the German viewpoint on ophthalmology will be found.

Presbyopia is Preventable and Curable

The truth about presbyopia is that it is not "a normal result of growing old." Presbyopia is both preventable and curable. It is not caused by hardening of the lens. Presbyopia is caused by a strain to see at the near point.

Presbyopia is not necessarily connected with age. It occurs in some cases as early as the age of ten. In others, it never occurs at all, even into the far reaches of old age. It is true that the lens does harden with advancing years, just as the bones become more brittle and the structure of the skin changes. But since the lens is not a factor in accommodation, its hardening is immaterial. True, in some cases the lens may become flatter or lose some of its refractive power with advancing years. But in other cases, it has been observed to remain perfectly clear and unchanged in shape up to the age of ninety.

Since the ciliary muscle is also not a factor in accommodation, its weakness or atrophy can contribute nothing to the decline of accommodative power. Presbyopia is, in fact, simply a form of farsightedness. The difference between the two conditions is not always clear. A person with farsightedness may or may not be able to read fine print. A person at the presbyopic age may be able to read fine print without apparent inconvenience and yet have imperfect sight for the distance. In both conditions, the sight at both distance and the near point is lowered, although the person may not be aware of it.

When the eyes strain to see at the near point, the near point is always pushed farther away in one or all meridians. By means of simultaneous retinoscopy, it can always be demonstrated that when a person with presbyopia tries to read fine print and fails, the near point is always pushed farther away than it was before the attempt was made. This shows that the failure was caused by strain.

Even the thought of making such an effort to focus up close will produce strain. With such a thought, the refraction changes, as seen by the retinoscope. Pain, discomfort and fatigue are then produced before even looking at the fine print.

Furthermore, when people with presbyopia rest the eyes by closing them or palming, their ability to see up close always improves. They become able to read fine print at six inches, for a few moments at least. This again shows that the previous failure was caused not by any fault of the eyes, but by a strain to see. When the strain is permanently relieved, the presbyopia is permanently cured. I have seen this happen in many cases. I have seen this happen at all ages, up to sixty,

seventy and even eighty years.

I First Cured Myself

The first person that I cured of presbyopia was myself. I had already demonstrated by means of experiments on the eyes of animals that the lens is not a factor in accommodation. I therefore knew that presbyopia must be curable. I also realized that I could not look for any general acceptance of my revolutionary conclusions so long as I wore glasses myself.

At that time, I was suffering from the maximum degree of presbyopia. I had no accommodative power whatsoever. With glasses that enabled me to read fine print at thirteen inches, I could not read fine print at either twelve inches or at fourteen. This made quite an array of eyeglasses necessary.

The retinoscope showed that when I tried to see anything at the near point without glasses, my eyes were focused for distance. It showed that when I tried to see anything at a distance, my eyes were focused for the near point. My problem was to find some way of reversing this condition and inducing my eyes to focus for the point I wished to see at the moment that I wished to see it.

I consulted various eye specialists, but my language was to them like that of St. Paul to the Greeks, namely, foolishness.

"Your lens is as hard as a stone," they said. "No one can do anything for you."

Then I went to a nerve specialist. He used the retinoscope on me and confirmed my own observations as to the peculiar contrariness of my accommodation. However, he had no idea what I could do about it. He would consult some of his colleagues, he said, and asked me

150

to come back in a month. I came back in a month, and he told me he had come to the conclusion that there was only one man who could cure me. That man, he said, was Dr. William H. Bates of New York.

"Why do you say that?" I asked.

"Because you are the only man who seems to know anything about it," he answered.

Thrown on My Own Resources

Thus thrown on my own resources, I was fortunate enough to find a non-medical gentleman who was willing to do what he could to assist me, the Rev. R. B. B. Foote, of Brooklyn. He kindly used the retinoscope through many long and tedious hours while I studied my own case. I persisted in trying to find some way of accommodating when I wanted to read, instead of when I wanted to see something at a distance.

One day, I was looking from a distance at a picture of the Rock of Gibraltar that hung on the wall. I noted some black spots on the face of the rock. I imagined that these spots were the openings of caves and that there were people in these caves moving about. When I did this, the retinoscope showed that my eyes were focused for the reading distance even though I was trying to see far away.

Then I came closer and looked at the same picture at the reading distance, still imagining that the spots were caves with people in them. The retinoscope then showed that I was focusing close up, and I was suddenly able to read the lettering beside the picture. I had, in fact, been temporarily cured of my presbyopia by the use of my imagination.

Later I found that when I imagined that the close up letters were black, I was able to see them as black. When I saw them as black, I was able to distinguish their form.

My progress after this was not what could be called rapid. It was six months before I could read newspapers with any kind of comfort. It was a year before I obtained my present accommodative range, which extends from four inches to eighteen inches. This is an accommodative range of fourteen inches.

[It's unclear here how Dr. Bates is defining "accommodative range." Here are the modern definitions:

[In terms of distance, the accommodative range is the distance from six meters away to the closest point at which a person can focus. They use the measurement of six meters as the "far point" because beyond six meters the eye does not change focus much at all.

[In terms of Diopters, the accommodative range is the number of Diopters by which the crystalline lens of the eye can change in order to focus up close. The normal accommodative range in Diopters is 15 D. Of course this assumes that the eye accommodates by changing the strength of the crystalline lens, which was not Dr. Bates's opinion. **MA]**

The experience was extremely valuable, for I experienced in pronounced form every symptom subsequently observed in my other presbyopic patients. Fortunately for them, it has seldom taken me as long to cure other people as it did to cure myself. In some cases, a complete and permanent cure was effected in a few minutes. Why, I do not know. I will never be satisfied till I find out.

CASE: A man who had worn glasses

for presbyopia for about twenty years was cured in less than fifteen minutes by the use of his imagination. When asked to read very small type, he said he could not do so because the letters were gray and looked all alike. I reminded him that the type was printer's ink and that there was nothing blacker than printer's ink. I asked him if he had ever seen printer's ink. He replied that he had. Did he remember how black it was? Yes. Did he believe that these letters were as black as the ink he remembered? He did, and then he was able to read the letters. Because the improvement in his vision was permanent, he said that I had hypnotized him.

CASE: In another case, a man had suffered from presbyopia for ten years. He was cured just as quickly by the same method. When reminded that the letters that he could not read were black, he replied that he knew they were black but that they looked gray.

"If you know they are black, and yet see them gray," I said, "you must be imagining them gray. Suppose you imagine that they are black. Can you do that?"

"Yes," he said, "I can imagine that they are black." He then proceeded to read them.

These extremely quick cures are rare. In nine cases out of ten, progress has been much slower, and it has been necessary to resort to all the methods of obtaining relaxation found useful in the treatment of other errors of refraction. In the more

difficult cases of presbyopia, the attempt to read fine print often results in illusions of color, size, form and number. This range of illusions is the same as those that occur when people with farsightedness, astigmatism and nearsightedness try to read the letters on a Snellen test chart from a distance.

Those with presbyopia are unable to remember or imagine even such a simple thing as a small black spot when trying to see at the near point. When they do not strain to see, then they can remember a small black spot perfectly. Their sight for the distance is often very imperfect and always below normal, although they may have thought it perfect. Just as in the case of other errors of refraction, improvement of distant vision improves vision at the near point. However, regardless of the difficulty of the case and the age of the patient, some improvement has always been obtained. If the treatment is continued long enough, the patient has been cured.

Reading Glasses
Make Presbyopia Worse

The idea that presbyopia is a normal result of growing old is responsible for much defective eyesight. When people who have reached presbyopic age experience difficulty in reading, they are very likely to resort at once to glasses. In some cases, such people may actually be presbyopic. In others, the difficulty may be something temporary. If they had been younger, they might have thought little about it. Such temporary difficulties in vision pass away on their own if Nature is left to herself. But in the great majority of cases, eyeglasses, once adopted, produce the very condition they were designed to relieve. If the condition already exists, the glasses make it worse, sometimes very rapidly. Every ophthalmologist knows this. People soon find that they can no longer read large print without glasses, although they could easily read it before. This sometimes happens in a couple of weeks. In from five to ten years of beginning to wear glasses for presbyopia, the accommodative power of the eyes is usually gone. If from this point, people do not go on to develop cataract, glaucoma or inflammation of the retina, they may consider themselves fortunate.

Only occasionally do eyes refuse to submit to the artificial conditions imposed on them. In such cases, they may keep up an astonishing struggle against the artificial conditions for long periods.

CASE: A woman of seventy had worn glasses for twenty years. Nevertheless, without glasses, she was still able to read very small type and had good distance vision. She said her glasses tired her eyes and blurred her vision. Because she had been told that it was necessary, she had persisted in wearing them in spite of a continual temptation to throw them off.

People should follow the example of Dr. Holmes's gentleman friend and make a practice of reading the finest print they can find. Then the idea that the decline of accommodative power as a normal result of growing old would soon die a natural death.

CHAPTER 21

Strabismus and Amblyopia: Their Cause

[If strabismus or amblyopia are not topics of interest to you, I encourage you to skip forward to another chapter. This current chapter is not important to the discussion of the errors of refraction (nearsightedness, farsightedness and astigmatism). **MA***]*

[Dr. Bates titled this chapter "Squint and Amblyopia." Technically, squint and strabismus are two words with the same meaning. However, the common meaning of "squint" is very different, meaning to narrow one's eyes in an attempt to see more clearly. For this reason, I have used the ophthalmological term "strabismus" throughout. **MA***]*

In strabismus, the eyes fail to coordinate their movements. Instead of both eyes pointing at the object of interest, each eye points in a different direction. If the eyes appear to point too much inward, this is termed convergent strabismus. The common term is "cross-eyed." If one eye seems to point too far outward, this is termed divergent strabismus. The common term is "wall-eyed."

Technically, amblyopia just means "vision loss without obvious physical cause." In practice, amblyopia refers to a process that occurs in children seven years old or younger. One eye sees poorly, and the developing brain begins to ignore the input from the weak eye. Eventually the part of the brain that should receive input from that eye shuts down completely. The eye is then essentially blind, although it may still be physically normal.

In healthy vision, both eyes create one image. Part of the process of creating one image is to have the eyes move and point in a coordinated way. Once the brain no longer experiences input from a weak eye, this coordination no longer occurs, and the eyes may point in different directions. Thus amblyopia is one cause of strabismus.

In a child with strabismus from causes other than amblyopia, the brain may have trouble fusing the two images. The brain may then begin to suppress one of the images. Thus strabismus is also one cause of amblyopia.

In the act of sight, two pictures are formed, one by each eye. To fuse these two pictures into one, there must be perfect harmony of action between the two eyes. In looking at a distant object, the two visual axes must be parallel. In looking at a closer object, which for practical purposes is any object less than twenty feet away, the eyes must point inward to exactly the same degree.

The absence of this harmony of action is known as strabismus. Strabismus is one of the most distressing of eye defects because the eyes, which are the most expressive feature of the face, lose their symmetry. This is disconcerting to others.

The Cause of Strabismus Is Unclear

Strabismus has long baffled ophthalmological science. The textbook theories as to its cause fit some cases. These theories fail completely in explaining many other cases. Whatever the theory, all methods of treatment are very uncertain in their results.

The idea that a lack of harmony in the movements of the eye is due to a corresponding lack of harmony in the strength of the muscles that turn the eyes in their sockets seems natural. This theory was almost universally accepted at one time. Surgeries based on it once were very popular. These days, such operations are considered a last resort. It is true that many people have benefited by them. However, at best, the correction is only approximate. In many cases, the operation fails and the condition is made worse. A return of the ability to fuse the two images from the eyes into one is scarcely even hoped for with surgery.

Then Dr. Donders advanced the idea that strabismus is caused by refractive errors. Farsightedness was held responsible for the production of convergent strabismus. Nearsightedness was put up as the cause of divergent strabismus. The earlier muscle weakness theory fitted the facts so poorly that it was immediately discarded, and this new theory was universally accepted.

Unfortunately, the refractive-error theory as the cause of strabismus also proved unsatisfactory. Currently *[in 1920 **MA**]*

medical opinion is divided between various theories. One school attributes the condition to a defect in the nerve supply, in the great majority of cases. Another suggests that the faculty of fusion of the images in the brain is defective. Another suggests that the shape of the eye sockets is to blame.

To make any of these theories appear consistent, it is necessary to explain away a great many troublesome facts. The uncertain results of operations on the eye muscles is sufficient to cast suspicion on the theory that amblyopia is due to any abnormality of those muscles. Furthermore, there are many cases in which marked paralysis of one or more of the extraocular muscles has been observed. Frequently, no strabismus occurs as a result of this paralysis. When paralysis and strabismus do occur together, relief of paralysis may not relieve the strabismus. Conversely, relief of the strabismus may occur without relief of the paralysis.

Errors of Refraction
Do Not Produce Strabismus

A multitude of facts shows that the state of the vision is not an important factor in the production of strabismus. It is true that strabismus is usually associated with errors of refraction, but some people with strabismus have only very slight errors of refraction. It is also true that many people with convergent strabismus are farsighted, but many others are not. Some people with convergent strabismus are nearsighted. A person with convergent strabismus may have normal vision in one eye and farsightedness in the other or may even be blind in one eye.

Usually the vision of the eye that turns in is weaker than that of the eye that is straight. Yet this is not always the case.

With two blind eyes, both eyes may be straight or one may turn in. With one good eye and one blind eye, both eyes may be straight. However, as a rule, the blinder the eye the more marked the strabismus. However, exceptions to this rule are frequent.

The behavior of strabismus is often completely unpredictable. In rare cases, an eye with nearly normal vision may turn in persistently. Strabismus may disappear and return again. Convergent strabismus can change into divergent strabismus and back again. With the same error of refraction, one person will have strabismus and another not. A third will have strabismus first with one eye and then with the other. In a fourth, the amount of the strabismus will vary. One person with strabismus may get well without glasses or other treatment. Another person will get well with glasses and other treatments. These cures may be temporary or permanent. When there are relapses, they may occur either with or without glasses.

However slight the errors of refraction, the vision of many eyes with strabismus is inferior to that of the straight eyes. No apparent or sufficient cause for this can be found in the constitution of the eye. Opinions vary as to whether the defect of vision is the cause or the result of the strabismus.

Amblyopia

It is believed that with strabismus, the mind suppresses the image of the deviating eye in order to avoid the annoyance of double vision. With disuse, the vision in that eye becomes weaker and weaker. This view has been crystallized in the name given to the condition: amblyopia ex anopsia. Literally, this means, "dimsightedness from non-use." There are many people with strabismus, however, who do not suffer from amblyopia. Conversely, amblyopia has been found in eyes that have never had strabismus.

The medical literature on amblyopia is full of the impossibility of a cure. People having the care of children are urged to have cases of strabismus treated early, so that the vision of the eye with strabismus may not be lost. According to one author, not much improvement can ordinarily be obtained in amblyopic eyes after the age of six. Another author says, "The function of the retina never again becomes perfectly normal, even if the cause of the visual disturbance is done away with."

Yet it is well known that if the sight of the good eye is lost at any period of life, the vision of the amblyopic eye will often become normal. Furthermore, an eye may be amblyopic at one time and not at another. When the good eye is covered, the amblyopic eye may be so amblyopic that it can scarcely distinguish daylight from darkness. Yet when both eyes are open, the vision of the amblyopic eye may be found to be as good as that of the straight eye, if not better. In many cases, too, the amblyopia will change from one eye to the other.

Double vision occurs very seldom in strabismus, and when it does, it often assumes very curious forms. When the eyes turn in, the image seen by the right eye should be to the right, according to all the laws of optics. The image seen by the left eye should be seen to the left. When the eyes turn out, the opposite should be the case. But often the position of the images is quite the reverse. Often the image of the right eye in convergent strabismus is seen to the left and that of the left eye to the right. Often in divergent strabismus, the opposite is the case. This condition is known as paradoxical diplopia. *[Diplopia just means double vision.* **MA]** Furthermore, people with almost normal vision may also have paradoxical diplopia.

Strabismus Is Always Accompanied by Strain

All the theories suggested earlier fail to explain the foregoing facts. It is a fact, however, that in all cases of strabismus a strain can be demonstrated. Moreover, it is a fact that the relief of the strain is in all cases followed by cure of the strabismus, the amblyopia and the error of refraction.

It is also a fact that all people with normal eyes can produce strabismus by a strain to see. It is not a difficult thing to do. Many children derive much amusement from the practice, while it gives their elders unnecessary concern that the temporary strabismus may become permanent.

It is comparatively easy to produce convergent strabismus. Children usually do it by straining to see the end of their noses. The production of divergent strabismus is more difficult. However, with practice, people with normal eyes become able to turn out either eye, or both, at will. They also become able to turn either eye upward and inward, or upward and outward, at any desired angle. Any kind of strabismus can be produced at will by the appropriate kind of strain. Some people retain the power to produce voluntary strabismus more or less permanently. Others quickly lose it if they do not keep in practice. There is usually a lowering of the vision when voluntary strabismus is produced. At the same time, accepted methods of measuring the strength of the extraocular muscles seem to show deficiencies corresponding to the direction of the strabismus.

CHAPTER 22

Strabismus and Amblyopia: Their Cure

The evidence is conclusive that strabismus and amblyopia, like errors of refraction, are purely functional troubles. They have no innate physical cause. Since they are always relieved by the relief of the strain with which they are associated, it follows that any of the methods that promote relaxation and central fixation may be employed for their cure. As in the case of errors of refraction, strabismus disappears and amblyopia is corrected just as soon as the person gains sufficient mental control to perfectly remember a perfectly black period. In this way, both conditions can be temporarily relieved in a few seconds. Their permanent cure is a mere matter of making this temporary state permanent.

One of the best ways of gaining mental control in cases of strabismus is to learn how to increase the strabismus, or produce other kinds of strabismus, voluntarily.

CASE: In one case, a woman had divergent vertical strabismus in both eyes. When the left eye was straight, the right eye turned out and up. When the right eye was straight, the left eye turned down and out. Both eyes were amblyopic and there was double vision, with the images sometimes on the same side and sometimes on opposite sides. She suffered

from headaches.

Having obtained no relief from glasses or other methods of treatment, she made up her mind to an operation. She consulted a surgeon. The surgeon, puzzled to find so many muscles apparently at fault, asked my opinion as to which of them should be operated on. I showed the patient how to make her strabismus worse and recommended that the surgeon treat her by eye education without an operation. He did so, and in less than a month, she had learned to turn both eyes in voluntarily. At first she did this by looking at a pencil held over the bridge of the nose. Later she became able to do it without the pencil. Ultimately she became able to produce every kind of strabismus at will.

The treatment was not pleasant for her, because the production of all these types of strabismus gave her pain. However, this approach effected a complete and permanent cure, both of the strabismus and the amblyopia. The same method has proved successful with other patients.

Some people do not know whether they are looking straight at an object or not. They may be helped by looking more nearly in the proper direction. When the deviating eye looks directly at an object, the strain to see is less. The vision is consequently improved.

The good eye may be covered with an opaque screen or ground glass. This encourages a more proper use of the amblyopic eye, especially if the vision of that eye is imperfect.

Children of six years or younger can usually be cured of strabismus by the use of atropine eye drops. This can take many months, a year or longer. The atropine makes it more difficult for the child to see and makes the sunlight disagreeable. In order to overcome this handicap, the eyes have to relax. The relaxation cures the strabismus.

The improvement resulting from eye education in cases of strabismus and amblyopia is sometimes so rapid as to be almost incredible.

A few of many examples follow:

CASE: A girl of eleven had convergent vertical strabismus of the left eye. The vision in the left eye was 3/200; at the near point, the vision was so bad she was unable to read. The vision of the right eye was normal both for the near point and the distance.

She was wearing glasses when she came to the office but had obtained no benefit from them. When she looked away from the largest C with the left eye from a distance of three feet, she saw it more clearly than when she looked directly at it. I then positioned my hand three feet away from the chart and asked her to count my fingers. This so attracted her attention that she was able to see the large C less clearly.

The fact was then impressed on her that she could at will see the chart better or worse when she was looking away from it. I also asked her to note that when she looked away from the chart and saw it less well, her vision improved. When she saw the chart more clearly when she looked away from it, her vision declined.

She practiced seeing the chart less well when she shifted her gaze three feet away from it. Her vision then improved to 10/200. Her ability to shift and see the periphery poorly improved so rapidly by practice that in less than ten days, her vision was normal in both eyes. In less than two weeks, her vision had improved to 20/10. She could read very small type with each eye at from three inches to twenty inches.

In less than three weeks, her vision for distance was 20/5. That is to say that she could see at twenty feet what a normal person could only see at five feet. She read photographic type reductions at two inches, tests being made with both eyes together and with each eye separately. She also read strange test charts as readily as familiar ones.

She was advised to continue the treatment at home to prevent a relapse. At the end of three years, none had occurred. During treatment at the office and practice at home, the good eye was covered with an opaque screen, but this was not worn at other times.

CASE: A very remarkable case was that of a girl of fourteen whom I treated. She had had strabismus from childhood. The internal rectus muscle of the right eye had been cut when she was two years old, but she still pulled the eye inward.

I prescribed glasses which blocked the vision in her good eye completely. The aim was to strengthen the weak eye by making it work. She objected to wearing these glasses because her friends teased her. She decided the odd-looking glasses made her more conspicuous than the strabismus. One day she lost her glasses in the snow. Her father, who was a man of strong character, immediately provided another pair. Then she announced that she was ill and couldn't go to school. I told the father that his daughter was hysterical. She was simply imagining she was ill to avoid treatment. He insisted that she continue treatment. As she did not consider herself well enough to come to see me, I called on her. With the assistance of her father, she was made to understand that she would have to continue treatment until she was cured. She at once went to work with such energy and intelligence that in half an hour, the vision of the eye with strabismus and amblyopia had improved from 3/200 to 20/30. She also became able to read fine print at twelve inches.

She went back to school wearing the ground glass over her good eye, but whenever she wanted to see, she looked over the top of it. Her father followed her to school and insisted that she use the weak eye instead of the strong one. She became convinced that the simplest way out of her troubles would be to follow my

instructions. Then, in less than a week, the strabismus was corrected and she had perfect vision in both eyes.

At the beginning of the treatment, she could not count fingers at three feet with the weaker eye. Three weeks later, including all the time that she had wasted, she had perfect sight.

CASE: A girl of eight had amblyopia and strabismus since childhood. The vision of the right eye was 10/40, while that of the left was 20/30. Glasses did not improve either eye.

She was seated twenty feet from a Snellen test chart and the weaker right eye was covered. She was directed to look with her better eye at the largest letter on the chart and to note its clarity. Next she was told to look at a point three feet to one side of the chart. Her attention was called to the fact that she did not then see the largest letter as well. The point of fixation was brought closer and closer to the letter, until she appreciated the fact that her ability to see the letter was less even when she looked only a few inches to one side of it.

At that point she was readily able to recognize that when looking at a small letter, an eccentric fixation of less than an inch decreased the clarity of vision.

I then taught her to increase the strabismus of the better eye. Once this was accomplished, the good eye was covered, and I taught her how to lower the vision of the weaker eye by increasing its eccentric fixation. This was accomplished in a few minutes.

She was told that the cause of her defective sight was her habit of looking at objects with a part of the retina to one side of the true center of sight. She was advised to see by looking straight at the Snellen test chart. In less than half an hour, the vision of the left eye became normal, and the right improved from 10/40 to 10/10. The cure was complete in two weeks.

CASE: The following case was unusually prolonged, because as soon as one eye had been cured the defect for which it had been treated appeared in the other eye.

The patient was a girl of ten. She had imperfect sight in both eyes but her sight was worse in the right than in the left. The vision of the right eye was restored after some weeks by eye education. At that point, the left eye turned in and became amblyopic. The right eye was then covered. After a few weeks of eye education, the left eye became normal. The right eye then turned in and the vision became defective.

It was necessary to educate the eyes alternately for about a year before both became normal at the same time. This patient had congenital paralysis of the external rectus muscle in both eyes, a condition that was apparently not relieved when the strabismus and amblyopia were cured.

CASE: The patient was a girl of six. She was first seen on December 11, 1914. She had had divergent strabismus of the left

eye for three years. She had worn glasses for this condition for two years without benefit.

Her prescription was convex +2.50 Diopters for the right eye. For the left eye it was +6.00 Diopters combined with a cylinder for astigmatism (+1.00 Diopter Cylinder, axis 90 degrees). The visual acuity of the right eye with glasses was 12/15 and of the left 12/200.

I prescribed atropine for the right eye to partially temporarily blind it. This would encourage proper function of the weaker left eye. The usual methods of securing relaxation, such as shifting, palming, memory, etc., were used.

On January 13, 1915, her vision without glasses had improved to 10/70 for the right eye and 10/50 for the left. On February 6, the vision of the right eye was 10/40 and of the left 10/30. The eyes were apparently straight. Testing showed that both eyes were being used at the same time (binocular single vision).

On April 17, after about four months of treatment, the vision in the left eye was normal and there was binocular single vision at six inches. On May 1, the vision of the left eye was still normal. At the beginning of treatment, she had been unable to read with the left eye at all, even with glasses. She now could read very small type without glasses at six inches.

On August 16, 1916, she had an attack of polio that was then epidemic. The sight of both eyes failed. The muscles that turned the eyes in and out (the medial and lateral recti muscles) were paralyzed. The eyelids twitched, and there was double vision. Various muscles of the head, left leg and left arm were also paralyzed.

When she left the hospital five weeks later, the left eye was turned in and the vision of both eyes was so poor that she was unable to recognize her mother. Later she developed alternate convergent strabismus. This is a condition where the eyes alternate in their ability to fix on objects and see them.

On November 2, the paralysis in the right eye subsided. Four weeks later, the paralysis in the left eye began to improve. On November 9, she returned for treatment without any conspicuous strabismus, but she was still suffering from double vision. The images were sometimes on the same side and sometimes on opposite sides.

On November 23, the eyes were straight and the vision normal.

On July 11, 1918, the eyes were still straight and the vision normal. There was binocular single vision at six inches. At that point, atropine had been used in the right eye every day for more than a year and been used intermittently for a much longer time. The pupil was dilated to the maximum. Nevertheless, the eye read fine print without difficulty at six inches, central fixation overcoming the paralyzing effect of the atropine. According to current theory, the accommodation should have been completely paralyzed by the atropine, making near vision quite impossible.

The patient also read fine print with the left eye as well as, or better than, with the right eye.

CHAPTER 23

Floaters: Their Cause and Cure

Floaters are a very common phenomenon of imperfect sight. They are also called muscae volitantes or flying flies. These floating specks are usually dark or black, but they sometimes appear like white bubbles. In rare cases, they may assume all the colors of the rainbow.

Floaters move somewhat rapidly, usually in curving lines. They always appear to be just beyond the point of fixation. If one tries to look at them directly, they seem to move a little farther away, hence their name of "flying flies."

The literature on the subject is full of speculations as to the origin of these floaters. Some have attributed them to the presence of floating specks in the vitreous humor, the clear jelly that fills the inside of the eyeball from the back of the lens to the front of the retina. These specks could be dead cells or the debris of dead cells.

Similar specks on the surface of the cornea have also been held responsible for floaters. It has even been surmised that they might be caused by the passage of tears over the cornea. Floaters are so common in nearsightedness that they have at times been considered to be one of its symptoms. In fact, floaters also occur with other errors of refraction as well as in eyes that are otherwise normal.

Floaters have been attributed to disturbances of circulation, digestion and the kidneys. Some people have considered floaters evidence of incipient insanity because so many mentally ill people have them.

The patent medicine business has thrived on floaters. It would be difficult to estimate the amount of mental torment floaters have caused, as the following cases illustrate.

CASE: A clergyman who was much annoyed by the continual appearance of floating specks before his eyes was told by his eye specialist that they were a symptom of kidney disease. The specialist said that disease of the retina may be an early symptom of kidney trouble. So at regular intervals, he went to the specialist to have his eyes examined.

When at length his eye specialist died, he looked around immediately for someone else to make his regular eye exams. His family physician directed him to me. I was by no means so well known as his previous ophthalmologist. However, it happened that I had taught the physician how to use the ophthalmoscope and he thought that I must know a lot about the use of the instrument. What the clergyman particularly wanted was someone capable of making a thorough examination of the interior of his eyes and detecting at once any signs of kidney disease that might make their appearance. So he came to me at least four times a year for ten years.

Each time, I made a very careful examination of his eyes. I took as much time over it as possible so that he would believe that it was careful. Each time he went away happy because I could find nothing wrong.

Once when I was out of town, he got a cinder in his eye and went to another oculist to get it out. When I came back late at night, I found him sitting on my doorstep on the chance that I might return. His story was a pitiable one. The strange doctor had examined his eyes with the ophthalmoscope and had suggested the possibility of glaucoma. The doctor described the disease as a very treacherous one that might cause him to go suddenly blind and would be agonizingly painful. This ophthalmologist emphasized what the patient had previously been told about the danger of kidney disease. In addition, he suggested that the liver and heart might also be involved. The doctor advised him to have all of these organs carefully examined.

I made another examination of the clergyman's eyes in general. I paid particular attention to checking the pressure inside his eyes, since increased pressure inside the eyes can presage glaucoma. When the pressure inside the eyes increases, this can be felt by gently pushing on the eyeballs through the closed eyelids.

I had him feel his eyeballs and compare them with my own, so that he might see for himself that they were not becoming hard as a stone. I finally I succeeded in reassuring him. I have no doubt, however, that he went at once to his family physician for an examination of his internal organs.

CASE: A man on a ship returning from Europe was looking at some white clouds one day when floating specks appeared before his eyes. He consulted the ship's doctor. The doctor told him that the symptom was very serious and that it might be the forerunner of blindness. It might also indicate incipient insanity, as well as other nervous or organic diseases. He advised him to consult his family physician as well as an eye specialist as soon as they landed, which the gentleman did. This was twenty-five years ago, but I shall never forget the terrible state of nervousness and terror the man had worked himself into by the time he came to me. It was even worse than that of the clergyman. The clergyman, at least, was always ready to admit that his fears were unreasonable.

I examined the patient's eyes very carefully and found them absolutely normal. The vision was perfect, both for the near point and distance. The color perception, the fields of vision, and the pressures inside the eyes were all normal. Under a strong magnifying glass, I could find no impurity in the gel that fills the eye. In short, there were absolutely no symptoms of any disease. I told the patient there was nothing wrong with his eyes. I also showed him an advertisement for a quack medicine in a newspaper. This advertisement gave a great deal of space to describing the dreadful things likely to follow the appearance of floating specks before the eyes. Of course, the ad said, these terrible things could be avoided if you began right away to take the medicine in question at one dollar a bottle. *[One dollar in 1920 was equivalent to about $12.50 in 2017. **MA]***

I pointed out that the advertisement, which was appearing in all the big newspapers of the city every day and probably in other cities as well, must have cost a lot of money. It must, therefore, be bringing in a lot of money. Evidently there must be a great many people suffering from floaters. If floaters were as serious as was generally believed, I argued, then there would be a great many more blind and insane people in the community than there actually were.

The patient went away somewhat comforted, but two hours later he was back again. He still saw the floating specks and was still worried about them. I examined his eyes again as carefully as before. Again I was able to assure him that there was nothing wrong with them. In the afternoon, I was not in my office, but I was told that he was there at three o'clock and again at five. At seven o'clock he came once more, bringing his family physician with him, who was an old friend of mine.

I said to the latter, "Please make this patient stay at home. I have to charge him for his visits because he is taking up so much of my time. It is a shame to take his money when there is nothing wrong with him."

What my friend said to him I do not know, but the patient did not come back again.

I did not know as much about floaters then as I know now. If I had, I might have saved both this gentleman and the clergyman a great deal of uneasiness. Back then I could tell them that their eyes were normal, but I did not know how to relieve them of the symptom.

Floaters are the Result of Mental Strain

Floaters are simply an illusion resulting from mental strain. The specks are associated to a considerable extent with markedly imperfect eyesight because people whose eyesight is imperfect always strain to see. People whose eyesight is ordinarily normal may at times see floaters. This is because no eye has normal sight all the time. Most people can see floaters when they look at the sun or at any uniformly bright surface, such as a sheet of white paper on which the sun is shining. This is because most people strain when they look at surfaces of this kind. In short, the specks are never seen except when the eyes and mind are under a strain. The floaters always disappear when the strain is relieved. If one can remember a small letter on the Snellen test chart by central fixation, the specks will immediately disappear or cease to move. If one tries to remember two or more letters equally well at one time, the floaters will reappear and move. Usually the strain that causes floaters is very easily relieved.

CASE: A school teacher who had been annoyed by floaters for years came to me because the condition had recently grown much worse. She was slightly nearsighted. I was able to improve her sight to normal in half an hour. At that point, the floaters disappeared. The next day, the floaters came back, but another visit to the office brought relief. After that, the patient was able to carry out the treatment at home and had no more trouble.

CASE: A physician who suffered constantly from headaches and floaters was able to read only 20/70 when he looked at the Snellen test chart. The retinoscope showed mixed astigmatism.

When he looked at a blank wall or a blank white chart, the retinoscope still showed mixed astigmatism, and he still saw the specks. However, when he remembered a black spot as well as he could see it, there were no floaters when looking at these surfaces. At that point, the retinoscope indicated no error of refraction. In a few days, he obtained complete relief from the astigmatism, the floaters and the headaches. His chronic conjunctivitis also went away. His eyes, which had been habitually partly closed, opened wide. The whites of his eyes became pure white and clear. He became able to read in moving trains with no

difficulty. What impressed him more than anything else was that he also became able to sit up all night with patients without having any trouble with his eyes the next day.

CHAPTER 24

Home Treatment

It is not always possible for people to go to a competent physician for relief. As the method of treating eye defects presented in this book is new, it may be impossible to find a physician in the neighborhood who understands it. People may not be able to afford the expense of a long journey and the inconvenience of being absent from home and work.

To such people I wish to say that it is possible for a large number of people to be cured of defective eyesight without the aid of either a physician or anyone else. They can cure themselves. For this purpose, it is not necessary to understand all that has been written in this book or in any other book. All that is necessary is to follow a few simple directions:

Place a Snellen test chart on the wall at a distance of ten feet.

[Snellen test charts can be downloaded free from the internet. Here is my favorite:

http://visionsofjoy.org/

pdfs/VoJeyechart.pdf **MA]**

Devote half a minute a day or longer to this exercise:

With each eye separately, covering the other completely but with no pressure on it, read the smallest letters you can see.

Keep a log, recording the date. Each day, for each eye, write down the fraction shown to the right of the line of the smallest letters you can read, substituting the "20" on the left to "10," to indicate that you are doing the test from a distance of 10 feet. The number to the right indicates the distance in feet at which that sized letter can be read by what is considered normal vision.

With continued practice, you should be able to read smaller and smaller letters. When you feel ready, consider increasing the distance by five or ten feet, and continue this sequence as long as you wish.

If your smallest clear vision was 10/200, it would mean that the largest E on the one line, which can be read by those with normal sight at 200 feet, cannot be seen by you at a greater distance than 10 feet.

A vision of 20/10 would mean that the ten line, which the normal eye is not ordinarily expected to read at a distance greater than ten feet, can be seen by you at twice that distance. This is better than normal vision—a standard commonly attained by people who have practiced my methods.

Another and even better way to test one's sight is to compare the blackness of a letter at the near point and at a distance. This can be done in both dim light and good light.

With perfect sight, black is not altered by illumination or distance. It appears just as black at a distance as at the near point and just as black in dim light as in good light. If it does not appear equally black to you under all these conditions, then your sight is imperfect.

Children under twelve years who have not worn glasses are usually cured of defective eyesight by my method in three months to a year. Adults who have never worn glasses are benefited in a very short time—a week or two. Adults whose vision is not very bad may be cured in the course of three to six months.

Children or adults who have worn glasses, however, are more difficult to relieve. They will usually have to practice the various methods of gaining relaxation described in other chapters. They will also have to devote considerable time to the treatment.

Glasses MUST Be Discarded

It is absolutely necessary that the glasses be discarded. No half-way measures can be tolerated if a cure is desired. Do not attempt to wear weaker glasses, and do not wear glasses for emergencies. People who are unable to do completely without glasses under all circumstances are not likely to be able to cure themselves.

Children and adults who have worn glasses will have to devote an hour or longer every day to practice with the test chart and with other objects. It will be well for such people to have two test charts, placing one at the near point where it can be seen best and the other at ten or twenty feet. People will find it a great help to shift from the near chart to the distant one. The unconscious memory of the letters seen at the near point helps to bring out those seen at a distance.

If the person can secure the aid of another with normal sight, it will be a great advantage. In fact, people whose cases are obstinate will find it very difficult, if not impossible, to cure themselves without the aid of a teacher. To benefit those embarking on this practice, the teachers must be able to derive benefit from the various methods recommended. If their vision is 10/10, they must be able to improve it to 20/10 or more. If they can read fine print at twelve inches, they must become able to read it at six inches or closer. They must also have sufficient control over their visual memory to relieve and prevent pain.

A person who has defective sight, either for distance or the near point, and who cannot remember black well enough to relieve and prevent pain, will be unable to be of any material assistance in obstinate cases. Nobody will be able to be of any assistance in the application of any method that they have not used successfully.

Parents who wish to preserve and improve the eyesight of their children should encourage them to read the Snellen test chart every day. In my opinion, there should be a Snellen test chart in every family. When properly used, the Snellen test chart always prevents nearsightedness and other errors of refraction. It always improves the vision, even when the vision is already normal. Furthermore, proper use of the Snellen test chart always benefits functional nervous troubles.

Parents should improve their own eyesight to normal so that their children will not imitate wrong methods of using the eyes and so that their children will not be subject to the influence of an atmosphere of strain. Parents should also learn the principles of central fixation sufficiently well to relieve and prevent pain in order that they may teach their children to do the same. This practice not only makes it possible to avoid suffering but is a great benefit to the general health.

CHAPTER 25

Correspondence Treatment

Correspondence treatment is usually regarded as quackery, and it would be manifestly impossible to treat many diseases in this way. Pneumonia and typhoid, for instance, could not possibly be treated by correspondence, even if the physician had a sure cure and the mails were fast enough for the purpose. In the case of most diseases, there are serious objections to correspondence treatment.

But nearsightedness, farsightedness and astigmatism are functional conditions. There are not, as the textbooks teach, any physical, anatomical defects that cause errors of refraction. These malfunctions are caused instead by the way we habitually move and focus our eyes. So treatment by correspondence does not have the drawbacks that exist in the case of most physical illnesses.

It is true that one cannot fit glasses as well by correspondence as when the patient is in the office. However, even the fitting of glasses can be done at a distance, as the following case illustrates.

CASE: An old woman of color in the wilds of Honduras, far removed from any physician or optician, was unable to read her Bible. Her son, a waiter in New York, asked me if I could do something for her.

The suggestion gave me a distinct shock, which I will remember as long as I live. I had never dreamed of the possibility of prescribing glasses for anyone I had not seen. Besides, I had some very disquieting recollections of women of color for whom I had tried to fit glasses at my clinic.

If I had so much difficulty in prescribing the proper glasses under favorable conditions, how could I be expected to fit a patient whom I could not even see? However, the waiter was deferentially persistent. He had more faith in my genius than had I. Also, as his mother was nearing the end of her life, he was very anxious to gratify her last wishes.

So, like the unjust judge of the parable in Luke: 18, I yielded at last to his importunity and wrote a prescription for +3.00 D. The young man ordered the glasses and mailed them to his mother. A very grateful letter came by return mail stating that the glasses were perfectly satisfactory.

A little later, the patient wrote that she couldn't see objects at a distance that were perfectly plain to other people. She asked if some glasses could be sent that would make her able to see at a distance as well as she now saw at the near point.

This seemed a more difficult proposition than the first one, but again the son was persistent. I myself could not get the old lady out of my mind. So again I decided to do what I could.

The waiter told me that his mother read her Bible long after the age of forty. Since nearsightedness delays the onset of symptoms of presbyopia, I knew she could not have much farsightedness and was probably slightly nearsighted. I knew also that she could not have much astigmatism, for in that case, her sight would have always been noticeably imperfect. Accordingly, I told her son to ask her to measure very accurately the distance between her eyes and the point at which she could read her Bible best with her glasses.

In due time, I received not numbers but a piece of string about a quarter of an inch in diameter and exactly ten inches long. Based on this measurement and the laws of optics, I was able to calculate her probable refraction: A person with presbyopia who has lost the ability to accommodate would read best at thirteen inches when wearing +3.00 reading glasses. But she saw best with her reading glasses at ten inches. Her refraction, then, must have been 4 Diopters. Subtracting from this the 3 Diopters of her reading glasses, I calculated that she had 1 Diopter of nearsightedness. I accordingly wrote a prescription for -1.00 D. and the glasses were ordered and mailed to Honduras.

The acknowledgment was even more grateful than in the case of the first pair of glasses. The mother wrote and said that

for the first time in her life, she was able to read signs and see other objects at a distance as well as other people did. She said that the whole world looked entirely different to her.

Would anyone venture to say that it was unethical for me to try to help this patient? Would it have been better to leave her in her isolation without even the consolation of Bible reading? I do not think so. What I did for her required only an ordinary knowledge of optics. If I had failed, I could not have done her much harm.

In the case of the treatment of imperfect sight without glasses, there can be even less objection to the correspondence method. It is true that in most cases, progress is more rapid and the results more certain when the patient can be seen personally. However, this is often impossible. I see no reason why patients who cannot have the benefit of personal treatment should be denied such aid as can be given them by correspondence. I have been treating patients in this way for years, often with extraordinary success.

CASE: Some years ago, an English gentleman wrote to me that his glasses were very unsatisfactory. They failed to give him good sight and increased the discomfort in his eyes. He asked if I could help him. Since relaxation always relieves discomfort and improves the vision, I did not believe that I was doing him an injury in telling him how to rest his eyes. He followed my directions with such good results that in a short time, he obtained perfect sight without glasses for both the distance and the near point. The pain in his eyes was completely relieved. Five years later, he wrote me that he had qualified as a sharpshooter in the army. Did I do wrong in treating him by correspondence? I do not think so.

CASE: After the United States entered the European war *[WW I* **MA***]*, an officer wrote to me from the deserts of Arizona that the use of his eyes at the near point caused him great discomfort. Glasses did not help, and the strain had produced blepharitis of the eyelids. *[Blepharitis is a condition in which the eyelids become inflamed, especially at the base of the eyelashes.* **MA***]*

As it was impossible for him to come to New York, I undertook to treat him by correspondence. He improved very rapidly. The inflammation of the lids was relieved almost immediately. After about four months, he wrote me that he had read one of my own reprints—by no means a short one—in a dim light, with no bad aftereffects. The glare of the Arizona sun, with the government thermometer registering 114 F, no longer annoyed him. He could read the ten line on the test chart almost perfectly at fifteen feet. Even at twenty feet, he was able to make out most of the letters on the ten line.

CASE: A third case was that of a forester in the employ of the U.S. Government. He had nearsighted astigmatism and suffered extreme discomfort. Glasses were no help. He was able to rest his eyes from close work during long summers in the mountains, but this was also no help.

He was unable to come to New York for treatment, and although I told him that correspondence treatment was somewhat uncertain, he said he was willing to risk it. It took three days for his letters to reach me and another three for my reply to reach him. As the letters were not always written promptly on either side, he often did not hear from me more than once in three weeks. Progress under these conditions was necessarily slow, but his discomfort was relieved very quickly. In about ten months, his sight had improved from 20/50 to 20/20.

In almost every case, the treatment of patients coming from a distance is continued by correspondence after they return to their homes. Although they do not get on so well as when they are coming to the office, they usually continue to make progress till they are cured.

At the same time, it is often very difficult to make patients understand what they should do when one has to communicate with them entirely by writing. Probably all would get on better if they could have some personal treatment.

At the present time, the number of doctors in different parts of the United States who understand the treatment of imperfect sight without glasses is altogether too few. My efforts to interest them in the matter have not been very successful. I would consider it a privilege to treat medical men without a fee. When cured, they would be able to assist me in the treatment of patients in their various localities.

CHAPTER 26

Prevention of Nearsightedness in Schools:

Methods That Failed

The cause and prevention of nearsightedness has been the subject of more discussion and investigation than any other area of ophthalmology. Even the question of accommodation takes second place.

In contrast, farsightedness was supposed to be due to a deformation of the eyeball. Astigmatism was also supposed until recently to be congenital in most cases. These conditions were not thought to call for any explanation. Nor did anyone feel that either could be prevented.

Nearsightedness, on the other hand, appears to be acquired. Children may start out with normal vision and later become nearsighted. Or they may start out slightly nearsighted and later become severely nearsighted. So nearsightedness presents a problem of immense practical importance to which many eminent men have devoted years of labor. Voluminous statistics have been and still are being collected regarding its occurrence [in 2018 as well as 1920. **MA**].

The subject of the prevention of nearsightedness has produced libraries of literature, but very little light is to be gained from the perusal of this material. For the most part the reader is left with an impression of hopeless confusion. It is even impossible to arrive at any conclusion as to its prevalence, because there has been no uniformity of standards and methods in diagnosing it. Furthermore, none of the investigators has taken into account the fact that the refraction of the eye is not constant; it continually varies.

There is no doubt, however, that most children are not nearsighted as they begin school. It is also clear that both the number of cases and the degree of nearsightedness steadily increase as the educational process progresses.

Education and Nearsightedness Go Hand in Hand

Hermann Cohen, a professor in Breslau, first called attention to this subject. He published a study of the eyes of around 10,000 children that showed that the higher the level of education the higher the frequency of nearsightedness. In it he found scarcely one per cent of nearsightedness in the village schools. By contrast he found twenty to forty per cent in the secondary schools, thirty to thirty-five per cent in the high schools, and fifty-three to sixty-four per cent in the colleges. His investigations were repeated in many cities of Europe and America. His observations were everywhere confirmed, with some minor differences in percentages.

These findings were unanimously attributed to the excessive use of the eyes for near work. In the context of the theory that nearsightedness is caused by the eyeball being too long, this makes no sense. Why should the eyeball become longer and longer just because the lens is holding focus at the near point?

On the other hand, these findings make perfect sense from the point of view that the eyeball normally elongates to see up close. The shape of the eyeball becomes fixed in the elongated form because that is the shape in which it is being most often used.

Many authorities have theorized that near work increases intraocular pressure and that this causes the soft pliable eyeballs of the young to elongate. Authorities have also theorized that when children are born with farsightedness or astigmatism, they must strain to see up close. This strain, they believe, produces irritation that leads to nearsightedness.

Authorities have developed other explanations for when nearsightedness does not develop until adulthood. The fact is that a considerable number of cases of nearsightedness are observed among peasants and others who do not use their eyes for near work. This has led some authorities to divide nearsightedness into two categories—one caused by near work and one unrelated to it. These authorities attribute the cases that are not caused by near work to hereditary tendencies.

Many Attempts to Protect the Vision From the Process of Education

Abandoning the educational system is not an option. Therefore, attempts have been made to minimize the supposed evil effects of the reading, writing and other near work that education demands. Careful and detailed rules have been laid down by various authorities regarding every aspect of a schoolbook's format: the sizes of type to be used, the length of the lines, the distance between lines, the distance at which the book should be held from the eyes, the amount and arrangement of the light, the construction of the desks, the length of time the eyes might be used without a change of focus, and so on. Face rests were even devised to hold the eyes at the prescribed distance from the desk and to prevent stooping. There was a theory that stooping could cause congestion of the eyeball and thus encourage elongation of the eyeball. The Germans, with characteristic thoroughness, actually used these instruments of torture. One authority never allowed his own children to write without one, "even when sitting at the best possible desk."

The results of all these preventive measures have been disappointing. Some observers reported a slight decrease in the incidence of nearsightedness. On the whole, however, "the injurious results of the educational process were not notably arrested."

Another authority examined the eyes of 1,229 of the pupils at two high schools of Zittau, Germany. In these schools the conditions for good vision were all that could be desired. He found, nevertheless, that "the excellent arrangements had not in any degree lessened the incidence of nearsightedness."

Current Thought
Does Not Implicate Education

Nowadays, the trend is toward absolving the schools of responsibility for nearsightedness As the American Encyclopedia of Ophthalmology points out, "the theory that nearsightedness is due to close work aggravated by town life and badly lit rooms is gradually giving ground before statistics."

In an investigation in London, for instance, the schools were carefully compared to reveal any differences that might arise from various influences and circumstances. The proportion of nearsightedness in the best lit building of the group was actually found to be higher than in the one where the lighting conditions were the worst. It has also been found that there is just as much nearsightedness in schools where little near work is done as in those where much more close work is required.

Moreover, only a minority of all children become nearsighted, yet all children are subject to practically the same influences. Even in the same child, one eye may become nearsighted while the other remains normal. How could a theory that assumes that nearsightedness arises from external conditions account for this?

There is now a growing disposition to attribute nearsightedness to hereditary tendencies, but no satisfactory evidence on this point has been brought forward. Indeed, indigenous peoples who have always had good eyesight become nearsighted just as quickly as any others when subjected to the conditions of civilized life. Even those who hold to these theories of nearsightedness consider the use of the eyes at the near point under unfavorable conditions a secondary cause, this despite the repeated failure of preventive measures.

Another authority, Dr. Sidler-Huguenin, has observed so little benefit from precautions to prevent nearsightedness that he believes that it makes no difference whether a nearsighted person studies to become an engineer or takes up farming and forestry. He also made a study of people who have nearsightedness in only one eye. He published a series of 150 cases in which the subjects used only one eye because the other was so nearsighted. The weaker eye, he reports, became gradually more and more nearsighted even though it was not being used. This is in open defiance of all the accepted theories that overuse of an eye would make it more nearsighted. Based on these results, Dr. Sidler-Huguenin suggests that the use of nearsighted eyes may possibly be more favorable to their well-being than their non-use.

The prevalence of nearsightedness, the unsatisfactoriness of all explanations of its origin, and the futility of all methods of prevention has led some writers of repute to the conclusion that the elongated eyeball is a natural physiological adaptation to the needs of civilization. Against this view two unanswerable arguments can be brought. First is that the nearsighted eye does not see as well at the near point as does the normal eye. Second, nearsightedness tends to progress with very serious results, often ending in blindness. If Nature has attempted to adapt the eye to civilized conditions by an elongation of the eyeball, She has done it in a very clumsy manner.

It is true that many authorities assume the existence of two kinds of nearsightedness. One is physiological and harmless, the other is pathological. But since it is impossible to say with certainty which is which, this is not a useful distinction.

The Truth Is Simple

The misdirected labors of a hundred years have thus led us into a slough of despond and contradiction! But in the light of truth, the problem turns out to be a very simple one. In view of the facts given in Chapters 5 and 9, it is easy to understand why all previous attempts to prevent nearsightedness have failed: They have all aimed at lessening the strain of near work on the eye. They have not addressed the strain to see distant objects, and they have totally ignored the mental strain that underlies the optical one.

There are huge differences in the experience of a child raised in an indigenous society compared with those of a child raised in an industrialized society. Reading and writing is only one such difference. Civilized children are shut up for hours every day within four walls. For much of their waking lives they are in the charge of teachers who are too often nervous and irritable. Children are even compelled to remain in the same position for long periods. The things they are required to learn may be incredibly boring to them. They are under a continual compulsion to think of better marks and prizes rather than the joy of acquisition of knowledge for its own sake.

Some children endure these unnatural conditions better than others. Many children cannot stand the strain and as a result become nearsighted. Schools thus become hotbeds of nearsightedness as well as all other errors of refraction.

CHAPTER 27

The Prevention and Cure of Nearsightedness in Schools:

A Method That Succeeds

You cannot see anything with perfect sight unless you have seen it before. When the eye looks at an unfamiliar object, it always strains to see that object. An error of refraction is thus always produced. When children look at unfamiliar writing, numbers or images on the blackboard, the retinoscope always shows that in that moment they are nearsighted. This occurs even among those children whose vision is absolutely normal under other circumstances. The same thing happens when adults look at unfamiliar distant objects.

Lessen Eye Strain by Looking at a Familiar Object

When the eye regards a familiar object, the effect is quite otherwise. A familiar object can be regarded without strain. In fact, the strain of looking at an unfamiliar object can be lessened by first looking at a familiar object.

This phenomenon furnishes us with a means of overcoming the mental strain to which children are subjected by the modern educational system. It is impossible to see anything perfectly when the mind is under a strain. If children become able to relax when looking at familiar objects, they can then become able to maintain their relaxation when looking at unfamiliar objects. This sometimes

occurs in an incredibly brief period of time.

I discovered this while examining the eyes of 1,500 school children in Grand Forks, North Dakota, in 1903. Many of these children could not read all of the letters on the Snellen test chart at the first test, but they could read them on the second or third test. After a class had been examined, the children who had failed would sometimes ask for a second test. Then it often happened that they would read the whole chart with perfect vision. So frequent were these occurrences that there was no escaping the conclusion that in some way, the vision was improved by reading the Snellen test chart.

CASE: In one class I found a boy who at first appeared to be very nearsighted. Yet after a little encouragement, he read all the letters on the test chart. The teacher asked me about this boy's vision, because she had found him to be very nearsighted. When I said that his vision was normal, she was incredulous. She suggested that he might have learned the letters by heart or been prompted by another pupil. She said the child was unable to read the writing or numbers on the blackboard or to see the maps, charts and diagrams on the walls. He did not even recognize people across the street.

The teacher asked me to test the child's sight again. I did this very carefully, under her supervision. The sources of error that she had suggested were clearly eliminated. Again the boy read all the letters on the chart.

Then the teacher tested the child's sight. She wrote some words and numbers on the blackboard and asked him to read them. He did so correctly. Then she wrote additional words and numbers, which he read equally well. Finally, she asked him to tell the hour by the clock, which was twenty-five feet away. He was able to read the clock correctly. It was a dramatic situation. Both the teacher and the children in the class were intensely interested.

Three other cases in the class were similar. Their vision, which had previously been very defective for distant objects, became normal in the few moments devoted to testing their eyes. It is not surprising that after such a demonstration, the teacher asked to have a Snellen test chart placed permanently in the room. The children were directed to read the smallest letters they could see from their seats at least once every day. This was to be done first with both eyes together and then with each eye separately.

Those whose vision was defective were encouraged to read the chart more frequently. In fact, they needed no encouragement to do so when they found that the practice not only helped them see the blackboard but also stopped the headaches or other discomforts that had previously resulted from the use of their eyes.

Many Other Successes

In another class of six- to eight-year-olds, thirty out of forty were cured later under the supervision of the teacher by exercises in distant vision with the test chart. This teacher had noted every year for fifteen years that at the opening of school in the fall, all the children could see the writing on the blackboard from their seats. Then, by the time school closed the following spring, all of them without exception complained that they could not see what was written on the blackboard at a distance of more than ten feet.

This teacher saw the benefits of the daily practice of distant vision with familiar objects. She then kept a Snellen test chart in her classroom continually. She directed the children to read it every day. The result was that for eight years, no more of the children under her care acquired defective eyesight.

Prior to my visit, this teacher had attributed the invariable deterioration of the children's eyesight during the school year to the fact that her classroom was in the basement and the light was poor. But teachers with well-lit classrooms had the same experience. In both well-lit and poorly lit rooms, if the children read the Snellen test chart every day, the deterioration of their eyesight ceased, and the vision of all improved. Vision that had been below normal improved to normal, in most cases. Children who already had normal sight (20/20) became able to read 20/15 or 20/10. Not only was nearsightedness cured, but vision for near objects improved as well.

When Applied in Schools the System Works

At the request of the superintendent of the schools of Grand Forks at the time, the system was introduced into all the schools of the city. Before the introduction of the system, the incidence of nearsightedness was six per cent. After the system was used continuously for eight years, the incidence of nearsightedness fell to less than one per cent.

In 1911 and 1912, the same system was introduced into some of the schools of New York City, with an attendance of about ten thousand children. Many of the teachers neglected to use the Snellen test charts, being unable to believe that such a simple method could accomplish the desired results. Others kept the charts in a closet except when they were needed for the daily eye drill, lest the children should memorize them. Thus they not only put an unnecessary burden on themselves but did what they could to defeat the purpose of the system. They failed to provide the children daily exercise in distant vision with a familiar object as the point of fixation.

A considerable number of teachers, however, used the system intelligently and persistently. In less than a year, reports showed that of three thousand children with imperfect sight, over one thousand had obtained normal vision. Some of these children were cured in a few minutes. Many of the teachers were

also cured, some of them very quickly. In some cases, the results of the system were so astonishing as to be scarcely credible.

There was a class of developmentally disabled children where the teacher had kept records of the eyesight for several years. These records showed that the vision grew steadily worse as the term advanced. As soon as the Snellen test chart was introduced, however, the children's vision began to improve. Then came a doctor from the Board of Health who tested the eyes of the children and put glasses on all of them, even those whose sight was fairly good. The use of the Snellen test chart was discontinued, as the teacher did not consider it proper to interfere while the children were wearing glasses prescribed by a physician. Very soon, however, the children began to lose, break, or discard their glasses. Some said that the spectacles gave them headaches or that they felt better without them. In the course of a month or so, most of the eyeglasses disappeared. The teacher then felt herself at liberty to resume the use of the Snellen test chart. Its benefits were immediate. The eyesight and the mentality of the children improved simultaneously. Soon they were all drafted into the regular classes because it was found that they were making the same progress in their studies as the other children.

Truancy Decreased When the System Was Used

Another teacher reported an equally interesting experience. She had a class of children who did not fit into the other grades. Many of them were backward in their studies. Some were persistent truants. All of them had defective eyesight. A Snellen test chart was hung in the classroom where all the children could see it, and the teacher carried out my instructions literally. At the end of six months, all but two had been cured. The two who still had a defect in vision had nevertheless improved very much. At the same time, the worst incorrigibles and the worst truants had become good students.

CASE: One incorrigible had previously refused to study because it gave him a headache to look at a book or the blackboard. He then found that the test chart, in some way, did him a lot of good. Although the teacher had asked him to read it but once a day, he read it whenever his eyes felt uncomfortable. The result was that in a few weeks, his vision had become normal, and his objection to studying had disappeared. This truant had been in the habit of remaining away from school two or three days every week. Neither his parents nor the truant officer had been able to do anything about it. To the great surprise of his teacher, he never missed a day after having begun to read the Snellen test chart. When she asked for an explanation, he told her that what had driven him away from school was the pain that came in his eyes whenever he tried to study or to read the writing on the blackboard. After reading the Snellen test chart, he said, his eyes and head were rested, and he was able to read without any discomfort.

To remove any doubts that might arise as to the cause of the improvement noted in the eyesight of the children, comparative tests were made with and without the Snellen test charts present. In one case, six pupils with defective sight were examined daily for one week without the use of the test chart. No improvement took place. The chart was then restored to its place, and the group was instructed to read it every day. At the end of another week, all had improved and five were cured.

In another group with learning disabilities, the results were similar: During the week that the chart was not used, no improvement was noted. Then, after a week of exercises in distant vision with the chart, they showed marked improvement. At the end of a month, all the children in this group were cured.

That there might be no question as to the reliability of the records of the teachers, some of the principals asked the Board of Health to send an inspector to test the vision of the pupils. Whenever this was done, the records were found to be correct.

One day I visited the city of Rochester, New York. While there, I called on the Superintendent of Public Schools and told him about my method of preventing nearsightedness. He was very much interested and invited me to introduce it into one of his schools. I did so, and at the end of three months, a report was sent to me showing that the vision of all the children had improved. Quite a number of the children had obtained normal vision in both eyes.

The method has been used in a number of other cities and always with the same result.

The vision of all the children improves, and many of them obtain normal vision in the course of a few minutes, days, weeks, or months.

Since this system improved the vision of all the children who used it, it follows that none could have grown worse. It is therefore obvious that this system must have prevented nearsightedness. This cannot be said of any previous attempt at preventing nearsightedness in schools. All other methods are based on the idea that it is the excessive use of the eyes for near work that causes nearsightedness. All methods based on this view have failed.

It is also obvious that my method must have prevented other errors of refraction. This is an area that has not even been considered previously because farsightedness and astigmatism are considered congenital. However, anyone who knows how to use a retinoscope may demonstrate in a few minutes that both farsightedness and astigmatism are actually acquired. We know this because no matter how farsighted or astigmatic an eye may be, its vision always becomes normal when it looks at a blank surface without trying to see.

Children Need Eye Education

When children are learning anything that requires close work with unfamiliar objects, farsightedness or farsighted astigmatism is always produced. The retinoscope shows this, no matter the nature of the activity. The same is true for adults.

So far as I am aware, these facts have not been reported before. They strongly suggest that children need eye education, first and foremost. By daily exercise in distant vision with the Snellen test chart, children become able to look at strange letters or objects at the near point without strain. Then they can really progress in their studies. In every case in which this method has been tried, it has worked. When distant vision improves by daily reading of the eye chart at a distance, children invariably become able to use their eyes without strain at the near point.

This method succeeds best when the teacher does not wear glasses. In fact, the effect on the children of a teacher who wears glasses is so detrimental that no such person should be allowed to teach. Since errors of refraction are curable, such a rule would work no hardship on anyone. Children imitate the visual habits of a teacher who wears glasses. Moreover, the nervous strain of which the defective sight is an expression produces a similar strain in the children. In classes of the same grade with the same lighting, the sight of children whose teachers did not wear glasses has always been found to be better than the sight of children whose teachers did wear them. In one case, I tested the sight of children whose teacher wore glasses. I found their sight to be very imperfect. The teacher went out of the room on an errand. After she was gone, I tested the children again. The results were very much better.

When the teacher returned, she asked about the sight of a particular boy who was a very nervous child. As I was proceeding to test him, she stood before him and said, "Now, when the doctor tells you to read the chart, do it." At that point, the boy couldn't see anything. Then she went behind him and the effect was the same as if she had left the room. The boy read the whole chart.

Reorganize the Educational System

Still better results would be obtained if we could reorganize the educational system on a rational basis. Then we might expect a general return of that wonderful acuity of vision that we read about in the memoirs of travelers visiting indigenous peoples. But even under existing conditions, it has been proven beyond a shadow of a doubt that errors of refraction are not a necessary part of the price we must pay for education.

There are at least ten million children in the schools of the United States who have defective sight. This condition prevents them from taking full advantage of their educational opportunities. It undermines the children's health and wastes the taxpayers' money. If allowed to continue, poor vision will be an expense and a handicap to them throughout their lives. In many cases, it will be a source of continual misery and suffering. And yet practically all of these cases could be cured and the development of new ones prevented by the daily reading of the Snellen test chart.

Why should our children be compelled to suffer and wear glasses for want of this simple measure of relief? The method costs practically nothing. Not only does it place almost no additional burden on the teachers, it makes their work easier by improving the eyesight, health, disposition and mentality of their pupils. Furthermore, no one would venture to suggest that it could possibly do any harm. Why, then, should there be any

delay about introducing it into the schools? If further investigation and discussion is needed, we can investigate and discuss just as well after the children get the charts as before. By adopting this course, we shall not run the risk of needlessly condemning another generation to that curse that heretofore has always dogged the footsteps of civilization: defective eyesight. I appeal to all who read these lines to use whatever influence they possess toward the attainment of this end.

Directions for Using the Snellen Test Chart for the Prevention and Cure of Imperfect Sight in Schools

Place the Snellen test chart permanently on the wall of the classroom.

Every day, have the children silently read the smallest letters they can see from their seats with each eye separately. Cover the other eye with the palm of the hand in such a way as to avoid pressure on the eyeball.

This takes no appreciable amount of time, and it is sufficient to improve the sight of all children in one week and to cure all errors of refraction after some months, a year, or longer.

Children with markedly defective vision should be encouraged to read the chart more frequently. Children wearing glasses should not be interfered with, as they are under the care of a physician. Using the test chart will do these children little or no good while the glasses are worn.

While not essential, it is a great advantage to have records made of the vision of each student annually or more frequently. This may be done by the teacher. Such records should include the name and age of the pupils, the vision of each eye tested at twenty feet, and the date.

A certain amount of supervision is absolutely necessary. At least once a year, someone who understands the method should visit each classroom for the purpose of answering questions, encouraging the teachers to continue the use of the method, and making some kind of a report to the proper authorities.

It is not necessary that anyone involved understand anything about the physiology of the eye.

CHAPTER 28

The Story of Emily

Almost all people, when they are cured, proceed to cure others.

At a social gathering one evening, a lady told me that she had met a number of my patients. When she mentioned their names, I found that I did not remember any of them and I said so.

"That is because you cured them by proxy," she said. "You didn't directly cure Mrs. Jones or Mrs. Brown, but you cured Mrs. Smith. It was Mrs. Smith who cured the other ladies. You didn't treat Mr. and Mrs. Simpkins or Mr. Simpkins's mother and brother, but you may remember that you cured Mr. Simpkins's boy of a strabismus, and he cured the rest of the family."

In schools where the Snellen test chart was used to prevent and cure imperfect sight many children have been cured. Many children, after they were cured themselves, often took to the practice of ophthalmology with the greatest enthusiasm and success. They cure their fellow students, their parents and their friends. They make a kind of game of the treatment, and the progress of each case is followed with the most intense interest by all the children. On a good day, when the patients saw well, there was great rejoicing. On a bad day there was corresponding depression.

One girl cured twenty-six children in six months. Another cured twelve in three months.

One girl named Emily developed quite a varied ophthalmological practice and did things of which older and more experienced practitioners might well be proud. One day I went to the school that Emily attended. I asked her about her sight, which had been very imperfect. She replied that it was now very good and that her headaches were quite gone. I tested her sight and found it normal. Then another child whose sight had also been very poor spoke up:

"I can see all right too," she said. "Emily cured me."

"Indeed!" I replied. "How did she do that?"

The second girl explained that at the beginning, she could not see the Snellen test chart at all from the back of the room. Emily had her read the chart at a distance of a few feet. The next day Emily moved it a little farther away, and so on, until the girl was able to read it from the back of the room, just as the other children did.

Emily now told her to cover her right eye and read the chart with her left. Both girls were considerably upset to find that the uncovered eye was apparently blind. The school doctor was consulted and said that nothing could be done. The eye had been blind from birth, and no treatment would do any good. Undaunted, however, Emily undertook the treatment. She told the girl to cover her good eye and go up close to the chart. At a distance of a foot or less, they found that the girl could read even the small letters with the "blind" eye. Emily then proceeded as confidently as with the other eye. After many months of practice, the girl became the happy possessor of normal vision in both eyes. The case had, in fact, been simply one of extreme nearsightedness. Not being a specialist, the school doctor had not detected the difference between this and blindness.

A Little Girl with Cataract

In the same classroom there had been a little girl with congenital cataract. By the time of my visit, however, the cataract had disappeared. This, too, it appeared, was Emily's doing. The school doctor had said that there was no help for this girl's eye except through surgery. Fortunately, the sight of the other eye was pretty good, so he did not think surgery necessary. Emily accordingly took the matter in hand.

Emily had this girl stand close to the chart. With the good eye covered, the girl was unable to see even the largest C. Emily now held the chart between the person and the light and moved it back and forth. At a distance of three or four feet, the person could see this movement indistinctly. Emily then moved the chart farther away. Soon the person became able to see it move at ten feet and to see some of the larger letters indistinctly at a closer distance. Finally, after six months, she became able to read the chart with the bad eye as well

as with the good one.

After testing this child's sight and finding it normal in both eyes, I said to Emily, "You are a splendid doctor. You beat them all. Have you done anything else?"

A Cure of Strabismus

Emily blushed. Turning to another of her classmates, she said, "Mamie, come here."

Mamie stepped forward, and I looked at her eyes. There appeared to be nothing wrong with them.

"I cured her," said Emily.

"What of ?" I inquired.

"Cross eyes," replied Emily.

"How?" I asked, with growing astonishment.

Emily described a procedure very similar to one I have adopted in other cases of strabismus. She found that the sight of the crossed eye was very poor and that Mamie could see practically nothing with it. To Emily, the obvious course of action seemed to be the restoration of its sight. Never having read any medical literature, she did not know that this was impossible. So she went at it. She had Mamie cover her good eye and practice with the bad one at home and at school. At last, the sight became normal and the eye straight.

The school doctor had wanted to have the eye operated on. Fortunately, Mamie was scared and would not consent. And here she was with two perfectly good, straight eyes.

A Cure of Pain

"Anything else?" I inquired, when Mamie's case had been disposed of.

Emily blushed again, and said,

"Here's Rose. Her eyes used to hurt her all the time, and she couldn't see anything on the blackboard. Her headaches used to be so bad that she had to stay away from school every once in a while. The doctor gave her glasses but they didn't help her. She wouldn't wear them. When you told us the chart would help our eyes, I got busy with her. I had her read the chart close up, and then I moved it farther away. Now she can see all right, and her head doesn't ache any more. She comes to school every day, and we all thank you very much."

This was a case of compound farsighted astigmatism.

Such stories might be multiplied indefinitely. It is true, Emily's astonishing record cannot be attained by most. But lesser cures by cured patients have been very numerous. They serve to show that the benefits of the method of preventing and curing defects of vision in the schools presented in Chapter 27 would be far-reaching. Errors of refraction as well as many more serious defects would be cured. The children would be helped, and they would go on to help their families and friends.

CHAPTER 29

Mind and Vision

There is much more involved in defective vision than a mere inability to see the blackboard. Defective vision is the result of an abnormal condition of the mind. When the mind is in an abnormal condition, it is obvious that education cannot proceed productively. In some cases, putting glasses on a child may neutralize the effect of the abnormal state of the mind on the eyes. Glasses may to some extent make the child more comfortable. This increased comfort may improve the child's mental faculties somewhat. But glasses do not fundamentally alter the condition of the mind. Instead, by confirming the mind in a bad habit, they may make the condition of the mind worse.

Poor sight is considered to be one of the most common causes of poor progress in school. Experts estimate that limitations in vision may reasonably be held responsible for a quarter of the children habitually left back. The common view is that this would be prevented by suitable glasses.

When vision is impaired, memory is impaired. This is easy to demonstrate. A large part of the educational process consists of storing facts in the mind. All the other mental processes depend on knowledge of facts. So it is easy to see how little is accomplished by merely putting glasses on children who have "trouble with their eyes."

The extraordinary memory of indigenous peoples has been attributed to necessity. Lacking written records, they had to depend on their memories, which were strengthened accordingly. My view is quite different: the excellent memory of indigenous peoples is due to the same cause as their keen vision—minds at rest.

Excellent memory and excellent vision can be found among civilized people as well. Testing would show that excellent vision and excellent memory always occur together. This principle was demonstrated by the child who could see the moons of Jupiter:

CASE: The subject was a girl of ten named Phebe. Phebe had such marvelous eyesight that she could see the moons of Jupiter with her naked eyes. This fact was confirmed when she drew them just as others see them through the telescope. Her memory was equally remarkable. She could recite the whole content of a book after reading it.

Phebe had a sister named Isabel who had 6 Diopters of nearsightedness. Phebe was able to learn more Latin in a few days without a teacher than Isabel had learned in several years with a teacher.

Recalling a visit to a restaurant five years earlier, Phebe remembered what she ate, the name of the waiter, and the street address of the building. She also remembered what she wore on that occasion and what everyone else in the party wore.

Phebe could demonstrate the same detailed memory of every other event that had awakened her interest in any way. It was a favorite amusement in her family to ask her what the menu had been and what people had worn on various occasions.

I have found that when the sight of two people is different, their memories differ in exactly the same degree.

CASE: For example, I had two other sisters as patients. One had ordinary good vision (20/20), while the other had excellent vision (20/10 in this case). I asked these two sisters to learn eight verses of a poem. We found that the time it took them to memorize the verses varied in almost exactly the same ratio as their sight. The one with excellent vision learned the verses of the poem in fifteen minutes. The one with normal vision required thirty-one minutes to do the same.

After palming, the one with normal vision learned eight more verses in twenty-one minutes, while the one with 20/10 vision was unable to reduce her time significantly. In other words, the mind of the child with excellent vision was already so relaxed that she could not improve appreciably by palming. The mind of the child with normal vision was under a strain, so she was able to gain relaxation and hence improve her memory by palming.

The correlation between memory and vision applies even where the difference in sight is between the two eyes of the same person. Memory is better with both eyes open and worse when the better eye is closed.

Under the present educational system, there is a constant effort to compel children to remember. These efforts always fail. They spoil both memory and sight. Memory cannot be forced any more than vision can. We remember without effort, just as we see without effort. The harder we try to remember or see, the less we are able to do either.

Boredom Impairs Eyesight

The sorts of things we remember are the things that interest us. Children have difficulty learning their lessons because they are bored by them. Boredom impairs eyesight because boredom is a condition of mental strain.

Incentives may awaken a child's interest. Betty Smith may become interested in winning a prize, for instance, or in merely getting ahead of Johnny Jones. This interest may even develop into a genuine interest in the acquisition of knowledge.

Unfortunately, teachers often try to motivate students with fear. This usually has the effect of completely paralyzing minds that are already numb. The effect on the vision is equally disastrous.

In short, our irrational and unnatural educational system is the fundamental reason for both poor memory and poor eyesight in school children.

Only Interested Children Can Learn

Montessori has taught us that it is only when children are interested that they can learn. It is equally true that only when they are interested can they see. This fact was strikingly illustrated by the example of Phebe and her sister. Phebe, of the keen eyes, could recite whole books if she happened to be interested in them. But Phebe disliked mathematics and anatomy extremely. She could not learn them, and she became nearsighted when she tried to do so. Phebe could read letters a quarter of an inch high at twenty feet in poor light. But when asked to read numbers one to two inches high in good light at ten feet, she miscalled half of them. When asked to tell how much two and three made, she said "four" before finally deciding on "five." The entire time that she was occupied with this disagreeable subject, the retinoscope showed that she was nearsighted. When I asked her to look into my eyes with the retinoscope, she was not interested. When she tried, she could see nothing. This despite the fact that a much lower degree of visual acuity is required to see inside the eye with a retinoscope than to see the moons of Jupiter.

Shortsighted Isabel, on the contrary, had a passion for mathematics and anatomy. She excelled in these subjects. Isabel learned to use the ophthalmoscope as easily as Phebe had learned Latin. Almost immediately, Isabel saw the optic nerve and noted that the center was whiter than the periphery. She saw the light-colored lines (which are the arteries) and the darker lines (which are the veins). She could even see the lights streaks that follow the course of the blood vessels at the back of the eyes. Some specialists never become able to see these light streaks, and no one could see them without normal vision. Therefore, Isabel's vision must have been temporarily normal when she did it. Her vision for numbers, although not normal, was better than for letters.

In these two, the level of interest determined both the ability to learn and the ability to see. Phebe could read a photographic reduction of the Bible and recite what she had read verbatim. She could see the moons of Jupiter and draw a diagram of them afterward. Why? Because she was interested in these things. But Phebe could not see the interior of the eye nor see numbers even half as well as she saw letters. Why? Because these things bored her.

Phebe's teachers were always reproaching her for her backwardness in mathematics. I suggested to her that it would be a good joke to surprise her teachers by taking a high mark in a coming examination. This awoke her interest in the subject, and she contrived to learn enough to get seventy-eight per cent.

In Isabel's case, letters were antagonistic. She was not interested in most of the subjects with which letters dealt. She was backward in those subjects and had become habitually nearsighted. But when asked to look at objects that aroused an intense interest, her vision became normal.

In short, when one is not interested, one's mind is not under control. Without mental control, one can neither learn nor see. Not only the memory but all other mental faculties are improved when the eyesight becomes normal. It is a common experience with patients cured of defective sight to find that their ability to do their work has improved.

Improved Teaching Skills

A teacher whose letter is quoted in Chapter 31 testified that after gaining perfect eyesight, she "knew better how to get at the minds of the pupils." She felt she was "more direct, more definite, less diffused, and less vague." In fact, she felt she possessed "central fixation of the mind." In another letter, this teacher said, "The better my eyesight becomes, the greater is my ambition. On the days when my sight is best, I have the greatest excitement to do things."

Another teacher reported that one of her pupils used to sit doing nothing all day long. He was apparently not interested in anything. After the test chart was introduced into the classroom, his sight improved. He became anxious to learn, and he speedily developed into one of the best students in the class. In other words, his eyes and his mind became normal together.

CASE: A bookkeeper nearly seventy years of age had worn glasses for forty years. When he gained perfect sight without glasses, he found that he could work longer, more rapidly, and more accurately than ever before in his life. During busy seasons, or when short of help, he worked for some weeks at a time from 7 a.m. until 11 p.m. He insisted that he felt less tired at night after he was

through than he did in the morning when he started. Previously, although he had done more work than any other man in the office, it always tired him very much. This gentleman also noticed an improvement in his temper. Having been so long in the office and knowing so much more about the business than his fellow employees, he was frequently appealed to for advice. Before his sight became normal, these interruptions were very annoying to him. They often caused him to lose his temper. Once his sight was normal, however, the interruptions caused him no irritation whatever.

CASE: In another man, symptoms of insanity were relieved when his vision became normal. The patient was a physician who had been seen by many nerve and eye specialists before he came to me. He consulted me at last, not because he had any faith in my methods, but because nothing else seemed to be left for him to do. He brought with him quite a collection of glasses prescribed by different men, no two of them alike. He told me he had worn glasses for many months at a time without benefit. He had left them off for months at a time and had been apparently no worse. Outdoor life had also failed to help him. On the advice of some prominent neurologists, he had even given up his practice for a couple of years to spend time on a ranch. The vacation had done him no good.

I examined his eyes and found no physical defects. He had no error of refraction as determined by the retinoscope. Yet his vision with each eye was only three-quarters normal. He suffered from double vision as well as all sorts of other unpleasant symptoms. He used to see people standing on their heads. He would see little devils dancing on the tops of high buildings. He also had other illusions too numerous to include. At night his sight was so bad that he had difficulty finding his way about. When walking along a country road, he believed that he saw better when he turned his eyes far to one side, viewing the road with the side of the retina instead of with the center. At variable intervals, without warning and without loss of consciousness, he had attacks of blindness. These caused him great uneasiness, for he was a surgeon with a large and lucrative practice. He feared that he might have an attack while operating.

His memory was very poor. He could not remember the color of the eyes of any member of his family, although he had seen them all daily for years. Neither could he recall the color of his house, the number of rooms on the different floors of his house, or other details. The faces and names of patients and friends he recalled only with difficulty or not at all.

His treatment proved to be very difficult. He had an infinite number of erroneous ideas about the optics of vision in general and his own case in particular. He insisted that all these should be discussed. While these discussions were going on, he received no benefit. He

would talk and argue every day for hours at a time. This went on for a long time. His logic was wonderful, apparently unanswerable, and yet utterly wrong.

He had a very high degree of eccentric fixation. When he looked at a point forty-five degrees to one side of the largest E on the Snellen test chart, he saw the letter just as black as when he looked directly at it. The strain to do this was terrific and produced a high degree of astigmatism. However, the patient was unconscious of both his eccentric fixation and the strain. He could not be convinced that there was anything abnormal in seeing the letter just as black in the peripheral vision as at the center of his vision. If he saw the letter at all, he argued, he must see it as black as it really was, because he was not colorblind.

Finally, he became able to look away from one of the smaller letters on the chart and see it less well than when he looked directly at it. It took eight or nine months to accomplish this. At that point, he said it seemed like a great burden had been lifted from his mind. He experienced a wonderful feeling of rest and relaxation throughout his whole body.

When asked to remember black with his eyes closed and covered, he said he could not do so. He saw every color but black. However, he had been an enthusiastic football player at college. Finally, he found that he could remember a black football. I asked him to imagine that this football had been thrown into the sea and that it was being carried outward by the tide, becoming constantly smaller but no less black. This he was able to do. The strain floated away with the football until by the time the football had been reduced to the size of a period in a newspaper, the strain was entirely gone. The relief continued as long as he remembered the black spot. Since he could not remember it all the time, I suggested another method of gaining permanent relief. This was to make his sight voluntarily worse. He protested against this plan with considerable energy.

"Good heavens!" he said. "Isn't my sight bad enough without making it worse?"

After a week of argument, however, he consented to try the method. The result was extremely satisfactory. Since he suffered from double, triple and multiple vision, I first had him learn to see two or more lights where there was only one. This was accomplished by straining to see a point above the light while still trying to see the light clearly. In this way, he became able to avoid the unconscious strain that had produced his double and multiple vision. He was not troubled by these superfluous images any more. In a similar manner, other illusions were dispelled.

One of the last illusions to disappear was his belief that an effort was required to remember black. His logic on this point was overwhelming. Finally, after many demonstrations, he was convinced that no effort was required. When he realized this, both his vision and his mental condition improved immediately. He became able to read the test chart down to the 20/10 line or more. Although he was more than fifty-five years of age, he also became

able to read very small type at from six to twenty-four inches. His night blindness was relieved. His attacks of day blindness ceased. He could tell me the colors of the eyes of his wife and children.

One day he said to me, "Doctor, I thank you for what you have done for my sight, but no words can express the gratitude I feel for what you have done for my mind." Some years later, he called with his heart full of gratitude because there had been no relapse.

From all these examples, it will be seen that problems of vision are far more intimately associated with problems of education than we had supposed. These problems can by no means be solved by putting concave, convex, or cylinder lenses before the eyes of the children.

CHAPTER 30

Normal Sight and the Relief of Pain

for Soldiers and Sailors

The Great War is over *[WWI.* **MA***]*. Millions of brave men laid down their lives in the cruel conflict. Among them were some who thought that by doing so, war would be no more. But the earth is still filled with wars and rumors of war. In the countries of the victorious Allies, the spirit of militarism is rampant. In the United States, we are being urged toward increased naval and military expenditure, and there is a strong demand for universal military training.

We need not enter here into the question of whether or not it is necessary for us as a nation to join in the militarization that has already resulted in such upheavals. But if we are going to do so, we may as well have soldiers and sailors with normal sight. If we attain this end, we shall not have borne the burdens of militarism and navalism altogether in vain.

After the United States entered the war, I had the privilege of making it possible for many young men to meet the visual requirements for military service. Seeing no reason why such benefits should be confined to the few, I supplied the Surgeon General of the Army with a plan. My plan was not acted on. I now present it, with some modifications, to the public. My hope is that enough people will see its military value to secure its adoption

by the military.

If we are to have universal military training, the recruits must have adequate eyesight. In the draft for the recent war, defective eyesight was initially the greatest single cause for rejection, as I mentioned in Chapter 1. The standards for visual acuity had to be lowered in order to get enough recruits. Even then, poor eyesight remained one of the top three causes for rejection. Yet there is no obstacle to the raising of an army that could be more easily removed.

We want our children to grow big and healthy enough to be soldiers. Every one of the advanced countries of Europe has programs in place to prevent childhood illness and encourage the growth of strong, healthy children. Here in the United States, we shall have to make such arrangements as well. We shall have to employ school physicians full time and pay them a physician's wage. We shall also have to see that the children are not sacrificed to the ignorance or poverty of their parents before they reach school age. These are huge projects.

But to preserve their eyesight, it is only necessary to place Snellen test charts in every school classroom and to see that the children read them every day. Using this simple system of eye education from kindergarten to university would assure that the young people of our country, on arrival at military age, were practically free from eye defects. But some years must elapse before this happy result can be achieved.

Eye Education for Training Camps and for the Front

Everyone's eyes are subject to visual lapses, especially under stress. Such lapses are particularly dangerous in military and naval operations. Moreover, all eyes, no matter how good their vision, are benefited by the daily practice of the art of seeing. By such practice, those visual lapses to which every eye is subject and that are particularly dangerous in military and naval operations, are either prevented or minimized. Therefore, a system of eye education for training camps and for the front should also be provided. A modified version of the method used in schools would serve this purpose well.

A Snellen test chart might be impracticable under conditions of actual warfare or on the parade grounds of training camps. However, there are other letters or small objects that would serve the purpose equally well. Letters or objects that require a vision of 20/20 should be selected by someone who has been taught what 20/20 means. The recruits should be required to regard these letters or objects twice a day. After reading the letters, they should be directed to palm and remember black for thirty seconds. Then they should view the objects again and note any improvement in vision.

The whole procedure would not take more than a minute. It should be made part of the regular drill, morning and night. Those with imperfect sight should be encouraged to repeat the procedure as many times a day as is convenient. They will need no urging, for imperfect vision is a bar to advancement in the military. Imperfect vision excludes one from the most desired branch of the service—aviation.

In each regiment, groups of ten should be under the supervision of one person who understands the method. These supervisors must possess normal vision without glasses. They should carry a pocket test chart consisting of a few of the smaller letters. They should test the vision of those under their direction at the beginning of the training and thereafter at intervals of three months. Results should be reported to the medical officer in charge.

No Soldier Should Wear Glasses

Since errors of refraction are curable, no soldier should be allowed to wear glasses. If the use of glasses is permitted, those wearing them should not be required to take part in the eye drills. Eye drills will do them no good if they wear glasses. When they see the benefits of eye education, however, they may wish to join them. They then will, no doubt, be willing to submit to the temporary inconvenience of going without glasses.

In military colleges, the same method could be used as in the schools. A daily eye drill should also form part of the maneuvers on the parade ground. This will prepare the students for using it later in training camps or at the front.

Eye Education for Pilots

Eye education is of particular importance to all types of pilots. Unexplained accidents to pilots are easily explained when one understands how quickly perfect vision may be lost amid unaccustomed surroundings, dangers and hardships.

It was formerly supposed that pilots maintained their equilibrium in the air by the aid of the internal ear. Not so. Equilibrium is maintained almost entirely, if not entirely, by the sense of sight. This is confirmed by the testimony of pilots who have found themselves emerging from a cloud with one wing down or even with their aircraft turned completely upside down. If the pilot loses his sight, he is lost. One of those "unaccountable" accidents may then occur. During the war, this was, unhappily, common in the Air Force.

All pilots, therefore, should make a daily practice of reading small, familiar letters at distances of ten feet or more. Observing other small objects in the same way may also suffice. They should have a few small letters painted on their aircraft visible from the cockpit at a distance of five, ten, or more feet from their eyes. They should be able to illuminate these letters while flying at night or in the fog. While in the air, pilots should read them. This would greatly lessen the danger of visual lapses and the accompanying loss of equilibrium and judgment.

Eye Education for Fatigue and Pain

Eye education not only improves the sight, it affords a means by which pain, fatigue, discomfort and other symptoms of disease can be relieved. For this purpose, it is of the greatest value to soldiers and sailors. Much suffering and many deaths during the recent war would have been prevented if this method had been well-known. If soldiers in a flooded trench can remember black perfectly, they will know the temperature of the water but will not suffer from the cold. Even if they succumb to weakness on the march, they will not feel fatigue. They may die of hemorrhage, but they will die painlessly.

The relief of pain by memory makes morphine unnecessary. Thus the danger of returning to civilian life under the handicap of a lifelong addiction can be averted. The problem of addiction assumed enormous proportions during the war. The Germans used a bullet that broke when it struck the bone and thus caused intense pain. Men often died of this pain before help arrived. When they were rescued, the surgeons would at once give them morphine. A few hours later, the injection was probably repeated. Then the drug would be given less frequently. However, in many cases, morphine was not discontinued entirely while the man was in the hospital. A Red Cross surgeon at a meeting of the New York County Medical Society stated that he had been responsible for producing morphine addiction in thousands of soldiers. He said that every physician at the front had done the same. By such a simple method as palming, all this might have been prevented.

If we are going to have universal military and naval training, an essential part of that training should be instruction in the art of relieving one's own pain. In the event of war, everyone who goes to the front, from the

generals and admirals down to the ambulance
drivers, should understand palming. Everyone
in the war zone, no matter how far behind the
lines, may need this knowledge to relieve his
own pain, and everyone may need it to relieve
the pain of others.

CHAPTER 31

Letters From Patients

The following letters have been selected almost at random from my mail-bag. They are only examples of many more that are equally interesting. I felt that people's personal stories, told in their own words, might be more interesting and helpful to many readers than the more formal presentations in the preceding chapters.

Army Office Cures Himself

The sight always improves when glasses are discarded, though this improvement may be so slight as not to be noticed. In a few unusual cases, people find out on their own how to avoid straining their eyes. They thus regain a degree of normal visual power.

The writer of the following letter was able to discover and put into practice the main principles presented in this book without any help from anyone. He thus became able to read without glasses. He is an engineer. At the time the letter was written, he was fifty-one years old. He had worn progressively stronger glasses since 1896. He suffered from astigmatism and later, from presbyopia. At one time, he asked his ophthalmologist and several opticians if his eyes could not be strengthened by exercises, thus making glasses unnecessary. They said, "No. Once started on glasses, you must keep to them."

When the war broke out, he was very nearly disqualified for service in the Expeditionary Forces by his eyes. He did manage to pass the required tests, after which he was ordered abroad as an officer in the Gas Service. While there, he saw a reference to my method of curing defective eyesight without glasses in the "Literary Digest" of May 2, 1918.

On May 11, he wrote to me in part as follows:

"At the front I found glasses a horrible nuisance. Also, they could not be worn with gas masks. After I had been about six months abroad I asked an officer of the Medical Corps about going without glasses. He said I was right in my ideas and told me to try it. The first week was awful, but I persisted and only wore glasses for reading and writing. I stopped smoking at the same time to make it easier on my nerves.

"Now I no longer use the lenses for presbyopia. I only use those for astigmatism. Three months ago I could not read ordinary headlines in newspapers without glasses. Today, with a good light, I can read ordinary book type at a distance of eighteen inches from my eyes.

"Since the first week in February, when

I discarded my glasses, I have had no headaches, stomach trouble or dizziness. I am in good health generally. My eyes are coming back, and I believe it is due to sticking it out. I ride considerably in automobiles and trains. Somehow the idea has crept into my mind that after every trip my eyes are stronger. This, I think, is due to the rapid changing of focus in viewing the scenery as it goes by so rapidly. Other men have tried this plan on my advice, but they gave it up after two or three days. Yet, from what they say, I believe they were not as uncomfortable as I was for a week or ten days. I now believe most people wear glasses because they 'coddle' their eyes."

The patient was right in thinking that the motor and train rides improved his sight. The rapid motion compelled rapid shifting.

A Teacher's Experiences

Imperfect vision is always associated with an abnormal state of mind. When the vision improves, the mental faculties also improve to a greater or lesser degree. The following letter is a striking illustration of this fact. The writer, a 40-year-old teacher, was first treated on March 28, 1919.

At that time she was wearing the following glasses:

Right eye:

+0.75 D

+4.00 D Cylinder at 105°

Left eye:

+0.75 D

+3.50 D Cylinder at 105°

[For an explanation of the degrees of cylinder, please see Appendix 1, page 232. **MA***]*

On June 9, 1919, she wrote:

"I will tell you about my eyes, but first let me tell you other things. You were the first to unfold your theories to me, and I was favorably impressed from the start. I did not take up the cure because other people recommended it but because I was convinced. First, I was convinced that you believed in your discovery yourself. Second, I was convinced that your theory as to the cause of eye trouble was true. I don't know how I knew these two things, but I did. After our short conversation, you and your discovery both seemed to me to bear the earmarks of the genuine article. As to my chances of success, I did have a little doubt. You might cure others, but you might not be able to cure me. However, I took the plunge and it has made a great change in me and my life.

"To begin with, I enjoy my sight. Like a child, I love to look at things and examine them in a leisurely, thorough way. I never realized it at the time, but it was irksome for me to look at things when I was wearing glasses. I did as little of it as possible. The other day, going down on the Sandy Hook boat, I enjoyed a most wonderful sky without that hateful barrier of misted glasses. I am positive I distinguished delicate shades of color that I never would have been able to see, even with clear glasses. Things seem to me now to have more form and more reality than when I wore glasses. Looking into the mirror you see a solid representation on a flat surface. The flat glass can't show you anything really solid. My eyeglasses, of course, never gave me this impression, but they did give one curiously like it. I can see so clearly without them that it is like looking around corners without changing position. I feel that I can almost do that.

"I very seldom have occasion to palm. Once in a great while I feel the necessity of it. The same with remembering a period. Nothing else is ever necessary. I seldom think of my eyes, but at times it is borne in on me how much I do use them and enjoy using them.

"My nerves are much better. I am more equable, more poised, and less shy. I never used to show that I was shy or that I lacked confidence. I used to go ahead with what was required, but it was hard. Now I find it easy. Glasses, or rather poor sight, made me self-conscious. It certainly is a great defect, and one people are sensitive to without realizing it. I mean the poor sight and the necessity for wearing glasses. I put on a pair of glasses the other day just as an experiment, and I found that they magnified things. My skin looked as if it were under a magnifying glass. Things seemed too near. The articles on my chiffonier looked so close I felt like pushing them away from me. I especially wanted to push away the glasses. They brought irritation at once. I took them off and immediately felt peaceful. Things looked normal.

"From the beginning of the treatment I could use my eyes pretty well, but they used to tire. I remember making a large

Liberty Loan poster two weeks after I took off my glasses. I was amazed to find that without glasses I could make the whole layout almost perfectly without a ruler. When I came to true it up with the ruler I found only the last row of letters a bit out of line at the very end. I couldn't have done better with glasses. However, this wasn't fine work. About the same time I sewed a hem at night in a black dress, using a fine needle. I suffered a little for this, but not much. I used to practice my exercises at that time and palm faithfully. Now I don't have to practice, or palm. I feel no discomfort, and I am absolutely unsparing in my use of my eyes. I do everything I want to with them. I shirk nothing, and I pass up no opportunity of using them. From the beginning of treatment I did all my school work, read every notice, and wrote all that was necessary, neglecting nothing.

"Now to sum up the school end of it: I used to get headaches at the end of the month from adding the columns of numbers necessary for reports and so on. Now I do not get headaches. I used to get flustered when people came into my room. Now I do not. I welcome them. It is a pleasant change to feel this way. And — I suppose this is most important really, though I think of it last — I teach better. I know how to get at the mind and how to make the children see things in perspective. I gave a lesson on the horizontal cylinder recently. This is not a thrillingly interesting subject. Yet it got a grip on every girl in the room, stupid or bright. What you have taught me makes me use the memory and especially the imagination more.

"To sum up the effect on my mind of my cured vision: I am more direct, more definite, less diffused and less vague. In short, I am conscious of being better centered. It is central fixation of the mind. I saw this in your latest paper, but I realized it long ago and knew what to call it."

A Mental Transition

A man of forty-four who had worn glasses since the age of twenty was first seen on October 8, 1917. He was suffering from very imperfect sight as well as from headache and discomfort.

He was wearing the following prescription:
Right eye:
-5.00D
-0.50D.C., 180°
Left eye:
-2.50D
-1.50D.C., 180°

[For an explanation of the degrees of cylinder, please see Appendix 1, page 232. **MA]**

As his visits were not very frequent and he often went back to his glasses, his overall vision improved only slowly. But his pain and discomfort were relieved very quickly, and almost from the beginning he had flashes of greatly improved or even normal vision. This encouraged him to continue. Currently his vision and his general condition are both greatly improved. His wife was particularly impressed with the improvement in his general condition.

In December, 1919, she wrote:

"I have become very much interested in the thought of renewing my youth by becoming like a little child. The idea of this mental transition is not unfamiliar. Yet the idea that this mental, or should I say spiritual, transition should produce a physical effect that would lead to seeing clearly, is a sort of miracle.

"In my husband's case, certainly, some such miracle was wrought. Yes, he was able to lay aside his spectacles after many years of constant use. He became able to read in almost any light. But more miraculous, I particularly noticed his serenity of mind after treatments. In this serenity he seemed able to do a great deal of work very efficiently. This was quite different from working under the high nervous pressure whose after-effect is the devastating scattering of the life forces.

"It did not occur to me for a long time that perhaps your treatment was quieting his nerves. But I think now that the quiet periods of relaxation, two or three times a day, during which he practiced with the Snellen chart, must have had a very beneficial effect. He is so enthusiastic by nature, and his nerves are so easily stimulated, that for years he periodically overdid things. Of course, his greatly improved eyesight and the reduced eye strain must be a large factor in this improvement. But I am inclined to think that the intervals of quiet and peace were wonderfully beneficial. And why shouldn't they be? We are living on stimulants, physical and mental stimulants of all kinds. The minute these stop, we feel we are merely existing. Yet, if we retain any of the normality of our youth, do you not think that we respond very happily to natural simple things?"

Relief After Twenty Five Years

While many people are benefited by the prevailing methods of treating vision, a minority gets little or no help from them. These people sometimes despair and give up the search for relief. But sometimes they continue the search with surprising tenacity. Despite the testimony of experience, they are simply unable to abandon the belief that somewhere in the world, someone has sufficient skill to fit them with the right glasses.

The rapidity with which these people respond to treatment by relaxation is often very dramatic. It affords a startling illustration of the superiority of relaxation to treatment by glasses and, in the case of strabismus, surgery.

In the following example, relaxation did in twenty-four hours what the old methods, as practiced by a succession of eminent specialists, could not do in twenty-five years.

CASE:

The patient was a man of forty-nine. His imperfect sight was accompanied by continual pain and misery. This pain and misery was so severe that, twenty years before I saw him, it culminated in a complete nervous breakdown. He was a writer, dependent on his pen for a living. His vision problems were a serious economic handicap. He consulted many specialists in the vain hope of obtaining relief.

Glasses did little to help his vision, his pain or his discomfort. The eye specialists talked vaguely about disease of the optic nerve and brain as a possible cause of his troubles. The neurologists, however, were unable to do anything to relieve him. One specialist diagnosed his case as muscular and gave him prisms for strabismus. This helped him a little. Since most of the problems remained, the same specialist later cut the external ocular muscles of both eyes. This also brought some relief, but not much.

At the age of twenty-nine, the patient suffered a nervous breakdown. For this he was treated unsuccessfully by various specialists. For nine years, he was compelled to live out of doors. This life, although it benefited him, failed to restore his health. When he came to me on September 15, 1919, he was still suffering from neurasthenia *[nervous exhaustion. MA]*. His distant vision was less than 20/40 and could not be improved by glasses. He was able to read with glasses but could not do so without discomfort. I could find no symptom of disease of the brain or of the interior of the eye. When he tried to palm, he saw gray and yellow instead of black. However, he was able to rest his eyes simply by closing them. By this means alone, he became able to read very small type and to make out most of the letters on the twenty line of the test chart at twenty feet in twenty-four hours. At the same time, his discomfort was materially relieved. He was under treatment for about six weeks. On October 25, he wrote as follows:

"I saw you last on October 6. At the end of that week I started off on a ten-day motor trip as one of the officials of the Cavalry Endurance Test for horses. The last hint of eye strain which used to affect me with stress was gone. On the trip I averaged but five hours sleep, rode all day in an open motorcar without goggles and wrote reports at night by bad light. Despite all this, I had no trouble. After the third day the universal slow swing seemed to establish itself, and I have never had a moment's discomfort since. I withstood fatigue and excitement better than I have ever done, and went with less sleep. My practicing on the trip was necessarily somewhat curtailed, yet there was noticeable improvement in my vision. Since returning I have spent a couple of hours a day in practice, and have at the same time done a lot of writing.

"Yesterday, the 24th, I made a test with very small type. I found that after twenty minutes' practice I could get the lines distinct. I could as well make out the capital letters and bits of the text at a scant three inches. At seven inches I could read the text readily, though I could not see it perfectly. This was by overcast daylight. In good daylight I can read the newspaper almost perfectly at a normal reading distance, say fifteen inches.

"I feel now that I am really out of the woods. I have done night work without suffering for it! This is a thing I have not

been able to do in twenty-five years. I can now work steadily for more hours than since my breakdown in 1899. All this occurs without any sense of strain or nervous fatigue. You can imagine my gratitude to you. Not only for my own sake, but for yours, I shall leave no stone unturned to make the cure complete and get back the child eyes that seem perfectly possible in the light of the progress I have made in eight weeks."

Seeking a Cure for Nearsightedness

Despite the emphatic denials of the possibility of curing errors of refraction, many people refuse to believe they are incurable. The author of the following statement is remarkable only in the persistency with which he searched for relief. He was first seen on June 27, 1919, at which time he was thirty-two years of age. His vision in each eye was 20/100.

After he had obtained almost normal vision, he wrote the following account of his experiences for Better Eyesight Magazine:

"When the Lusitania was sunk I knew that the United States was going to get into trouble. I wanted to be in a position to join the Army. I was suffering from a high degree of nearsightedness, and I knew they wouldn't take me with glasses. Later on they took almost anyone who wasn't blind, but at that time I couldn't possibly have measured up to the standard. So I began to look about for a cure. I tried osteopathy, but didn't go very far with it.

I asked the optician who had been fitting me with glasses for advice. He said that nearsightedness was incurable.

"I dismissed the matter for a time, but I didn't stop thinking about it. I am a farmer. I knew from the experience of outdoor life that health is the normal condition of living beings. I knew that when health is lost it can often be regained. I knew that when I first tried to lift a barrel of apples onto a wagon I could not do so, but that after a little practice I became able to do it easily. I did not see why, if one part of the body could be strengthened by exercise, others could not also be strengthened. I could remember a time when I was not nearsighted. It seemed to me that if a normal eye could become nearsighted, it ought to be possible for a nearsighted eye to regain normality.

"After a while I went back to the optician and told him that I was convinced that there must be some cure for my condition. He replied that this was quite impossible, as everyone knew that nearsightedness was incurable. The assurance with which he made this statement had quite the opposite effect from that which he intended. When he said that the cure of nearsightedness was impossible I knew that it was not. I resolved never to give up the search for a cure until I found it.

"Shortly after, I had the good fortune to hear of Dr. Bates. I lost no time in going to see him. At the first visit I was able, just by closing and resting my eyes, to improve my sight considerably by the measure of the Snellen test chart. After a few months of intermittent treatment I became able to read 20/10, but only in flashes. I am still improving. When I can see a little better I mean to go back to that optician and tell him what I think of his ophthalmological learning."

Facts Versus Theories

Reading fine print is commonly supposed to be an extremely dangerous practice. Reading print of any kind on a moving vehicle is thought to be even more dangerous. Looking away to the distance, however, and not seeing anything in particular is believed to be very beneficial to the eyes. In the light of these superstitions, the information contained in the following letter is particularly interesting:

"On reaching home Monday morning I was surprised and pleased at the comments of my family regarding the appearance of my eyes. They all thought they looked so much brighter and rested, and that after two days of riding on the railroad. I didn't spare my eyes in the least on the trip. I read magazines and newspapers, and looked at the scenery. In fact, I used my eyes all the time. My sight for the near point is splendid now. I can read for hours without tiring my eyes. However, I went downtown today and my eyes were very tired when I got home. The fine print on the practice chart helps me so much that I would like to have your little Bible. *[He is referring to Dr. Bates's photographic reduction of the Bible with very small type.* **MA]** I'm sure the very fine print has a soothing effect on one's eyes, regardless of what my previous ideas on the subject were."

It will be observed that the eyes of this patient were not tired by her two days journey on the railroad, although she read constantly during the trip. They were not tired by hours of reading after her return. Her eyes were rested by reading extremely fine print. But her eyes were very much tired by a trip downtown, during which they were not called on to focus on small objects. Later I sent her a leaf from the tiny print Bible, and she wrote,

"The effect even of the first effort to read it was wonderful. If you will believe it, I haven't been troubled by having my eyes feel "crossed" since. While my actual vision does not seem to be any better, my eyes feel a great deal better."

Cured Without Personal Assistance

I am constantly hearing of patients who have been able to improve their sight by following the instructions in my writings. The writer of the following letter, a physician, is a remarkable example. He was able not only to cure himself but to relieve some very serious cases of defective vision among his patients.

"I first tried central fixation on myself and had marvelous results. I threw away my glasses and can now see better than I have ever seen. I read very fine type (smaller than newspaper type) at a distance of six inches. I can hold the same type out to full arm's length and still read it without blurring.

"I have instructed some of my patients in your methods, and all are getting results. One case who has a partial cataract of the left eye could not see anything on the Snellen test chart at twenty feet. She could see the letters only faintly at ten feet. Now she can read 20/10 with both eyes together, and also with each eye separately. The left eye, though, does seem to be looking through a little fog.

"I could cite many other cases that have benefited by central fixation, but this one is the most interesting to me."

CHAPTER 32

Reason and Authority

Someone—perhaps it was Bacon —said, "You cannot by reasoning correct a man of an ill opinion which by reasoning he never acquired." He might have gone a step further and stated that neither by reasoning nor by actual demonstration of the facts can you convince some people that an opinion that they have accepted on authority is wrong.

There is an ophthalmologist whose name I do not care to mention. He is a professor and a writer of books well known in this country and in Europe. This gentleman saw me perform one of the experiments described in this book. This experiment demonstrates beyond any possibility of error that the lens is not a factor in accommodation. Others who have witnessed it agree.

At each step of the operation, this gentleman testified to the facts. Yet at the conclusion, he preferred to discredit the evidence of his own senses rather than accept the conclusion that these facts demanded.

First he examined the eye of an animal's cadaver with the retinoscope. He found it normal, and this fact was written down.

Then the eye was stimulated with electricity, and he agreed that it accommodated. This fact was also written down.

I then cut the superior oblique muscle, and the eye was again stimulated with electricity. The doctor observed the eye with the retinoscope as this was being done and said, "You failed to produce accommodation." This fact, too, was written down.

The doctor now used the electrode himself but again failed to observe accommodation, and these facts were written down.

I then sewed the cut ends of the muscle together, and once more stimulated the eye with electricity. The doctor said, "Now you have succeeded in producing accommodation," and this was written down.

At that point, I asked, "Do you think that the superior oblique muscle had anything to do with producing accommodation ?"

"Certainly not," he replied.

"Why?" I asked.

"Well," he said, "I have only the testimony of the retinoscope. I am getting on in years, and I don't feel the confidence in my ability to use the retinoscope that I once had. I would rather you wouldn't quote me on this."

While the operation was in progress, however, he gave no indication whatever of doubting his ability to use the retinoscope. He was very positive that I had failed to produce accommodation after the cutting of the oblique muscle, and his tone suggested that he considered the failure ignominious.

It was only after he found himself in a logical trap, with no way out except by discrediting his own observations, that he appeared to have any doubts as to the value of those observations.

Demonstration of Cure Did Not Change Belief

People whom I have cured of various errors of refraction have frequently returned to the specialists who prescribed glasses for them. By reading the Snellen test chart with normal vision, they demonstrated the fact that they were cured. These demonstrations have in no way shaken the faith of these practitioners in the doctrine that such cures are impossible.

The woman with progressive nearsightedness whose case was mentioned in Chapter 15 was cured. She returned after her cure to the specialist who had prescribed her glasses. This specialist had told her both that there was no hope of improvement and that the condition would probably progress until it ended in blindness. She told him the good news of her cure. As he was an old friend of her family, she felt he had a right to know. He was unable to deny that her vision was now normal without glasses. But he still maintained that it was impossible that she was cured of nearsightedness because nearsightedness was incurable. He was unable to make clear to her how he reconciled this statement with her recovery.

A lady with compound nearsighted astigmatism suffered from almost constant headaches that were very much worse when she took her glasses off. The theater and the movies caused her so much discomfort that she feared to indulge in these recreations. I told her to take off her glasses and advised, among other things, going to the movies. I instructed her to look first at the corner of the screen, then off to the dark, then back to the screen a little nearer to the center, and so forth. She did so, and soon became able to look directly at the pictures without discomfort. After that, nothing troubled her.

One day she called on her ophthalmologist and told him of her cure. The facts seemed to make no impression on him whatsoever. He only laughed and said, "I guess Dr. Bates is more popular with you than I am."

Sometimes patients themselves, after they are cured, allow themselves to be convinced that it was impossible that such a cure could have happened. They go back to their glasses. This happened with a man already mentioned in the chapter on presbyopia. He was cured in fifteen minutes by the aid of his imagination. He was very grateful for a time. Then he began to talk to eye specialists whom he knew. Straightway he grew skeptical as to the value of what I had done for him. One day I met him at the home of a mutual friend. In the presence of a number of other people, he accused me of having hypnotized him, adding that to hypnotize a patient without his knowledge or consent was to do him a grievous wrong.

Some of the listeners protested that whether I had hypnotized him or not, I had done him no harm but in fact had greatly benefited him. They said he ought to forgive me. He was unable to take this view of the matter, however. Later he called on a prominent eye specialist who told him that the presbyopia and astigmatism from which he suffered were incurable. This specialist told him that if he persisted in going without his glasses, he might do himself great harm. The fact that his sight was perfect without glasses both at the distance and at the near point had no effect on the specialist. The man allowed himself to be frightened into disregarding this fact as well. He went back to his glasses. So far as I know, he has been wearing them ever since.

The story obtained wide publicity, for the man had a large circle of friends and acquaintances. If I had destroyed his sight, I could scarcely have suffered more than I did for curing him.

The Cure of Cataracts

Fifteen or twenty years ago, the same specialist read a paper on cataracts at a meeting of the Ophthalmological section of the American Medical Association in Atlantic City. He asserted there that anyone who said that a cataract could be cured without the knife was a quack. At that time, I was Assistant at the New York Eye and Ear Infirmary. It happened that I had been collecting statistics on the spontaneous cure of cataracts at the request of the executive surgeon of this institution, Dr. Henry G. Noyes, Professor of Ophthalmology at the Bellevue Hospital Medical School. As a result of my inquiry, I had secured records of a large number of people who had recovered from cataracts, not only without the knife but without any treatment at all.

I also had records of cases that I had sent to Dr. James E. Kelly of New York. Dr. Kelly had cured these cases of cataract largely by hygienic methods. *[I believe this refers to methods of internal cleansing and diet. MA]*

Dr. Kelly is not a quack. At that time, he was Professor of Anatomy in the New York Post Graduate Medical School and Hospital and attending surgeon to a large city hospital.

In the five minutes allotted to those who wished to discuss the paper, I was able to tell the audience enough about these cases to make them want to hear more. My time was therefore extended, first to half an hour and then to an hour. Later, both Dr. Kelly and myself received many letters from men in different parts of the country who had tried his treatment with success.

The physician who wrote the paper saying cataracts never resolve without surgery had blundered. However, he did not lose any prestige because his theory was discredited. He is still a prominent and honored ophthalmologist. In his latest book, he gives no hint of having ever heard of any successful method of treating cataract other than by operation. He was not convinced by my record of spontaneous cures nor by Dr. Kelly's record of cures by hygienic treatments. A few men were sufficiently impressed to try the treatment recommended. When they did, satisfactory results were obtained. But all these facts made no impression on the profession as a whole and did not modify in the least what is taught in the medical schools.

That spontaneous cures of cataract do sometimes occur cannot be denied, but they are supposed to be very rare. People who suggest that the condition can be cured by treatment still expose themselves to the suspicion of being quacks.

Facts Versus Authority

Between 1886 and 1891, I was a lecturer at the New York Post Graduate Hospital and Medical School. The head of the institution was Dr. D. B. St. John Roosa. He was the author of many books and was honored and respected by the whole medical profession. At the school, they had gotten into the habit of putting glasses on the nearsighted doctors, and I had gotten into the habit of curing them so that they did not need glasses. It was naturally annoying to a man who had put glasses on a student to have him appear at a lecture without them and say that Dr. Bates had cured him. Dr. Roosa found it particularly annoying, and the trouble reached a climax one evening at the annual banquet of the faculty. In the presence of one hundred and fifty doctors, he suddenly poured out the vials of his wrath upon my head. He said that I was injuring the reputation of the Post Graduate Hospital and Medical School by claiming to cure nearsightedness. Everyone knew that Dr. Donders *[a great authority on the subject; see Ch. 2.* **MA***]* said it was incurable, and I had no right to claim that I knew more than Dr. Donders.

I reminded him that he himself had fitted with glasses some of the men I had cured. He replied that if he had said they were nearsighted, he had made a mistake.

I suggested further investigation: "Fit some more doctors with glasses for nearsightedness," I said, "and I will cure them. It is easy for you to examine them afterwards and see if the cure is genuine."

This method did not appeal to him, however. He repeated that it was impossible to cure nearsightedness, and to prove that it was impossible, he expelled me from the Post Graduate Hospital and Medical School. Even the privilege of resigning was denied to me.

It remains true that, except in rare cases, human beings are not reasoning beings. We are dominated by authority. When the facts are not in accord with the view imposed by authority, so much the worse for the facts. The facts may, and indeed must, win in the long run. In the meantime, the world gropes needlessly in darkness and endures much suffering that might have been avoided.

APPENDIX 1

Astigmatism

Regardless of distance, when a person with astigmatism looks at an object, their eyes are unable to focus it into a clear image on the retina. In this respect, astigmatism is fundamentally different from the other errors of refraction. With nearsightedness and farsightedness, the eye can create a clear image of an object, as long as the object is the right distance away. Not so with astigmatism.

Astigmatism can cause discomfort or even severe pain. Other symptoms may include eye strain, eye pain, headache, dry eyes, sensitivity to light, frequent blinking, tilting the head when looking, and half closing the eyelids when looking.

The word "astigmatism" was coined in 1849. "Stigma" is from the Greek, meaning a

point or dot. "A" means without. So the literal meaning of astigmatism is "a condition of being without a clear dot or point" – no clear focal point

A cornea with astigmatism is not symmetrically rounded. It is shaped more like a squashed contact lens, or like the back of a spoon, or like the side of an egg shell. (Figure A1.1)

A cornea with astigmatism, then, will have a long axis and a short axis. (Figure A1.2). In the world of ophthalmology, the convention is that if "long" or "short" is not specified, the word "axis" standing alone refers to the long axis.

Astigmatism is best illustrated with lines. Take the simplest case, where the axis (i.e. the long axis) is horizontal and the eye is looking at two

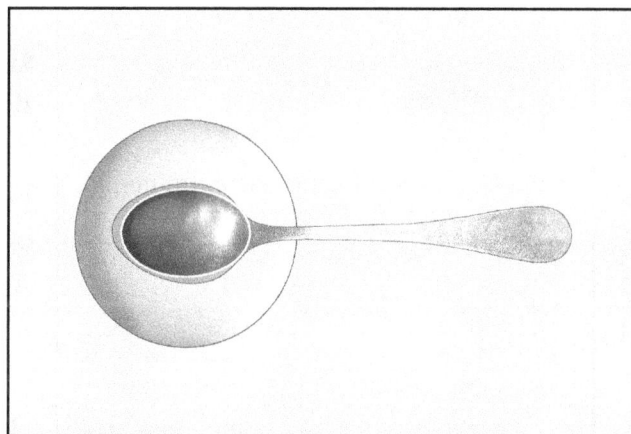

Figure A1.1: The Astigmatic Cornea Is Shaped Like the Back of a Spoon.

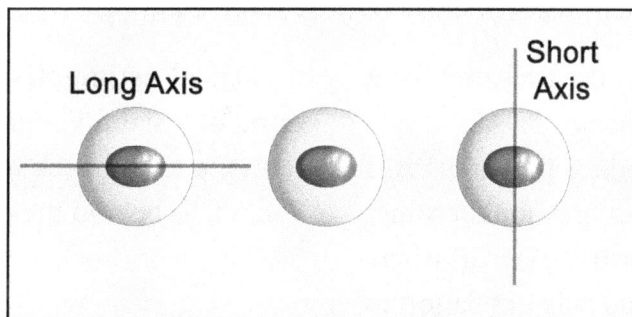

Figure A1.2: Long and Short Axes

crossed lines, one vertical and one horizontal. When an astigmatic eye brings one line into focus, the other must be blurred. (Figure A1.3)

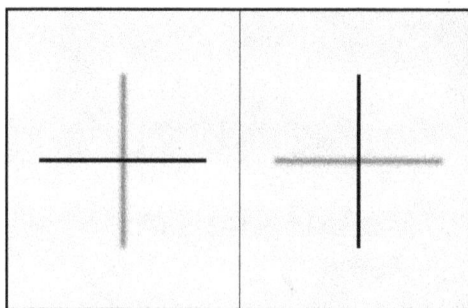

It's easy to understand why: The focal length of a lens depends on how sharply the surface curves. The sharper the curve, the shorter the focal length. Since the curve is more gentle along the long axis, the focal length of that axis is longer. By contrast, the curve is sharper along the short axis. This makes the focal length of the short axis shorter. (Figure A1.4).

The line that engages the weaker axis will come into focus farther away from the cornea. The line that engages the stronger axis will come into focus nearer to the cornea. If the eye focuses on one line, the other line must be blurred.

The two different focal lengths of the axis and the short axis define the back and front of the Zone of Partial Focus.

Now the meaning of the different types of astigmatism that Dr. Bates mentions becomes clear. All the different terms just tell us where the Zone of Partial Focus falls in relation to

Figure A1.3: Crossed Lines Can't Both Be in Focus.

In the long axis, the curve is more gentle, so the focal length is longer.

In the short axis, the curve is sharper, so the focal length is shorter.

Figure A1.4: Two Different Curves

the retina.

Simple nearsighted astigmatism: The front of the Zone of Partial Focus falls in front of the retina, and the back of the Zone of Partial Focus falls on the retina (Figure A1.5).

Simple farsighted astigmatism: The front of Zone of Partial Focus falls on the retina, and the back of the Zone of Partial Focus falls behind the retina (Figure A1.6).

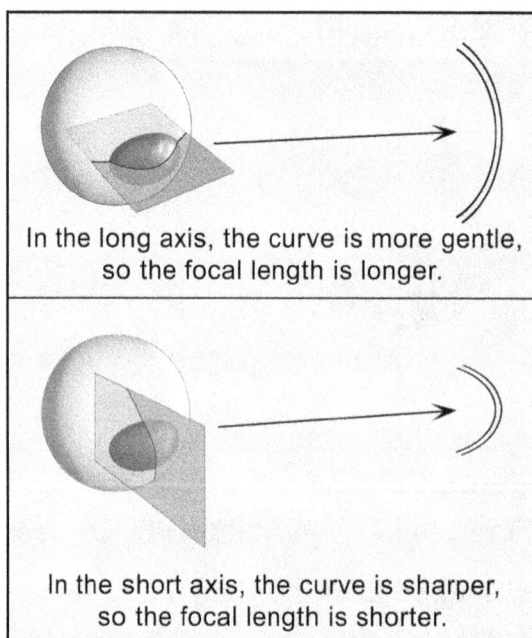

Compound nearsighted astigmatism: Both the front and the back of the Zone of Partial Focus fall in front of the retina (Figure A1.7).

Compound farsighted astigmatism: Both the front and the back of the Zone of Partial Focus fall behind the retina (Figure A1.8).

Mixed astigmatism: The front of the Zone of Partial Focus falls in front of the retina, and the back of the Zone of Partial Focus falls behind the retina (Figure A1.9).

Five Types of Astigmatism

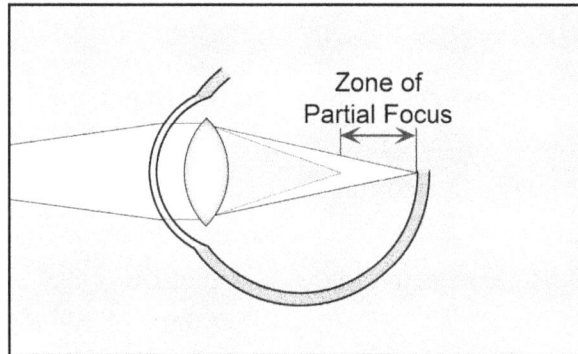

Fig. A1.5: Simple Nearsighted

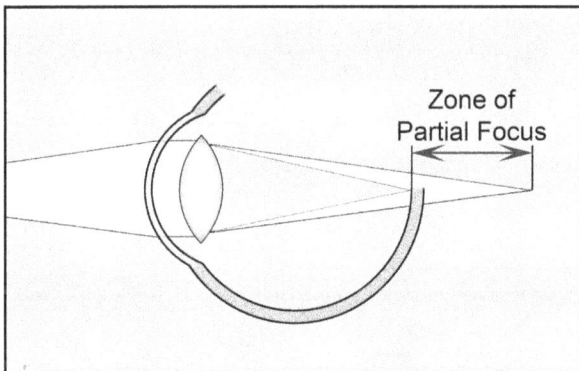

Fig. A1.6: Simple Farsighted

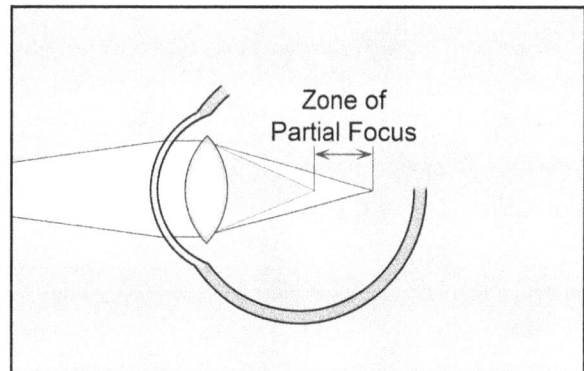

Fig. A1.7: Compound Nearsighted

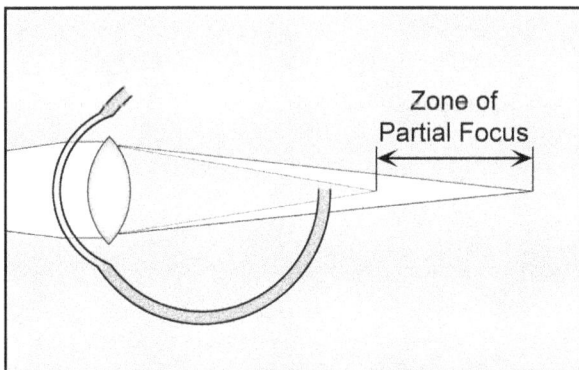

Fig. A1.8: Compound Farsighted

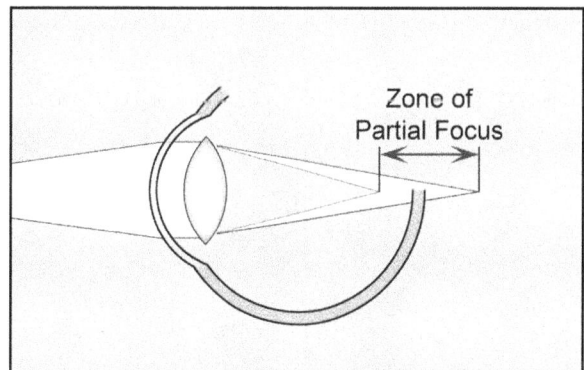

Fig. A1.9: Mixed

Axis of Astigmatism
and
Degrees of Cylinder

There is one more aspect of astigmatism that comes up in this book. So far, I have shown the axis of astigmatism as horizontal. Actually the long axis could be at any angle. The phrase "axis of astigmatism" refers to that orientation.

Similarly, the phrase "degrees of cylinder" describes how to turn the cylinder lens so that it corrects the astigmatism and creates one clear plane of focus.

The axis of the astigmatic cornea could be horizontal, vertical or anywhere in between. Figures A1:1.10, 1.11, and 1.12 show some examples. The axis of astigmatism varies from person to person.

During an eye exam, if there is astigmatism, the examiner measures both the severity of the astigmatism and the axis of its orientation.

All the possible orientations are described by imagining a protractor superimposed on the eye. For example, if the axis of astigmatism is horizontal, they call that 180 degrees. If it is perfectly vertical, they call that 90 degrees.

The correct way to orient the cylinder lens for each individual is expressed in the same way – degrees of cylinder.

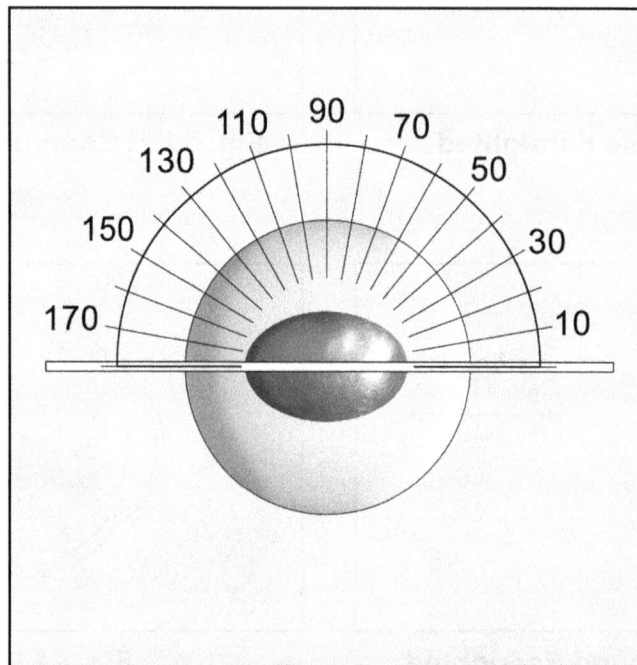

Figure A1.10: Axis 180 Degrees

232

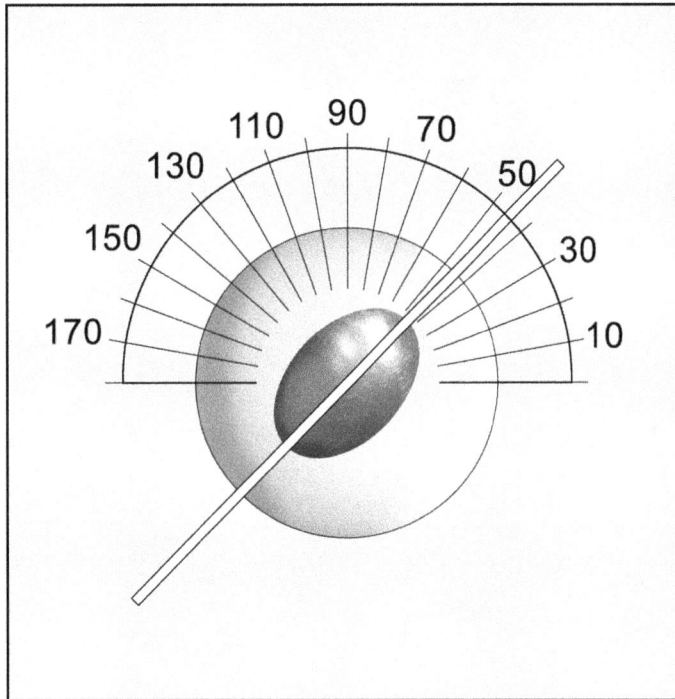

Figure A1.11: Axis 45 Degrees

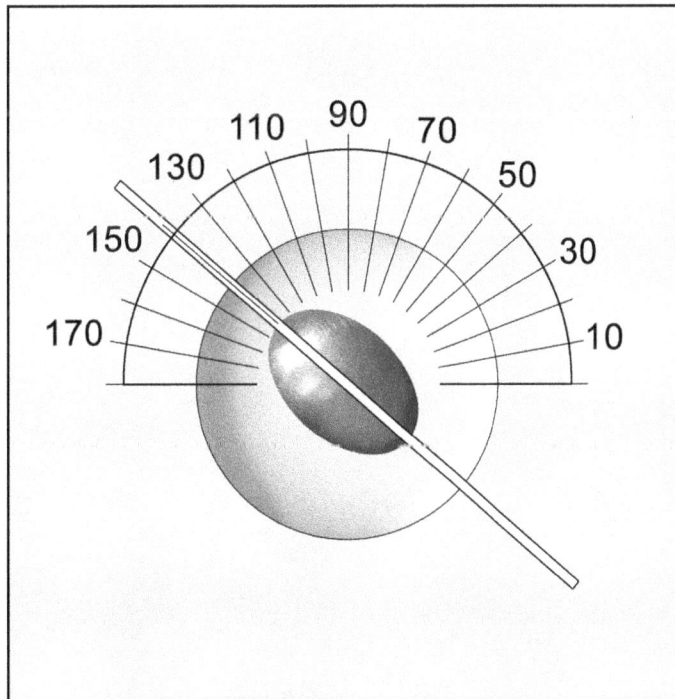

Figure A1.12: Axis 140 Degrees

Glossary

accommodation. The process by which the eye changes focus from far away to close up.

amblyopia. Decreased vision in one eye that develops in childhood because the brain, for various reasons, is ignoring the input from that eye. If not treated amblyopia can become permanent.

amblyopia ex anopsia. Literally "dim vision from not looking." The full name for amblyopia, which is defined above.

astigmatism. A condition in which the eye cannot focus clearly because the cornea is not properly and symmetrically shaped.

astigmatism, compound nearsighted. See Appendix 1, p. 230–231.

astigmatism, axis of. See Appendix 1, p. 232–233.

astigmatism, compound. See Appendix 1, p. 230-231.

astigmatism, compound farsighted. See Appendix 1, p. 230-231.

astigmatism, farsighted. See Appendix 1, p. 230-231.

astigmatism, mixed. See Appendix 1, p. 230-231.

atropine. A medicine which blocks the nerve transmitter. Atropine has many uses. In ophthalmology, atropine eye drops were used to dilate the pupil in order to better examine the inside of the eye. Atropine eye drops were also used as a treatment for amblyopia. Put in the good eye they make the vision blurry, forcing the brain to use the other eye to see.

axis of astigmatism. See Appendix 1, p. 232.

blepharitis. Inflammation of the eyelids from any cause (usually allergy, infection or irritation).

cataract. Clouding of the crystalline lens of the eye causing impaired vision or blindness. Usually due to aging or trauma.

cataract, incipient. The beginnings of a cataract. The crystalline lens shows mild clouding. Incipient cataracts can "ripen" into actual cataracts.

ciliary muscle. A muscle which encircles the crystalline lens and is attached to it by tiny, hair-like fibers. The conventional theory is that when the ciliary muscle contracts, it produces accommodation by loosening the stretch on the crystalline lens, allowing the lens to become more rounded.

compound nearsighted astigmatism. See Appendix 1, p. 230-231.

compound farsighted astigmatism. See Appendix 1, p. 230-231.

compound astigmatism. See Appendix 1, p. 230-231.

cones. A type of photoreceptor in the retina that allows the eye to distinguish color.

cranial nerves. Nerves that exit the brain and go directly to their target site without first passing down the spinal cord.

cranial nerve, fourth. A cranial nerve that goes to the superior oblique muscle of the eyes.

crystalline lens. The lens in the human eye that, with the help of the cornea, focuses an image onto the retina.

cylinder, degrees of. A system of describing how to orient a cylinder lens for making eyeglasses or contact lenses (see Appendix 1, p. 232).

cylinder lens. A lens shaped like a slice off a cylinder parallel to the cylinder's long axis. Used in the treatment of astigmatism.

degrees of cylinder. A system of describing how to orient a cylinder lens for making eyeglasses or contact lenses.

divergent strabismus. A form of strabismus ("cross-eyed") in which one eye looks away (laterally) from straight forward.

eccentric fixation. Normally, one moves the eyes in such a way as to place the image of the object of interest directly on the fovea. The fovea is the area of the retina which captures the most clarity and detail. Eccentric fixation is a term coined by Dr. Bates to describe how people with visual problems place the image on some part of the retina other than the fovea.

error of refraction. Any error in the way the eye focuses an image onto the retina. This includes nearsightedness, farsightedness and astigmatism.

extraocular muscles. Six muscles that attach to the outside of the eyeball and are responsible for moving the eye around in the eye socket.

farsightedness. An error of refraction in which the eye has trouble focusing on close-up objects.

farsighted astigmatism. See Appendix 1, p. 230-231.

farsightedness, latent. A condition in which at rest the eye is farsighted, but the eye can compensate by accommodating. The constant effort of this often leads to headache.

floaters. Small, translucent spots or threads that drift through one's field of vision.

flying flies. Another term for floaters.

fovea. The area of the retina that sees with the most clarity and detail. The fovea is very small. It lies at the center of the macula. The diameter of the fovea is about 1.5 mm. (For comparison, the thickness of a credit card is 0.75 mm.)

incipient cataract. The beginnings of a cataract. The crystalline lens shows mild clouding. Incipient cataracts can "ripen" into actual cataracts.

inferior rectus. One of the six extraocular muscles around the outside of the eye. The inferior rectus attaches to the bottom of the eyeball. When it contracts the eye looks downward.

iris. The colored disc at the front of the eye with a black hole (the pupil) at the center. The iris can contract or relax, which controls the size of the pupil, which controls how much light enters the eye.

iritis. Inflammation of the iris from any cause.

latent farsightedness. Farsightedness that is not immediately evident because the eye is constantly but successfully struggling to adjust for it. This constant adjustment may cause eye strain.

latent nearsightedness. Nearsightedness that is not immediately evident because the eye is constantly but successfully struggling to adjust for it. This constant adjustment may cause eye strain.

lateral rectus. One of the six extraocular muscles around the outside of the eye. The lateral rectus attaches to the lateral side of the eyeball. When it contracts, the eye looks off to the side.

lazy eye. A common term for strabismus ("cross-eyed").

macula. A small yellow spot near the center of the retina. In the center of the macula is the fovea. The macula and the fovea account for the clearest, most detailed image that the retina can produce. The diameter of the macula is on average 5.5 mm, which is about the diameter of the erasers one finds attached to the end of a pencil.

medial rectus. One of the six extraocular muscles around the outside of the eye. The medial rectus attaches to the medial side of the eyeball. When it contracts, the eye looks toward the bridge of the nose.

mixed astigmatism. See Appendix 1, p. 230, 231.

Montessori. An unusual approach to childhood education that regards the child as an eager learner ready and willing to explore and achieve if only given the freedom and environment to do so. The Montessori method was developed by Maria Montessori, MD, and first entered the United States around 1912.

morphine. An extract of the poppy flower. Morphine is used for pain. It is an opioid like codeine, oxycodone and heroin. Morphine is addictive. Historically, morphine has the distinction of being the first drug isolated from a plant (1803).

muscae volitantes. Floaters.

muscles of accommodation. The muscles in the eye that allow the eye to change focus from far away to close up. In the conventional view this is the ciliary muscle. In Dr. Bates's view these are the extraocular muscles.

near point. The nearest point at which the eyes can focus.

nearsightedness. An error of refraction in which the eye cannot focus on far away objects.

nearsightedness, latent. Nearsightedness that is not immediately evident because the eye is constantly but successfully struggling to adjust for it.

nystagmus. A neurological condition in which the eyes rapidly twitch back and forth very subtly.

ophthalmometer. An instrument used to measure how the surface of the cornea curves. This is especially useful in determining the degree and orientation of astigmatism. "Keratometer" is a synonym. The ophthalmometer was invented by the legendary Dr. Helmholtz in 1851.

ophthalmoscope. An instrument for examining the retina by looking through (and shining light through) the pupil.

optic nerve. The nerve that goes from the back of the eye to the brain, carrying all the information that the retina has gathered.

optic nerve atrophy. A condition in which, for various possible reasons, the optic nerve starts to shrivel up.

optimum. A term coined by Dr. Bates to describe any object that the individual likes seeing and therefore sees with better vision. That which is an optimum varies from individual to individual.

palming. A technique developed by Dr. Bates in which one rests and relaxes the eyes by placing the palms over the eyes without putting any pressure on the eyes themselves.

pessimum. A term coined by Dr. Bates to describe any object that the individual dislikes seeing and therefore sees with worsened vision. That which is an pessimum varies from individual to individual.

presbyopia. A form of farsightedness that reliably develops in most people as we age.

prism. A type of lens that does not change the image, but simply displaces where the image appears. The displacement could be in any direction — up, down, left, right and so forth. Prism lenses are most commonly used in the treatment of strabismus and double vision.

pupil (of the eye). The round black opening at the center of the iris through which light enters the eye.

Purkinje images. A number of images reflected from the front and back of both the cornea and the crystalline lens.

rectus muscles. Six muscles which attach to the outside of the eyeball and move the eyes about.

refract. 1. To bend light. A lens refracts light to form an image on the other side of the lens. 2. To determine what type and strength of lens a person needs in order to correct their nearsightedness, farsightedness or astigmatism.

refraction, errors of. Defects in the way the lenses of the eye (cornea and crystalline lens) bend light. These defects prevent a clear image from forming on the retina. There are three basic errors of refraction – nearsightedness, farsightedness and astigmatism.

retina. The inside back of the eyeball which translates light received into nerve impulses that go to the brain.

retinoscopy. The act of using a retinoscope in order to look into the eye and see the retina.

retinoscopy, simultaneous. The act of looking into the eye as an individual looks about or performs some activity. In this way the individual's refraction can be determined at any moment, and is seen to vary moment by moment.

rods. A type of light receptor in the retina that sees only black and white, but is more sensitive to light than the receptors that see color (that are called cones).

shifting. A vision improvement practice developed by Dr. Bates in which one restores the normal movements of the eyes by consciously looking from one object to another.

simultaneous retinoscopy. The act of looking into the eye as an individual looks about or performs some activity. In this way the individual's refraction can be determined at any moment, and is seen to vary moment by moment.

squint. In Dr. Bates's usage, strabismus.

strabismus. A condition in which the eyes fail to point together toward the object at which one is looking. Commonly known as being "cross-eyed."

strabismus, divergent. A form of strabismus ("cross-eyed") in which one eye looks away (laterally) from straight forward.

superior rectus muscle. The extraocular muscle that attaches to the top of the eyeball. When it contracts the eyeball looks upward.

swinging. A vision improvement practice developed by Dr. Bates in which one becomes conscious that when the eyes move, the scene or object at which one is looking appears to move in the opposite direction.

swinging, universal. The experience that when the eyes move, the entire world appears to be move in the opposite direction.

third cranial nerve. Also called the "oculomotor nerve," the third cranial nerve goes to many of the extraocular muscles of the eye and is responsible for many aspects of eye movement. It also goes to the muscles which lift the eyelids and control the size of the pupils. The third cranial nerve also goes to the ciliary muscle. This makes it, from the conventional point of view, responsible for accommodation because of this.

universal swing. See "swinging, universal."

vitreous humor. The clear, jelly-like substance that fills the inside of the eyeball.

white of the eye. The white coating on the outside of the eye. The anatomical term is "sclera."

Zone of Partial Focus. The area near the retina in which the astigmatic eye can somewhat bring an image into focus.

Index

M

macula 79–80, 88

medial rectus 35, 37, 64

memory 88, 90–91, 95–106, 108, 115, 117, 141–144, 164, 174, 199–203, 209, 216

memory as an aid to vision **95–100**

mental control 76, 84, 103, 105, 112, 125, 134, 161, 201

mental relaxation 71

microscopic vision 71, 101

military 20, 59, 207–209

mind and vision **199–204**

mixed astigmatism 43, 58, 143, 170, glossary

Montessori 73, 201

morphine 209

movie 74, 112, 133, 224

moving picture 19, 74, 112

muscae volitantes 123, 167

muscles of accommodation 54

nearsightedness, prevention of in schools **181–193**

N

near point 32, 50, 70, 95, 98, 114, 116–118, 121–122, 139, 147–150, 152, 162, 168, 173–174, 179, 182–183, 191, 219, 225

nearsightedness 9, 13, 15, 20–23, 25, 27, 35, 39, 43, 48, 53–54, 57–58, 62, 64, 67–70, 89, 75, 98–99, 105, 108, 116–117, 122, 134, 149, 152, 155–156, 167, 174, 177–178, 181–184, 187, 189–191, 196, 199, 218–219, 224, 226

nearsightedness, latent 53, glossary

nerves 42, 44, 54, 74, 92, 107–108, 213, 215–216

nystagmus 82

O

oblique muscle 38–39, 40 (Fig. 4.7), 42–44, 223

ophthalmology 19, 30, 32, 63, 149, 181, 183, 195, 225, glossary

ophthalmometer 51, glossary

ophthalmoscope 29, 81, 111, 201, 167–168, glossary

optic nerve 36 (Fig. 4.1), 38, 44, 74–76, 81, 83, 108, 131, 201, 217

optic nerve atrophy 108

optimum 91, **137–139**, 148, 235

P

pain 9, 59, 61, 64, 68, 75, 81, 83, 84, 87, 90, 92, 107, 111, 118, 134, **141–144**, 161, 174, 175, 179, 190, 209, 210, 216, 217

palming 87–93, 97, 113–114, 117, 143–144, 150, 164, 200, 209–210

perfect black 87–89, 92, 95, 96

perfect sight 19, 57–59, 71–74, 81, 87, 90, 100–101, 105, 107, 111–114, 121–126, 129, 131, 133, 141, 143, 147–148, 150, 163–164, 167, 173, 178–179, 187, 189, 193, 195, 202, 208, 216–217

period 32, 43, 55, 58, 88–89, 91, 96–101, 105–106, 108, 112, 114, 123, 129, 132, 153, 157, 161, 184, 187, 203–204, 205–216

permanent cure 55, 71, 83, 114, 151, 161

www.ingramcontent.com/pod-product-compliance
Lightning Source LLC
Chambersburg PA
CBHW080803300326
41914CB00056B/1149